Optimizing IUI Results

Optimizing
IUI Results

Second Edition

Editor

Sunita Tandulwadkar
MD (Obs & Gyne) FICS (Gynae-Endoscopy) FICOG
Gynecological Endoscopist and ART, IVF Specialist
Chief and Medical Director
IVF and Endoscopy Center, Ruby Hall Clinic
Dr DY Patil IVF and Endoscopy Center, Pune
Director, Solo Clinic IVF—Center for Excellence in Infertility
Founder and Medical Advisor
Solo Stem Cells—Stem Cell Research and Application Center
Pune, Maharashtra, India

Foreword

Rajesh Tandulwadkar

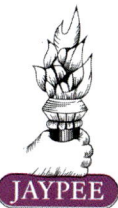

JAYPEE BROTHERS MEDICAL PUBLISHERS
The Health Sciences Publisher
New Delhi | London

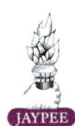 **Jaypee Brothers Medical Publishers (P) Ltd**

Headquarters
Jaypee Brothers Medical Publishers (P) Ltd
EMCA House, 23/23-B
Ansari Road, Daryaganj
New Delhi 110 002, India
Landline: +91-11-23272143, +91-11-23272703
+91-11-23282021, +91-11-23245672
Email: jaypee@jaypeebrothers.com

Corporate Office
Jaypee Brothers Medical Publishers (P) Ltd
4838/24, Ansari Road, Daryaganj
New Delhi 110 002, India
Phone: +91-11-43574357
Fax: +91-11-43574314
Email: jaypee@jaypeebrothers.com

Overseas Office
JP Medical Ltd
83 Victoria Street, London
SW1H 0HW (UK)
Phone: +44 20 3170 8910
Fax: +44 (0)20 3008 6180
Email: info@jpmedpub.com

Website: www.jaypeebrothers.com
Website: www.jaypeedigital.com

© 2024, Jaypee Brothers Medical Publishers

The views and opinions expressed in this book are solely those of the original contributor(s)/author(s) and do not necessarily represent those of editor(s) or publisher of the book.

All rights reserved. No part of this publication may be reproduced, stored or transmitted in any form or by any means, electronic, mechanical, photocopying, recording or otherwise, without the prior permission in writing of the publishers.

All brand names and product names used in this book are trade names, service marks, trademarks or registered trademarks of their respective owners. The publisher is not associated with any product or vendor mentioned in this book.

Medical knowledge and practice change constantly. This book is designed to provide accurate, authoritative information about the subject matter in question. However, readers are advised to check the most current information available on procedures included and check information from the manufacturer of each product to be administered, to verify the recommended dose, formula, method and duration of administration, adverse effects and contraindications. It is the responsibility of the practitioner to take all appropriate safety precautions. Neither the publisher nor the author(s)/editor(s) assume any liability for any injury and/or damage to persons or property arising from or related to use of material in this book.

This book is sold on the understanding that the publisher is not engaged in providing professional medical services. If such advice or services are required, the services of a competent medical professional should be sought.

Every effort has been made where necessary to contact holders of copyright to obtain permission to reproduce copyright material. If any have been inadvertently overlooked, the publisher will be pleased to make the necessary arrangements at the first opportunity.

Inquiries for bulk sales may be solicited at: jaypee@jaypeebrothers.com

Optimizing IUI Results

First Edition: 2010

Second Edition: **2024**

ISBN: 978-93-5696-627-7

Printed in India at Rajkamal Electric Press, Kundli, Haryana.

Dedication

I dedicate this book to
My Guru
Param Pujya Swami
Shree Gagangiri Maharaj

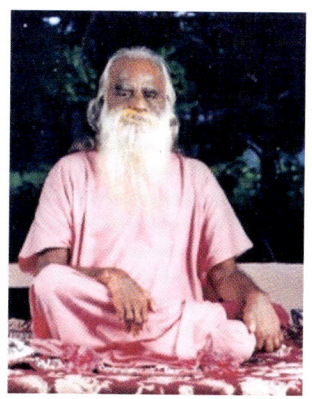

Guru Brahma, Guru Vishnu, Guru Devo Maheshwara.
Guru Sakshath Parambrahma, Tasmai Shri Gurave Namaha

(Tr: Guru is the creator Brahma, Guru is the preserver Vishnu,
Guru is the destroyer, Siva. Guru is directly the supreme spirit—
I offer my salutations to this Guru)

CONTRIBUTORS

Aanchal Garg
MBBS DGO DNB FRM Masters in Reproductive Medicine, London UK
Director and Fertility & IVF Consultant
Colors IVF and Fertility
Lucknow, Uttar Pradesh, India

Akhila MV MBBS MS (Obs & Gyne)
Senior Consultant
Department of Reproductive Medicine
and Obstetrics & Gynecology
Gunasheela Surgical and Maternity Hospital
Bengaluru, Karnataka, India

Ameet Patki
MD DNB FCPS FRCOG
Medical Director (Fertility Associates)
Reliance Life Sciences
Infertility and High-risk Pregnancy
Mumbai, Maharashtra, India
President, ISAR

Anshu Dhar
MBBS MD (Obs & Gyne) FNB (Reproductive Medicine)
Consultant IVF
Department of Obstetrics and Gynecology
Gunjan IVF World
Noida, Uttar Pradesh, India

Anshu Jindal MD DNB MNAMS FICMCH
Medical Director and IVF Specialist
High-risk Obstetrician and Gynecologist
Jindal Hospital and Fertility Center
Meerut, Uttar Pradesh, India

Ashish Kale MD DNB FICOG FICMCH DEPS FICS
Founder Director and Chief IVF Consultant
Department of Obstetrics and Gynecology
Ashakiran Hospital and Asha IVF Centre
Pune, Maharashtra, India

Ashwini M MBBS MS (Obs & Gyne) FIRM
Senior Consultant
Department of Reproductive Medicine and
Obstetrics & Gynecology
Gunasheela Surgical and Maternity Hospital
Bengaluru, Karnataka, India

Ashwini Yelikar Kale DGO DNB FICMCH
Director
Department of Obstetrics and Gynecology
Ashakiran Hospitals and Asha IVF Centre
Pune, Maharashtra, India

Bushra Khan MBBS MS (Obs & Gyne) FRM
IVF Consultant and Gynecologist
Department of IVF and Endoscopy
Dr DY Patil Medical College
Pune, Maharashtra, India

Chaitanya Nagori MD DGO
Director
Department of Reproductive Medicine
Dr Nagori's Institute for Infertility and IVF
Ahmedabad, Gujarat, India

Darshan SM
MBBS MS (Obs & Gyne) DNB FNB FNB (Reproductive Medicine)
Department of IVF and Endoscopy
Ruby Hall Clinic
Pune, Maharashtra, India

Devika Gunasheela MBBS MRCOG (Lond) FIRM
Managing Director
Department of Reproductive Medicine
and Obstetrics & Gynecology
Gunasheela Surgical and Maternity Hospital
Bengaluru, Karnataka, India

Fessy Louis T MBBS DGO DNB MNMAS FICOG
Professor and Head
Department of Reproductive Medicine
and Surgery
Amrita Institute of Medical Sciences
Kochi, Kerala, India

Gunjan Gupta Govil
MD (Obs & Gyne) FRCOG (London, UK) Advanced Diploma in Reproductive Medicine (Kiel, Germany)
Director and Founder
Department of Obstetrics and Gynecology
Gunjan IVF World
Ghaziabad, Uttar Pradesh, India

Contributors

Keshav Malhotra MBBS MCE
Lab Director
Department of Reproductive Medicine
ART Rainbow IVF
Agra, Uttar Pradesh, India

Kuldeep Jain
MD (Obs & Gyne) Fellowship ART (Singapore)
Director
Department of Reproductive Medicine
KJIVF and Laparoscopy Center
New Delhi, India

Lavanya Kiran
MBBS MS (Obs & Gyne) Dip Repro Med (Germany) Fellow Repro Med (RGUHS) Fellowship in Regen Med, Fellowship in Cosmetic Gyne, PGDMLE (NLS) MBA (Hosp Mang)
Lead Consultant
Department of Obstetrics & Gynecology,
Reproductive Medicine, and Robotic Surgery
Kauvery Hospitals
Bengaluru, Karnataka, India

Maansi Jain
MS (Obs & Gyne) Diploma ART Fellowship ART and Gynae Endoscopy
Endoscopy and ART Consultant
Department of Reproductive Medicine
KJIVF and Laparoscopy Center
New Delhi, India

Madhuri Patil MD DGO DFP FCPS FICOG
Clinical Director
Reproductive Endocrinology
ART and Endoscopy
Dr Patil's Fertility and Endoscopy Clinic
Bengaluru, Karnataka, India

Mily Pandey
MBBS MS (Obs & Gyne) DNB (Obs & Gyne)
FNB Reproductive Medicine
2nd year FNB Reproductive Medicine Fellow
IVF and Endoscopy
Ruby Hall Clinic
Pune, Maharashtra, India

Mounika Jampala MCh
Resident
Department of Reproductive Medicine and Surgery
Amrita Institute of Medical Sciences
Kochi, Kerala, India

Mrinmayi Dharmadhikari
MS MRCOG DNB (Obs & Gyne)
Consultant
Department of Obstetrics and Gynecology
Silver Lining IVF and Endoscopy Centre
Pune, Maharashtra, India

N Sanjeeva Reddy MD DGO
Professor
Reproductive Medicine and Surgery
Sri Ramachandra Medical College and Research and Institute
Chennai, Tamil Nadu, India

Neena Malhotra MD DNB FRCOG (UK)
Professor
Department of Obstetrics and Gynecology
All India Institute of Medical Sciences
New Delhi, India

Nikita Banerjee
MBBS MS (Obs & Gyne) DNB Fellowship Reproductive Medicine
Director
Department of Obstetrics and Gynecology
Hatch Fertility Center
New Delhi, India

Pinkee Saxena MD FICOG FICMCH
Senior Specialist
Department of Obstetrics and Gynecology
Deen Dayal Upadhyay Hospital
New Delhi, India

Noushin Abdul Majid
MD MRCOG MRCPI FRM
Senior Consultant (Reproductive Medicine)
Department of Reproductive Medicine
Craft Hospital and Research Centre
Thrissur, Kerala, India

Prashanth K Adiga
MBBS MD (Obs & Gyne)
Professor
Department of Reproductive Medicine and Surgery
Kasturba Medical College
Manipal, Karnataka, India

Pratap Kumar MBBS MD (Obs & Gyne) FICOG FICS
Professor and Head
Department of Reproductive Medicine and Surgery
Kasturba Medical College
Manipal, Karnataka, India

Radha Vembu MBBS DGO DNB PhD
Professor and Head
Department of Reproductive Medicine and Surgery
Sri Ramachandra Medical College and
Research Institute
Chennai, Tamil Nadu, India

Rajendra Shitole MBBS DGO DNB FRM
IVF Consultant and Endoscopic Surgeon
Department of Obstetrics & Gynecology,
Infertility and Gyne-Endoscopy
Dr DY Patil Hospital and Research Center
Pune, Maharashtra, India

Rashmika Gandhi
MBBS MS (Obs & Gyne) DNB Fellowship in Reproductive Medicine, Fellowship in Gynae Endoscopy
IVF and Laparoscopy Consultant
Department of IVF and Endoscopy, Obstetrics & Gynecology
Sukhmani Hospital
New Delhi, India

Rita Bakshi MD (Gyne) Fellow ART
Chairperson (Infertility and Gynecology)
RiSAA IVF
New Delhi, India

Riva Kiran KC MD (Obs & Gyne)
IVF Consultant
Department of Obstetrics and Gynecology
RISAA IVF
New Delhi, India

Rohit Gutgutia MBBS DGO
Medical Director
Nova IVF
Kolkata, West Bengal, India

Sandeep Talwar MBBS DNB (Obs & Gyne)
Senior Consultant
Nova Southend Fertility and IVF Clinic
New Delhi, India

Seema Pandey MBBS MD (Obs & Gyne)
Infertility Specialist, Gynecologist, Reproductive Endocrinologist (Infertility)
Seema Hospitals and Eva Fertility Clinic
and IVF Center
Azamgarh, Uttar Pradesh, India

Sonal Panchal MD PhD
Ultrasound Consultant
Dr Nagori's Institute for Infertility and IVF
Ahmedabad, Gujarat, India

Sonal Vaidya MSc (Zoology)
Chief Embryologist
ESHRE Certified Senior Clinical Embryologist
(First Indian)
Ruby Hall IVF and Endoscopy Centre
Pune, Maharashtra, India

Sonia Malik
MBBS MD FICOG FIAMS DGO (Obs & Gyne)
Chief Mentor
Nova IVF Fertility
New Delhi, India

Sowparnika SN DGO DNB FRM
Consultant
Department of Reproductive Medicine
Milann Fertility Center
Bengaluru, Karnataka, India

Spondita Banerjee
MSc (Clinical Embryology)
Research Embryologists
All India Institute of Medical Sciences
New Delhi, India

Subhashini S MD DNB (Obs & Gyne)
FNB 1st Year Resident
Department of Reproductive Medicine
Craft Hospital and Research Centre
Thrissur, Kerala, India

Sunil Jindal MS DNB MNAMS
Scientific Director and Andrologist,
Endo-Laparo-Micro Surgeon
Andrology and Reproductive Medicine
Jindal Hospital and Fertility Center
Meerut, Uttar Pradesh, India

Contributors

Sunita Tandulwadkar
MD (Obs & Gyne) FICS (Gynae-Endoscopy) FICOG
Gynecological Endoscopist and ART, IVF Specialist
Chief and Medical Director
IVF and Endoscopy Center
Ruby Hall Clinic
Dr DY Patil IVF and Endoscopy Center, Pune
Director, Solo Clinic IVF—Center for Excellence in Infertility
Founder and Medical Advisor
Solo Stem Cells—Stem Cell Research and Application Center
Pune, Maharashtra, India

Surveen Ghumman MD (Gynecology)
Senior Director and Head
Department of IVF and Reproductive Medicine
Max Superspecialty Hospital
New Delhi, India

Tejas Gundewar
MCh Reproductive Medicine & Surgery MRCOG
MS (Obs & Gyne)
Chief (Male & Female) Fertility Consultant
Department of IVF
Ruby Hall Clinic
Pune, Maharashtra, India

FOREWORD

It is with great pleasure and admiration that I introduce the second edition of *"Optimizing IUI Outcomes"* authored by the distinguished Dr Sunita Tandulwadkar. Dr Tandulwadkar, a luminary in Obstetrics and Gynecology, has left an indelible mark on the landscape of women's healthcare in India through her tireless pursuit of innovation and compassion.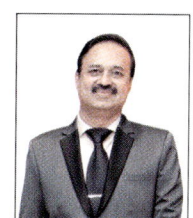

This book reflects not only her exceptional expertise but also her deep commitment to advancing the field.

"Success is not final, failure is not fatal: It is the courage to continue that counts."

–Winston Churchill

This profound quote by Winston Churchill resonates with the essence of Dr Tandulwadkar's journey and the importance of this book. In the dynamic realm of reproductive medicine, where challenges and successes coexist, Dr Tandulwadkar's courage to persist in her pursuit of excellence shines through. The insights shared in these pages are a testament to her resilience, expertise, and unyielding dedication to providing the best possible care to those seeking to build their families.

May this book serve as a guidepost for practitioners, offering not only knowledge but also encouragement to continue in the face of challenges, with the belief that the journey toward successful outcomes is a continuous, courageous endeavor.

Warm regards

Rajesh Tandulwadkar
MS FICS Dip in Endoscopy and HPB Surgery and Liver Transplants (UK)
Director, Solo GI Clinic
Director, Solo Stem Cells
Hon Consultant
Poona Hospital and Research Centre
Pune, Maharashtra, India

PREFACE TO THE SECOND EDITION

Welcome to the enhanced and refined world of *"Optimizing Intrauterine Insemination (IUI) Outcomes,"* now in its eagerly anticipated 2nd edition. As we embark on this journey once again, we find ourselves at the forefront of advancements in assisted reproductive technologies, armed with updated insights and a commitment to maximizing success in IUI.

In the ever-evolving landscape of reproductive medicine, this edition strives to bridge the gap between tradition and innovation. Our understanding of fertility has deepened, and breakthroughs in research have illuminated new pathways to success. This edition not only builds upon the foundations laid in the previous one but also embraces the latest scientific revelations, ensuring you have the most comprehensive guide at your fingertips.

As we delve into the intricacies of optimizing IUI outcomes, we explore cutting-edge strategies and evidence-based practices that have emerged since our last edition. From refined protocols to personalized approaches and a deeper understanding of pathophysiology, the landscape of fertility enhancement has seen remarkable shifts. The pages that follow will equip you with the knowledge and tools needed to navigate this dynamic field with confidence.

In the spirit of progress, we extend our gratitude to the pioneers who paved the way for advancements in reproductive medicine. Their contributions inspire us to continually strive for excellence and push the boundaries of what is possible. We hope this book serves as a beacon of knowledge, guiding you toward optimized IUI outcomes and, ultimately the realization of your dreams.

Let this second edition be your companion on the path to success, offering a contemporary perspective on fertility optimization and a source of inspiration as we collectively advance in the pursuit of building families.

Sunita Tandulwadkar

PREFACE TO THE FIRST EDITION

Infertility as a specialty has grown by leaps and bounds to surpass even endoscopy. It is today the fastest growing superspecialty. Although the incidence of infertility remains around 10–15% of the population, more and more couples are now seeking help.

IVF, ICSI, GIFT, ZIFT and all these fancy acronyms may be glamor gals, but the time tested and real workhorse of infertility is the simple and elegant IUI.

This is a procedure that is easy, safe, has a small learning curve and can form part of the clinical armamentarium of the general gynecologist.

As primary care providers for our patients, we need to develop our skills in the practice of IUI to give maximum benefit to them. So that when the need comes to refer to an ART clinic both parties are very sure and satisfied that they put in their best efforts.

In this book, *Optimizing IUI Results: A Guide to Gynecologists,* I have tried to provide a step-by-step orientation to IUI.

It is my hope that many more of my gynecology colleagues will start this procedure. For those who are doing it, my humble wish is that this book will help them improve their results.

Starting from the basics of ovulation induction and sperm preparation to the procedure itself, we have to try to keep it simple and easy to follow.

The important tips and advice are the result of many cycles of experience and trials. We hope that all of you will benefit from them, and your patients will have more pregnancies.

Putting it together was a labor of love. All of us have worked to make the book interesting, useful, and informative.

We hope that you will do many successful IUI cycles and that will be the best reward, for then the hard work will have been worthwhile.

No person can know everything for knowledge is ever evolving. We will welcome feedback and reaction so that we will learn from our collective experience.

I wish to thank all my team members in the Department of IVF and Endoscopy, Ruby Hall Clinic, Pune, for providing valuable suggestions and special thanks to Dr Sabrina Bokil who has taken efforts to read all the chapters carefully for grammatical correction.

I wish to thank all my gynecologist friends who have given me this suggestion of pen suing down years of experience and come out with a book which will help to decrease the learning curve of beginners.

Most of all, thanks go to my family. My husband, Dr Rajesh Tandulwadkar, Surgeon, Gastroenterologist and GI Endoscopist and my son Rishi, all took notes for me that found their way into the pages of my book. And as for my earlier writings, my husband continues to be my first reader and key critic apart from my great assistant in difficult situations.

Sunita Tandulwadkar

ACKNOWLEDGMENTS

In the creation of this work, I have been fortunate to collaborate with a cadre of distinguished authors whose timely contributions and profound knowledge have immeasurably enriched this volume. Their dedication and expertise have provided invaluable insights, reflecting the latest advancements in our field.

I am profoundly indebted to my peers in gynecology. Their recommendation to distill my years of professional experience into a written form has been a guiding light in this endeavor. This book, I hope, will serve as an essential resource for those embarking on their careers, helping to expedite their professional development.

My deepest gratitude is extended to my family, the bedrock of my support. To my husband, Dr Rajesh Tandulwadkar, an eminent Surgeon Gastroenterologist and GI Endoscopist, and my son Rishi, whose diligent note-taking has been a cornerstone in the compilation of this manuscript. Dr Rajesh, ever my first reader and astute critic, continues to provide invaluable feedback and unwavering support in the most challenging of circumstances.

I extend my heartfelt thanks to M/s Jaypee Brothers Medical Publishers, whose exceptional skill in bringing this book to fruition cannot be overstated. A special acknowledgment to Shri Jitendar P Vij (Group Chairman), Mr Ankit Vij (Managing Director), Mr MS Mani (Group President), Ms Chetna Malhotra (Senior Director—Professional Publishing, Marketing, and Business Development), Ms Pooja Bhandari (Director—Production) and Asmi Bharati (Development Editor), their insightful and creative input has been paramount in enhancing the academic rigor and presentation of our book. Their meticulous attention to detail has been a driving force in ensuring the highest standards of quality and precision in our content.

CONTENTS

SECTION 1: Basics

1. **Endocrinology of Follicular Phase in Unstimulated Cycle** 3
   Rashmika Gandhi, Sunita Tandulwadkar

2. **Endocrinology of Follicular Phase in Stimulated Cycle** 12
   Rashmika Gandhi, Sunita Tandulwadkar

3. **Endocrinology of Luteal Phase in Unstimulated Cycle** 21
   Rashmika Gandhi, Sunita Tandulwadkar

4. **Endocrinology of Luteal Phase in Stimulated Cycles** 30
   Madhuri Patil

5. **Endocrinology of Ovulation and Its Clinical Application** 42
   Tejas Gundewar

SECTION 2: Investigations and Counseling

6. **Evaluation of Female Partner** 51
   Nikita Banerjee

7. **Evaluation of Male Partner to Optimize Intrauterine Insemination Success** 61
   Sunil Jindal, Anshu Jindal

8. **Selection and Counseling of Couple for Intrauterine Insemination** 68
   Surveen Ghumman, Pinkee Saxena

SECTION 3: Ultrasonography in Intrauterine Insemination

9. **Monitoring of Intrauterine Insemination Cycles and Dopplers in Intrauterine Insemination** 77
   Sonal Panchal, Chaitanya Nagori

SECTION 4: Ovulation Induction Protocols: Oral Ovulogens

10. **Selective Estrogen Receptor Modulators** 93
    Gunjan Gupta Govil, Anshu Dhar

11. **Aromatase Inhibitors in Ovulation Induction** 108
    Lavanya Kiran, Sowparnika SN

12. **Insulin Sensitizers: Where We Stand?** 117
    Bushra Khan

SECTION 5: Ovulation Induction Protocols: Gonadotropins

13. Gonadotropins in Intrauterine Insemination 129
    Ameet Patki, Mrinmayi Dharmadhikari

14. Use of Gonadotropin-releasing Hormone: Analogs in
    Intrauterine Insemination 136
    Seema Pandey, Aanchal Garg

SECTION 6: Ovulation Trigger

15. Ovulation Trigger: Dose and Timing 147
    Rajendra Shitole

SECTION 7: Andrology and Laboratory Aspect

16. Semen Analysis 155
    Sunita Tandulwadkar, Darshan SM

17. Sperm Functional Assay 165
    Spondita Banerjee, Neena Malhotra

18. Optimizing Sperm Preparation for Intrauterine Insemination 176
    Keshav Malhotra

19. Setting Up an Intrauterine Insemination Laboratory 184
    Sonal Vaidya

20. Assisted Reproductive Technology Act 2022: Level 1 Clinic 194
    Ashwini Yelikar Kale, Ashish Kale

SECTION 8: Techniques

21. Procedure of Intrauterine Insemination 201
    Sunita Tandulwadkar, Darshan SM

SECTRION 9: Luteal Phase Support

22. Luteal Phase Support 207
    Pratap Kumar, Prashanth K Adiga

SECTION 10: Analyzing Results

23. Intrauterine Insemination Results and Coping with Failure 215
    N Sanjeeva Reddy, Radha Vembu

SECTION 11: Intrauterine Insemination in Special Situations

24. **Intrauterine Insemination in Female Subfertility** 225
    Fessy Louis T, Mounika Jampala

25. **Intrauterine Insemination in Endometriosis** 238
    Kuldeep Jain, Maansi Jain

26. **Intrauterine Insemination in Polycystic Ovarian Syndrome** 243
    Devika Gunasheela, Ashwini M, Akhila MV

27. **Intrauterine Insemination in Human Immunodeficiency
    Virus Serodiscordant Couples**..258
    Noushin Abdul Majid, Subhashini S

28. **Intrauterine Insemination in Unexplained Infertility** 268
    Sandeep Talwar, Rohit Gutgutia, Sonia Malik

29. **Cost-effective Intrauterine Insemination** 276
    Rita Bakshi, Riva Kiran KC

SECTION 12: Recent Updates

30. **Artificial Intelligence and Intrauterine Insemination** 289
    Rashmika Gandhi, Sunita Tandulwadkar

31. **Intrauterine Insemination Guidelines**...295
    Mily Pandey

SECTION 13: Frequently Asked Questions

32. **Frequently Asked Questions**...303
    Sunita Tandulwadkar, Mily Pandey

Index 305

SECTION 1

Basics

1. **Endocrinology of Follicular Phase in Unstimulated Cycle**
   Rashmika Gandhi, Sunita Tandulwadkar

2. **Endocrinology of Follicular Phase in Stimulated Cycle**
   Rashmika Gandhi, Sunita Tandulwadkar

3. **Endocrinology of Luteal Phase in Unstimulated Cycle**
   Rashmika Gandhi, Sunita Tandulwadkar

4. **Endocrinology of Luteal Phase in Stimulated Cycles**
   Madhuri Patil

5. **Endocrinology of Ovulation and Its Clinical Application**
   Tejas Gundewar

CHAPTER 1

Endocrinology of Follicular Phase in Unstimulated Cycle

Rashmika Gandhi, Sunita Tandulwadkar

■ INTRODUCTION

This chapter delves into the intricacies of the follicular phase in an unstimulated cycle, unraveling the orchestrated interplay of hormones, cellular interactions, and regulatory loops that define the normal physiological processes leading to ovulation.

The female reproductive process is a meticulously orchestrated sequence of events crucial for a well-functioning ovulatory menstrual cycle. To effectively address reproductive challenges, it is imperative for gynecologists to comprehend the intricacies of normal physiology encompassing menstruation, anatomy, and the interplay of hormonal components.

For clarity, we categorize the menstrual cycle into three distinct phases:
1. *Follicular phase:* This marks the initial stage of the menstrual cycle, characterized by the development of follicles in the ovaries. Follicle-stimulating hormone (FSH) plays a pivotal role in fostering the growth of these follicles, which house the maturing oocytes.
2. *Ovulation:* The midpoint of the menstrual cycle is marked by ovulation, where a matured oocyte is released from the ovary. This critical event is orchestrated by a surge in luteinizing hormone (LH) and signifies the fertile window for conception.
3. *Luteal phase:* Following ovulation, the ruptured follicle transforms into a structure known as the corpus luteum. This structure produces progesterone, preparing the uterine lining for potential implantation of a fertilized egg. If fertilization does not occur, the corpus luteum degenerates, leading to the onset of menstruation and the beginning of a new cycle.

This division into phases facilitates a comprehensive understanding of the menstrual cycle's dynamic processes and sets the foundation for effective management of reproductive issues by gynecologists.[1]

■ FOLLICULAR PHASE

The "follicular phase" unfolds as a dynamic and continuous process, persisting from the onset of menarche to the cessation of menopause. This period of follicular development, known as "folliculogenesis," is a meticulously organized sequence of events designed to ensure the availability of an appropriate number of follicles poised for ovulation. The ultimate objective of this intricate process is the emergence of a single resilient mature oocyte, ready for potential fertilization.

Gonadotropin-independent Folliculogenesis

Gonadotropin-independent folliculogenesis represents a phase where the initiation of follicle growth appears to be linked to the size of the residual pool of inactive primordial follicles. The specific mechanism governing the selection and number of follicles entering the growth phase within a given cycle remains elusive. The journey from the primordial follicle to the preantral stage spans approximately 10 weeks and occurs independently of gonadotropins, indicating a gonadotropin-independent phase.

At this stage, typically during the preantral stage, follicles transition to a phase where they become responsive to gonadotropins. It is crucial to note that, as gynecologists, we lack control over the determination of cohort size during this phase—it is preestablished in each individual. Predominantly dictated by age, ovarian reserve plays a pivotal role, and individuals may experience early ovarian failure, especially before the age of 40 years, due to factors such as diminished follicular endowment or accelerated follicular atresia. Various causes contribute to this phenomenon including chromosomal factors, iatrogenic influences (such as radiation or chemotherapy), surgical alterations affecting ovarian blood supply, infections, autoimmune diseases, galactosemia, smoking, among others.

Despite the diverse array of potential causes, the etiology of ovarian failure may remain undetermined in a majority of cases. Assessing ovarian reserve becomes a critical aspect, and gynecologists utilize parameters such as age, body mass index, day 2/3 serum FSH and estradiol levels, antral follicular count, ovarian volume, anti-müllerian hormone, inhibin, and other markers for a rough estimation of ovarian reserve. This multifaceted evaluation aids in understanding and managing the intricacies of gonadotropin-independent folliculogenesis and its implications for reproductive health.

Gonadotropin-dependent Folliculogenesis

Gonadotropin-dependent folliculogenesis unfolds over a span of 10–14 days, orchestrated by a sequential interplay of hormones, autocrine signals, and paracrine peptides.

In the absence of pregnancy, the corpus luteum from the preceding cycle regresses, resulting in a decline in estrogen and progesterone levels. This decline triggers an increase in FSH, initiating the growth of another cohort of preantral follicles, a process predetermined in each individual. These preantral follicles commence estrogen synthesis. By approximately the 6th day, one of these follicles emerges as the dominant follicle, generating escalating levels of estrogen. This surge in estrogen exerts negative feedback on FSH production, leading to a decrease in FSH levels. The reduction in FSH, in turn, contributes to the atresia of less developed follicles that were part of the growing cohort. This intricate regulatory mechanism ensures the dominance of a single, well-developed follicle, preparing the ovary for ovulation.

Two-cell Two-gonadotropin Theory

The "Two-Cell, Two-Gonadotropin Theory" elucidates the collaboration between granulosa cells and theca cells in the intricate process of estrogen synthesis.

In this theory, granulosa cells rely on theca cells to provide the essential androgen substrate required for estrogen production. LH plays a pivotal role by stimulating theca cells, prompting them to produce androgens, with androstenedione being a primary component. Subsequently, these androgens are transported to the granulosa cells. Under the influence of FSH, the granulosa cells initiate aromatization, a biochemical process that transforms androgens into estrogen. This marks the onset of estrogen synthesis, a crucial element in the regulation of the female reproductive system. The orchestrated interaction between LH-stimulated theca cells and FSH-driven aromatization in granulosa cells exemplifies the intricate coordination inherent in the "Two-Cell, Two-Gonadotropin Theory."

Role of Estrogen and Androgen

The pivotal roles of estrogen and androgen in orchestrating sustained follicular growth are crucial for understanding the intricate dynamics of the reproductive process.

FSH and estrogen dominance emerges as a prerequisite for maintaining continuous follicular development. Androgens serve as the substrate for FSH-induced aromatization, exhibiting a dual role in this context. At lower levels, androgens enhance aromatase activity, facilitating the conversion of androgens to estrogen. However, elevated levels of androgens can lead to the production of more potent 5α-reduced androgens, impeding aromatization and inhibiting the expression of FSH receptors on granulosa cells. In this androgenic microenvironment, the follicle is propelled toward atresia, emphasizing the delicate balance required for optimal follicular development.

In the absence of FSH, androgen assumes dominance in the follicular fluid, promoting degenerative changes within the follicle. The fate of the antral follicle is intricately tied to its estrogen concentration and the androgen-estrogen ratio. An antral follicle with the highest estrogen concentration and the lowest androgen-estrogen ratio is more likely to house a healthy oocyte. The successful conversion of androgen to estrogen in the dominant follicle signifies the selection of the follicle destined for ovulation.

This selection process is governed by estrogen's dual influence on FSH. Firstly, it establishes a negative feedback relationship with FSH at the hypothalamopituitary level, resulting in the withdrawal of gonadotropin support for less developed follicles. Simultaneously, estrogen exerts a positive influence on FSH action within the maturing follicle, showcasing a synergistic action that further propels the follicle toward ovulation. The delicate interplay between estrogen, androgen, and FSH underscores the intricacies of follicular selection and maturation.

Negative Feedback Effect of Estrogen for Follicle-stimulating Hormone at Hypothalamopituitary Level

The negative feedback effect of estrogen on FSH at the hypothalamopituitary level demonstrates the intricate regulatory mechanisms governing follicular development.

As the dominant follicle undergoes growth, the heightened production of estrogen exerts a negative feedback influence on pituitary FSH secretion. Remarkably, despite the decline in FSH levels, the dominant follicle maintains its growth momentum, showcasing several advantages in this process:

- *Higher FSH receptor content:* The dominant follicle possesses an elevated content of FSH receptors, enhancing its responsiveness to gonadotropins.
- *Enhanced FSH action:* The presence of a high intrafollicular estrogen concentration, along with local autocrine and paracrine peptides, synergistically amplifies FSH action within the dominant follicle.
- *Increased thecal vascularity:* The dominance is further reinforced by the higher

thecal vascularity of the follicle, facilitating preferential delivery of gonadotropins. This enables continued development even in the face of declining gonadotropin levels.

As FSH values decrease, the other developing follicles experience a wave of atresia, marked by their inability to progress. This wave of atresia occurs concurrently with the escalating levels of estrogen. The intricate interplay between estrogen and FSH allow development of dominant follicle.

Synergistic Effect of Estrogen with Follicle-stimulating Hormone

The "synergistic effect of estrogen" with FSH underscores the cooperative actions that govern granulosa cell function and follicular development.

- *Granulosa cell stimulation:* FSH, in conjunction with estrogen, orchestrates the stimulation of granulosa cell proliferation, differentiation, and estrogen synthesis. This collaborative effort ensures the dynamic growth and maturation of the follicle.
- *Enhanced FSH receptor expression:* Estrogen plays a pivotal role in increasing the expression of FSH receptors on granulosa cells. This action is further potentiated by the presence of autocrine and paracrine factors, creating a robust environment for follicular responsiveness.
- *Cell signaling through gap junctions:* While not every cell within the follicle may contain FSH receptors, signaling mechanisms are facilitated through gap junctions. This unique feature allows the transmission of hormonal signals across the follicular cell population, even if only a subset of cells directly binds the hormone.
- *Coordinated follicular performance:* The ability to transmit hormone-initiated actions throughout the follicle, despite receptor distribution variations, promotes a coordinated and synchronous performance across the entire follicular structure. This synchronization is crucial for the orderly progression of folliculogenesis.

Role of Luteinizing Hormone in Late Follicular Phase

- Establishing an estrogenic environment by promoting increased estrogen production from granulosa cells.
- FSH exerts its activity during the early follicular phase, stimulating small follicles, while LH takes charge in the mid- to late-follicular phase, promoting the growth of large follicles and inducing atresia in smaller ones.
- Improving oocyte quality and enhancing their competence.
- LH directly influences the endometrium, and disruptions in endometrial maturation are observed in women with low endogenous LH. This can be remedied by midcycle LH receptor stimulation using exogenous human chorionic gonadotropin (HCG) in the absence of ovarian activity.[2]

Oocyte-granulosa Cells Regulatory Loop

The "oocyte-granulosa cells regulatory loop" is a sophisticated network of bidirectional communication that significantly influences follicular development, involving various autocrine and paracrine factors and gap junctions.

Key components of autocrine and paracrine regulation:

- *Inhibin:* Granulosa cells release inhibin, with inhibin B predominant in the follicular phase and inhibin A in the luteal phase. Inhibin inhibits the synthesis

and release of FSH, contributing to the intricate feedback mechanisms.
- *Activin:* Also secreted by granulosa cells, activin stimulates FSH release, playing a role in the regulatory feedback loop governing gonadotropin dynamics.
- *Epidermal growth factors (EGF-L):* The EGF-L group, including epiregulin, amphiregulin, and β-cellulin, is rapidly induced in mural granulosa cells shortly after the LH surge. These factors serve as major secondary signals transmitting the ovulatory signal to the cumulus complex.
- *Transforming growth factor (TGF):* Experimental evidence supports the key roles of TGFs in various aspects of follicle development, encompassing primordial follicle recruitment, cell proliferation/atresia in granulosa and theca cells, steroidogenesis, gonadotropin receptor expression, oocyte maturation, ovulation, luteinization, and corpus luteum formation.
- *Oocyte maturation inhibitor (OMI):* Oocytes are held in the diplotene stage until just before ovulation, and OMI, a low molecular weight peptide found in follicular fluid, has been identified as an inhibitor of oocyte maturation.
- *Additional regulatory factors:* Renin-angiotensin, fibroblast growth factor, interleukin-1, tissue necrosis factor, follistatin, insulin-like growth factors, among others, contribute to the intricate regulation of follicular growth, highlighting the multifaceted nature of the regulatory environment.

This dynamic interplay of factors within the "oocyte-granulosa cells regulatory loop" emphasizes the active role of the oocyte as a fundamental regulator, shaping somatic cell differentiation and function throughout folliculogenesis.

■ OVULATORY PHASE

The preovulatory follicle has a fluid-filled antrum and the oocyte cumulus complex (OCC).

Biphasic Regulation of Estrogen on Luteinizing Hormone: Decoding the Dynamics

The impact of estrogen on LH release reveals a nuanced biphasic regulation, characterized by distinct effects depending on the concentration and duration of exposure:
- *Low-level influence:* At lower concentrations, estrogen establishes a negative feedback relationship with LH, contributing to the regulatory mechanisms governing hormonal dynamics.
- *High-level impact:* Conversely, at elevated concentrations, estrogen exerts a positive stimulatory feedback effect on LH release. This transition from suppression to stimulation unfolds notably during the midfollicular phase of the menstrual cycle.

Critical Determinants of Luteinizing Hormone Surge

Two pivotal features of estrogen play a crucial role in orchestrating the LH surge:
1. *Concentration of estradiol:* To initiate a positive feedback loop, the concentration of estradiol must reach 200 pg/mL or more, signifying a threshold for eliciting the desired hormonal response.
2. *Duration of estradiol elevation:* Sustaining the elevated estradiol concentration for an extended period is equally vital. This sustained elevation, lasting >48 hours, is a key factor in ensuring the progression

from LH suppression to the initiation of the surge.

The attainment of such elevated and sustained estradiol levels is typically associated with the maturation of the dominant follicle, usually reaching a diameter of 17 mm or more. Importantly, this heightened estrogenic environment must persist beyond the onset of the LH surge, ensuring its completeness and preventing premature cessation.

Understanding these intricate dynamics sheds light on the delicately balanced interplay between estrogen and LH, unraveling the nuanced orchestration of events leading to the timely and precise occurrence of the LH surge in the menstrual cycle.

Luteinizing Hormone Surge Unveiled: Orchestrating Ovulation and Hormonal Dynamics

As the peak level of estradiol is achieved, heralding the culmination of the follicular phase, the LH surge takes center stage in the menstrual cycle. The intricate dance of local estrogen-FSH interactions within the dominant follicle plays a pivotal role in inducing LH receptors on granulosa cells, initiating a cascade of events.

Key elements of the luteinizing hormone surge:
- *Initiation of LH surge:* The surge in LH serves as the ovulatory stimulus for the selected dominant follicle, marking a decisive moment in the cycle. Simultaneously, it seals the fate of the remaining follicles, characterized by lower estrogen and FSH content, by accentuating the androgen superiority in this population.
- *Promotion of luteinization and ovulation:* LH takes the reins in promoting the luteinization of granulosa cells within the dominant follicle, orchestrating the onset of ovulation. Typically, ovulation occurs approximately 12 hours after the peak of LH or around 34–36 hours following the initial rise in midcycle LH.
- *Progesterone production:* LH not only triggers ovulation but also stimulates the production of progesterone. This modest yet significant increase in progesterone during the preovulatory period holds immense physiological importance.

Physiological Significance of Luteinizing Hormone-induced Progesterone Rise

- *Positive feedback loop:* When introduced after sufficient estrogen priming, the rise in progesterone facilitates the positive feedback response of estrogen on LH, ensuring the robustness of the LH surge.
- *Second FSH peak:* Additionally, LH-induced progesterone production is responsible for the emergence of a second FSH peak in the late follicular phase. This ensures the completion of FSH action on the follicle, contributing to the overall orchestration of the complex hormonal interplay.

Understanding these intricacies provides insights into the finely tuned regulatory mechanisms that govern the transition from the follicular phase to ovulation, underscoring the physiological significance of the LH surge in the menstrual cycle.[2]

Unveiling the Significance of the Second Follicle-stimulating Hormone Peak: Orchestrating Ovulatory Perfection

The second FSH peak emerges as a crucial player in the intricate symphony of hormonal dynamics, ensuring the flawless execution of ovulation and the subsequent events in the menstrual cycle.

Key roles of the second FSH peak:
- *Completion of LH receptors:* FSH takes center stage in ensuring the comprehensive development of LH receptors on granulosa cells. Cycles characterized by low FSH levels may experience a shortened or insufficient luteal phase, underscoring the pivotal role of FSH in this process.
- *Plasminogen activator production:* FSH orchestrates the production of plasminogen activator, collaborating with LH and growth factors. This concerted effort facilitates the transformation of the oocyte cumulus cell mass into a free-floating entity within the antral fluid.

Understanding the nuanced role of the second FSH peak sheds light on its indispensable contributions to the intricacies of ovulation, emphasizing its role in ensuring the seamless transition from follicular development to the orchestrated release of the oocyte cumulus complex.[3]

Midcycle Luteinizing Hormone Surge and Ovulatory Cascade

- *Prostaglandins and proteolytic enzymes:* The midcycle LH surge triggers a remarkable surge in the local concentration of prostaglandins and proteolytic enzymes. This surge is instrumental in creating a breach in the follicular wall.
- *Expulsion of oocyte cumulus complex:* Through this meticulously orchestrated breach, the free-floating oocyte cumulus complex is expelled, marking the culmination of the ovulatory process.[3]

Follicle-stimulating Hormone Threshold and Window

The initiation and maintenance of follicular growth are governed by the FSH threshold, indicating the minimum FSH level needed for this process, and the FSH window, representing the range above the threshold where follicular growth is sustained. The variations in FSH threshold among follicles within the same cohort contribute to the asynchrony in their development. As long as the FSH values remain above the threshold, the FSH window is considered open, and follicular growth persists. Conversely, a decline in plasma FSH, often influenced by feedback from elevated estrogen produced by a dominant follicle, results in the preservation of the follicle with the lowest threshold, leading to atresia in others **(Fig. 1)**.

Luteinizing Hormone Ceiling

For the optimal growth of follicles during the early folliculogenesis phase, a minimum level of LH is essential (LH threshold). However, once LH surpasses a specific upper limit, it can hinder granulosa proliferation and trigger the atresia of less mature follicles (LH ceiling). Within the range defined by the LH threshold and LH ceiling, LH support appears sufficient for androgen synthesis, estrogen secretion, and effective control of follicular growth.

Following ovulation, the residual follicular structure transforms into the corpus luteum. Granulosa cells within the corpus luteum accumulate lipids and lutein, giving it a yellow hue. This structure releases hormones like progesterone, estrogen, and inhibin A. Angiogenesis and the dissolution of the basement membrane enable the systemic circulation of these steroids. They, in turn, suppress the development of new follicles, providing negative feedback to FSH and LH secretion.

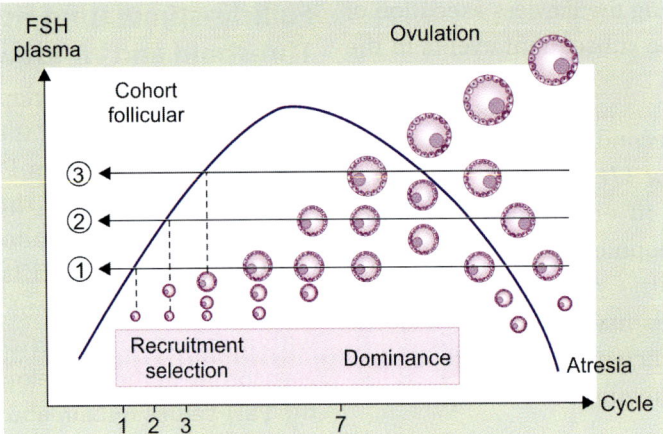

Fig. 1: Follicle-stimulating hormone (FSH) threshold and window concept.

In the event of pregnancy, placental hCG takes over this role until the luteal-placental shift around 7–9 weeks. In the absence of pregnancy, the corpus luteum regresses over 12–16 days, triggering menstruation. The decline in estrogen-progesterone levels prompts a rise in FSH and LH, initiating the growth of another cohort of follicles.

■ CONCLUSION

In conclusion, the menstrual cycle is a highly orchestrated and dynamic process characterized by distinct phases that are essential for successful reproduction. The follicular phase, encompassing gonadotropin-independent and -dependent folliculogenesis, plays a crucial role in preparing the ovary for ovulation. The "Two-Cell, Two-Gonadotropin Theory" highlights the collaboration between granulosa and theca cells in estrogen synthesis, emphasizing the delicate balance required for sustained follicular growth. The interplay between LH and estrogen in the late follicular phase is pivotal, ensuring an estrogenic milieu, promoting follicular growth, and influencing oocyte quality. The "Oocyte-Granulosa Cells Regulatory Loop" introduces bidirectional communication involving various autocrine and paracrine factors, shaping folliculogenesis. Additionally, the biphasic regulation of estrogen on LH reveals nuanced dynamics, emphasizing the critical role of estrogen concentration and duration in LH surge initiation. The LH surge marks the culmination of the follicular phase, orchestrating ovulation, and hormonal dynamics. The second FSH peak contributes to complete LH receptor development and facilitates the release of the oocyte cumulus complex. The FSH threshold and window concept, along with the LH ceiling, provide insights into the regulatory mechanisms governing follicular growth. Following ovulation, the corpus luteum emerges, releasing hormones that suppress new follicle development through negative feedback on FSH and LH. The luteal-placental shift in pregnancy maintains this suppression, while in the absence of pregnancy, the corpus luteum regresses, leading to menstruation. Understanding these intricacies is vital for gynecologists, providing insights into the normal physiological processes crucial for reproductive health. The delicate balance and orchestrated interplay of hormones, cellular interactions, and regulatory loops underscore the complexity of the menstrual cycle, paving the way for effective management of reproductive challenges.

■ KEY LEARNING POINTS

- *Dynamic folliculogenesis:* The orderly sequence of events in folliculogenesis ensures the preparation of an optimal number of follicles for ovulation, culminating in the survival of a mature oocyte.
- *Gonadotropin-independent folliculogenesis:* The initiation of follicular growth is influenced by the size of the residual pool of inactive primordial follicles. The ovarian reserve, largely determined by age, plays a pivotal role in follicular initiation.
- *Gonadotropin-dependent folliculogenesis:* This 10–14 days process involves hormonal and paracrine actions. Following corpus luteum regression, rising FSH stimulates preantral follicles for estrogen synthesis. Dominant follicle development, estrogen production, and FSH suppression contribute to the selection of the ovulatory follicle.
- *Two-cell two-gonadotropin theory:* LH stimulates theca cells to produce androgens, transferred to granulosa cells for estrogen synthesis. The delicate balance of FSH, estrogen, and androgens is essential for sustained follicular growth. Successful conversion of androgens to estrogen marks the selection of the follicle destined for ovulation.
- *Oocyte-granulosa cells regulatory loop:* Bidirectional communication between oocytes and somatic cells via gap junctions and soluble factors. Various factors, including inhibin, activin, EGF, TGF, OMI, and others, play critical roles in folliculogenesis.

■ ACKNOWLEDGMENTS

- Gardner DK. Assisted Reproductive Techniques: Laboratory and Clinical Perspectives; 3rd edition, 2001.
- Speroff L, Fritz MA. Clinical Gynecologic Endocrinology and Infertility, 7th edition, by 2005.
- Berek JS. Berek and Novak's Gynaecology, 14th Edition. United States: Lippincott Williams & Wilkins; 2007.

■ REFRENCES

1. Barbieri RL. The endocrinology of the menstrual cycle. Methods Mol Biol. 2014; 1154:145-69.
2. Gardner DK, Lane M. Towards a single embryo transfer. Reprod Biomed Online. 2003;6(4):470-81.
3. Holesh JE, Bass AN, Lord M. Physiology, Ovulation. In: StatPearls [Internet]. Treasure Island (FL): StatPearls Publishing; 2023.

CHAPTER 2

Endocrinology of Follicular Phase in Stimulated Cycle

Rashmika Gandhi, Sunita Tandulwadkar

■ INTRODUCTION

Ovarian stimulation is a pivotal element in assisted reproduction technology (ART) cycles, strategically designed to facilitate the development of multiple preovulatory follicles, ultimately leading to successful oocyte collection. The conventional ART stimulation cycle comprises three fundamental components:

1. *Induction of multifollicular growth with exogenous gonadotropins:* The initiation of a robust follicular phase involves the administration of exogenous gonadotropins, orchestrating the development of multiple follicles within the ovaries. This meticulous process is crucial for optimizing the yield of mature oocytes.
2. *Prevention of endogenous luteinizing hormone (LH) surge through gonadotropin-releasing hormone (GnRH) analogs:* To safeguard against premature ovulation, (GnRH) analogs are employed. These agents effectively suppress the endogenous LH surge, ensuring precise control over the timing of ovulation and enhancing the chances of successful oocyte retrieval.
3. *Inducing or mimicking LH surge with exogenous human chorionic gonadotropin (hCG) for oocyte maturation:* The final stage of the follicular phase involves triggering an endogenous LH surge or replicating it with the administration of exogenous human chorionic gonadotropin (hCG). This step is paramount for promoting the maturation of oocytes within the follicles, preparing them for subsequent retrieval and fertilization.

In the subsequent sections of this chapter, we will delve into a concise yet comprehensive exploration of the intricacies of the follicular phase in stimulated cycles. This will encompass a nuanced understanding of the physiological processes involved, potential challenges encountered, and contemporary approaches to optimizing outcomes in ARTs.

■ INDUCTION OF MULTIFOLLICULAR GROWTH WITH EXOGENOUS GONADOTROPINS

In the context of ovarian stimulation for ART cycles, it is essential to acknowledge the foundational understanding of follicular dynamics. Reproductive-aged women possess a finite number of primordial follicles within their ovaries. These primordial follicles undergo a process known as "primary recruitment," wherein a cohort initiates random and continuous growth. Antral stage development ensues independently of gonadotropin stimulation.

For further progression beyond the antral stage, follicle-stimulating hormone (FSH) becomes a crucial factor. The absence of adequate FSH, typical before puberty, results in atresia of antral follicles before reaching the preovulatory stage. The FSH threshold, the minimum level required for continued growth, varies among follicles at different stages. In a natural menstrual cycle, the rise in endogenous FSH production follows the decline of the corpus luteum, associated with decreased progesterone, estradiol, and inhibin A levels. This increase in FSH surpasses the threshold, allowing antral follicles to undergo "secondary" or "cyclic, gonadotropin-dependent recruitment." Approximately 10 antral follicles per ovary are recruited during the luteofollicular transition in a healthy young woman.[1] Growing antral follicles produce estradiol and inhibin B, initiating negative feedback on the hypothalamus and pituitary. This feedback leads to a reduction in pituitary FSH production below the threshold. While FSH-dependent antral follicles undergo atresia, the dominant follicle, expressing LH receptors, can sustain independent growth. This phase of FSH supply exceeding the threshold is termed the "FSH window." The purpose of ovarian stimulation in ART is to enhance the quantity of follicles progressing to the preovulatory stage, necessitating an extension of the FSH window. This extension is achieved through either administering exogenous FSH or utilizing antiestrogenic agents that disrupt negative feedback mechanisms, such as selective estrogen receptor modulators or aromatase inhibitors. In conventional ART cycles, exogenous FSH administration commences in the early follicular phase, a time when endogenous FSH levels dip below the threshold for existing antral follicles, facilitating the growth of this cohort up to the preovulatory stage. Follicular response to FSH stimulation is monitored through ovarian ultrasound examinations, and serum estradiol measurements offer a rough estimate of follicular growth during ovarian stimulation. Serum estradiol levels below 100 pg/mL on the 6th day of FSH stimulation suggest an insufficient follicular response, while levels exceeding 500 pg/mL indicate overstimulation. The trajectory of serum estrogen levels mirrors follicular growth throughout stimulation. Diminishing estradiol levels before triggering oocyte maturation are linked to reduced pregnancy rates. Inhibin-B, produced by granulosa cells of early antral follicles, can serve as a marker for follicular growth. Previous studies have demonstrated an association between serum inhibin-B levels between the 4th and 6th days of FSH stimulation and the number of mature oocytes collected. However, the routine practice of measuring inhibin-B levels over ultrasound and serum estradiol monitoring is questionable. Serum FSH levels lack informativeness concerning follicular growth. This is likely because the limiting factor for follicular response is the number of available antral follicles rather than the FSH level itself, if FSH is above the threshold. Additionally, the threshold varies among individual follicles, and there is a notable overlap in serum FSH levels between anovulatory women who responded, or did not respond, to exogenous FSH stimulation with follicular growth.[2]

PREVENTION OF ENDOGENOUS LUTEINIZING HORMONE SURGE AND FOLLICLE RUPTURE

Promoting multifollicular growth through exogenous FSH stimulation carries the inherent risk of triggering a premature LH surge, potentially resulting in the untimely rupture of follicles before oocyte collection. To avert this, interference with GnRH action on pituitary gonadotrophs becomes imperative. Two distinct approaches for pituitary suppression have been established:

1. *Pituitary Desensitization:* This method involves inducing pituitary desensitization through prolonged exposure to exogenous GnRH. Two protocols are commonly employed: (1) The long luteal GnRH agonist, where GnRH agonist administration begins either from the mid-luteal phase of the preceding cycle or concurrently with gonadotropin injections, and (2) the short GnRH agonist protocol, where these actions are taken simultaneously. The aim is to downregulate pituitary responsiveness to GnRH, thus mitigating the risk of an untimely LH surge.

2. *GnRH antagonist administration:* Alternatively, daily administration of a GnRH antagonist serves as a preventive measure when an endogenous LH surge is anticipated, typically in the late follicular phase. GnRH antagonists act by competing with endogenous GnRH at the pituitary receptor level, swiftly obstructing GnRH activity. Unlike GnRH agonists, which initially induce a "flare effect" by releasing FSH and LH from the pituitary, GnRH antagonists maintain endogenous gonadotropin production until their initiation in the late follicular phase. Consequently, the overall FSH consumption in GnRH antagonist cycles is lower compared to GnRH agonist cycles.

Moreover, it is important to note that GnRH agonist injections, despite their initial stimulatory effect, eventually lead to a hypogonadotropic state due to the internalization of GnRH receptors on gonadotrophs after prolonged exposure. In contrast, GnRH antagonist protocols maintain unaltered endogenous gonadotropin production until the initiation of the antagonist in the late follicular phase. This nuanced understanding of pituitary suppression strategies not only prevents premature LH surges but also influences the dynamics of FSH consumption in the context of assisted reproductive techniques.

■ ROLE OF LUTEINIZING HORMONE

The "two-cell, two-gonadotropin theory" proposes that ovarian steroidogenesis results from the distinct actions of FSH and LH on granulosa and theca cells, respectively, through specific receptors for each gonadotropin. LH stimulates the conversion of cholesterol to androstenedione in theca cells, which then diffuses into granulosa cells. Under FSH influence, androstenedione is aromatized to estrogens, highlighting the essential role of LH in estradiol production.[3] The concept of a therapeutic LH window, introduced by Balasch and Fabregues, emphasizes that maintaining LH levels above a certain threshold is crucial for optimal follicular maturation. Below this threshold, inadequate theca cell androgen synthesis and reduced aromatization of androgens to estrogens may lead to incomplete oocyte maturation.[4] GnRH analogs, used in ovarian stimulation, create an LH-deficient environment, potentially impacting follicle growth and maturity. Abnormal levels of LH, whether too low or too high, present challenges. Excess LH can lead to receptor downregulation and impaired granulosa cell proliferation, resulting in follicular atresia and premature luteinization. LH may also contribute to the deselection of subordinate follicles, suggesting a concept of an "LH ceiling" for optimal stimulation.[5] While LH is deemed necessary for optimal follicular growth, steroid environment, and implantation, the question of whether excessive LH is detrimental remains debated. Clinical trials on LH supplementation in ovarian stimulation yield conflicting results. Three commercially available gonadotropin preparations containing LH activity include urinary human menopausal gonadotropins (hMGs), LH glycoprotein produced by recombinant technology, and a combination of recombinant FSH (rFSH) and LH glycoproteins. Retrospective evaluations show no clear association between endogenous LH levels and ART outcomes, with equivalence observed between rFSH and hMG. Although rFSH stimulates more follicles and yields higher oocyte numbers, ovarian hyperstimulation syndrome incidence remains similar. Adding recombinant LH (rLH) to rFSH shows no significant difference in live birth rates, and endocrine profiles indicate comparable steroid hormone levels between rFSH and hMG. Routine LH administration's impact on ART outcomes, including implantation and pregnancy rates, lacks sufficient evidence. However, there is some indication of potential benefits in subsets of patients, particularly older women and those with diminished ovarian reserve. Amid uncertainties, routine monitoring of serum LH levels during stimulation cycles appears unwarranted. Plasma LH levels decline rapidly after GnRH antagonist administration, and the relevance of an isolated LH surge in GnRH antagonist cycles remains controversial, with no significant impact on cycle management.[6]

PROGESTERONE DURING OVARIAN STIMULATION FOR ASSISTED REPRODUCTIVE TECHNOLOGY

Menstrual bleeding ensues following the decline of the corpus luteum, a vital source of progesterone. In a natural cycle, serum progesterone levels remain below 1 ng/mL until the onset of an LH surge. However, in the long GnRH agonist protocol, the initial flare effect of the GnRH agonist on LH secretion can rescue the corpus luteum, leading to increased progesterone levels. If elevated progesterone levels coincide with the presence of an ovarian cyst at the commencement of gonadotropin injections, it signals an active corpus luteum. Managing this situation may involve extending downregulation with the GnRH agonist, delaying the start of gonadotropins until after the corpus luteum demise, or aspirating the cyst before initiating gonadotropin injections **(Figs. 1A and B)**.

While the routine measurement of serum progesterone levels is not necessary for confirming pituitary downregulation when ultrasound reveals a thin endometrium without an ovarian cyst exceeding 10 mm, high progesterone levels early in the cycle are often attributed to incomplete luteolysis. Research indicates that a serum progesterone level above 1.5 ng/mL on the 2nd day of a spontaneous menstrual cycle occurs in 4–13% of women scheduled for ovarian stimulation in a GnRH antagonist cycle. Studies consistently demonstrate a noteworthy reduction in pregnancy rates among women with elevated early follicular-phase progesterone levels. However, due to the relatively low incidence of elevated progesterone on the 2nd day of the cycle and the absence of established interventions to restore pregnancy rates, routine screening of serum progesterone levels before initiating stimulation is not recommended in GnRH antagonist cycles.[7-9]

LATE FOLLICULAR-PHASE SERUM PROGESTERONE LEVELS

The impact of late follicular serum progesterone elevation on IVF outcomes has garnered

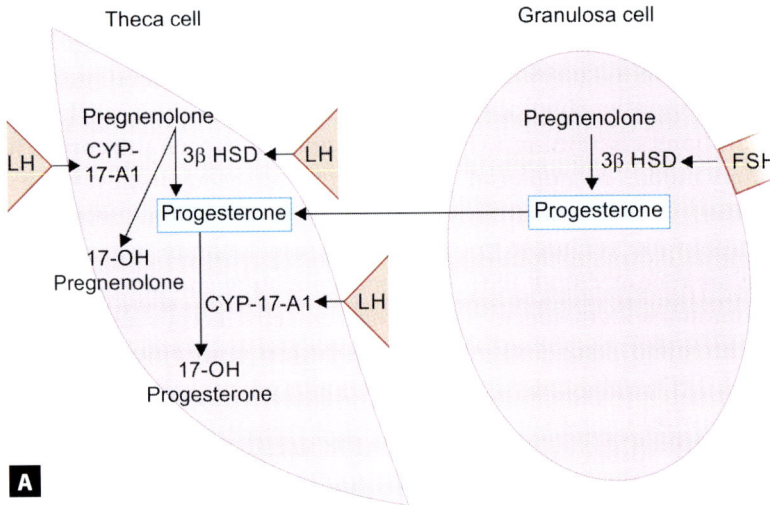

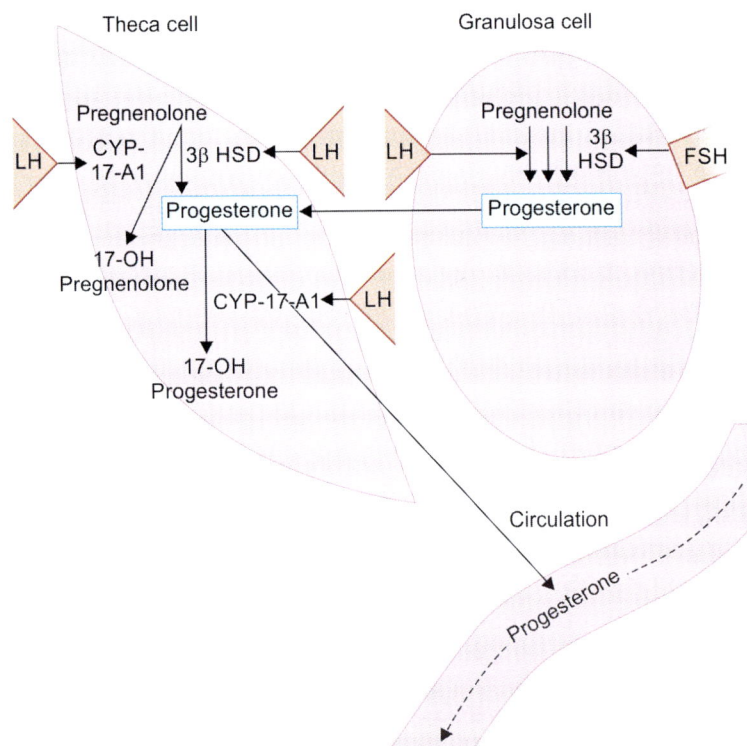

Figs. 1A and B: Progesterone synthesis and processing in the follicular phase involve distinct activities. The enzyme CYP-17-A1 (C17 hydroxylase) operates solely in the theca cells, leading to the migration of progesterone generated by granulosa cells into the theca cells for hydroxylation. (A) In the early follicular phase, LH selectively influences the theca cells, promoting 3β-hydroxysteroid dehydrogenase to transform pregnenolone into progesterone. Additionally, LH stimulates CYP-17-A1, converting progesterone into 17-hydroxylated progesterone; (B) As the late follicular phase unfolds, granulosa cells prominently express LH receptors. The impact of LH on progesterone production in granulosa cells is notably three times more potent than that of FSH. Excessively produced progesterone in granulosa cells may enter the bloodstream. (FSH: follicle-stimulating hormone; LH: luteinizing hormone).

significant attention since its initial report by Schoolcraft et al. in 1991.[10] The risk associated with this elevation is notably linked to the intensity of ovarian stimulation, including factors such as FSH dose consumption, serum estradiol concentration, and the number of retrieved oocytes. These findings underscore the pivotal role of the granulosa cell "mass" in influencing the likelihood of premature progesterone elevation, particularly in hyper-responder patients.

Interestingly, even in poor ovarian responders, an increase in serum progesterone can be observed, although the mechanism remains uncertain. Excessive FSH stimulation may still be a contributing factor in such cases. Furthermore, the choice of GnRH analog can impact the risk of progesterone elevation. Specifically, serum progesterone levels on the trigger day tend to be higher in cycles cotreated with GnRH agonists compared to those with GnRH antagonists. This discrepancy is primarily attributed to the retrieval of approximately one to two more oocytes and a higher endogenous LH concentration during the final days of stimulation in GnRH agonist cotreated cycles.[11]

TRIGGERING OF FINAL OOCYTE MATURATION

In the natural menstrual cycle, the mid-cycle LH surge plays a crucial role in inducing the release of the oocyte and subsequent follicle rupture. However, in stimulated ART cycles, the intentional suppression of the LH surge using GnRH analogs is a common practice to prevent follicle rupture before oocyte retrieval.

In the earlier days of ART, the norm was to mimic LH activity using hCG for two primary reasons: firstly, rLH was not readily available, and secondly, GnRH agonist protocols inhibited the induction of a spontaneous LH surge. Various dosages of hCG, ranging from 2,500 to 10,000 IU, are employed to trigger oocyte maturation. Notably, the plasma half-life of hCG is nearly 10 times longer than that of LH, not only facilitating oocyte maturation and release but also providing a sustained luteotropic effect.[12] The implications of this prolonged luteotropic effect on luteal-phase endocrinology are explored in the following section.

While it is technically feasible to trigger oocyte maturation using currently available rLH, extremely high dosages are required, making this approach impractical in clinical practice. The introduction of GnRH antagonists has revolutionized the process by enabling the induction of an endogenous LH surge with a single administration of GnRH agonist. Like the natural cycle, an endogenous FSH surge accompanies the GnRH agonist-induced LH surge. The benefits of this simultaneous FSH surge are currently a topic of controversy.[13]

Comparative analysis indicates that, in contrast to hCG triggering, the GnRH agonist-induced LH surge results in similar numbers of oocytes collected, fertilization rates, and embryo quality. However, it is important to note that the LH surge induced with GnRH agonists has a shorter duration compared to the natural cycle. This leads to rapid luteolysis, potentially impairing ongoing pregnancy rates when luteal phase support relies solely on progesterone.[14]

UNCONVENTIONAL OVARIAN STIMULATION

Traditional practice in ovarian stimulation adheres to the classical dogma of initiating stimulation in the early follicular phase. The underlying rationale is the simultaneous stimulation of a synchronized cohort of antral follicles recruited during the luteofollicular transition. However, emerging evidence challenges the concept of a single recruitment episode during the follicular phase, suggesting the existence of multiple waves of antral follicles within a menstrual cycle.

The wave theory, which posits that antral follicles develop in successive waves during the luteal phase, forms the basis for ovarian stimulation during this phase. While the dominant follicle from the final wave typically reaches ovulation, anovulatory waves precede and follow this ovulatory wave. Notably, a dominant follicle may also be selected during anovulatory waves in certain women, prompting the practice of initiating ovarian stimulation at any point in the menstrual cycle, termed "random start ovarian stimulation."[15]

Initially, employed for fertility preservation in cancer patients, random start stimulation has shown promising outcomes in women with normal or poor ovarian reserve. Another alternative strategy involves stimulating the ovaries twice within a single menstrual cycle. The initial stimulation begins in the follicular phase, and a subsequent cycle of stimulation is initiated after egg collection.

Given that some follicles recruited at the start of the luteofollicular transition may have already reached the preovulatory stage early in the follicular phase, it becomes possible to collect mature oocytes early in the follicular phase, capable of leading to a live birth.[16]

In essence, these unconventional approaches challenge the established dogma of universal follicular-phase stimulation, opening possibilities for alternative strategies in ovarian stimulation. However, the adoption of such strategies into common practice in reproductive endocrinology requires further extensive studies to validate their efficacy and safety.

■ CONCLUSION

In conclusion, the endocrine dynamics in a stimulated ART cycle deviate significantly from those in a natural cycle across both the follicular and luteal phases. Essential for the induction of multifollicular growth is the clear necessity to overshoot the FSH threshold. However, routine monitoring of serum FSH values is deemed unnecessary, as they do not reliably predict the extent of multifollicular growth.

Despite the acknowledged requirement for some LH activity in fostering proper follicle growth, a defined LH threshold remains elusive, and current evidence does not advocate for the routine monitoring of serum LH levels during stimulation. Elevated serum estradiol levels, reflective of extensive multifollicular growth, distinguish ART cycles from natural cycles. While distinct estradiol patterns during stimulation can offer insights into treatment outcomes, the existing evidence does not conclusively favor monitoring serum estradiol levels over ultrasound-only assessments.

In cases where ultrasound examination fails to confirm pituitary suppression in the long luteal GnRH agonist protocol, measuring serum levels of LH, estradiol, and progesterone can be considered for confirmation. While routine measurement of progesterone levels at the start of the GnRH antagonist cycle is not warranted due to its low incidence, elevated progesterone levels in the late follicular phase present informative considerations for treatment outcomes, influencing clinical decision-making.

In summary, the intricacies of endocrine profiles in ART cycles underscore the complexity of reproductive interventions. While certain markers offer insights into treatment outcomes, the overall landscape requires nuanced and individualized considerations. Further research is warranted to refine and expand our understanding of these endocrine dynamics, ultimately guiding more tailored and effective approaches in the realm of assisted reproductive techniques.

KEY LEARNING POINTS

- The primary goal of ovarian stimulation in ART cycles is to induce the development of multiple preovulatory follicles, facilitating the retrieval of oocytes for subsequent fertilization.
- Ovarian stimulation typically involves three main components—induction of multifollicular growth with exogenous gonadotropins, prevention of endogenous LH surge using GnRH analogs, and triggering an endogenous or exogenous LH surge for oocyte maturation.
- The natural follicular phase involves the growth of primordial follicles, and FSH plays a pivotal role in this process. Understanding the dynamics of follicular growth, FSH thresholds, and the interplay with hormonal changes in a natural cycle is crucial for comprehending the stimulated cycle.
- Routine monitoring of serum FSH and LH levels during stimulation cycles faces challenges, as serum FSH values are not indicative of multifollicular growth, and a defined LH threshold remains elusive. The chapter explores alternative monitoring strategies and their significance.
- Beyond the conventional approach, the chapter delves into alternative strategies challenging the dogma of universal follicular-phase stimulation. This includes insights into random start ovarian stimulation, luteal-phase initiation, and even dual stimulations within a single menstrual cycle.
- These keypoints set the stage for a comprehensive exploration of the pathophysiology of the follicular phase in stimulated ART cycles, providing a foundation for understanding the complexities and nuances involved in assisted reproductive techniques.

REFERENCES

1. Pache TD, Wladimiroff JW, de Jong FH, Hop WC, Fauser BC. Growth patterns of nondominant ovarian follicles during the normal menstrual cycle. Fertil Steril. 1990;54:638-42.
2. van Weissenbruch MM, Schoemaker HC, Drexhage HA, Schoemaker J. Pharmacodynamics of human menopausal gonadotrophin (HMG) and follicle-stimulating hormone (FSH). The importance of the FSH concentration in initiating follicular growth in polycystic ovary-like disease. Hum Reprod. 1993;8:813-21.
3. Loumaye E, Engrand P, Shoham Z, Hillier SG, Baird DT. Clinical evidence for an LH "ceiling" effect induced by administration of recombinant human LH during the late follicular phase of stimulated cycles in World Health Organization type I and type II anovulation. Hum Reprod. 2003;18:314-22.
4. Balasch J, Fabregues F. Is luteinizing hormone needed for optimal ovulation induction? Curr Opin Obstet Gynecol. 2002;14:265-74.
5. Shoham Z. The clinical therapeutic window for luteinizing hormone in controlled ovarian stimulation. Fertil Steril. 2002;77:1170-7.
6. Wong PC, Qiao J, Ho C, Ramaraju GA, Wiweko B, Takehara Y, et al. Current opinion on use of luteinizing hormone supplementation in assisted reproduction therapy: an Asian perspective. Reprod Biomed Online. 2011; 23:81-90.
7. Hamdine O, Macklon NS, Eijkemans MJ, Laven JS, Cohlen BJ, Verhoeff A, et al. Elevated early follicular progesterone levels and in vitro fertilization outcomes: A prospective intervention study and meta-analysis. Fertil Steril. 2014;102:448-54, e1.

8. Kolibianakis EM, Zikopoulos K, Smitz J, Camus M, Tournaye H, Van Steirteghem AC, et al. Elevated progesterone at initiation of stimulation is associated with a lower ongoing pregnancy rate after IVF using GnRH antagonists. Hum Reprod. 2004;19:1525-9.
9. Christophe B, Miriam B, De Vos M, Greta V, Paul D. Administration of GnRH antagonists in case of elevated progesterone at initiation of the cycle: a prospective cohort study. Curr Pharm Biotechnol. 2011;12:423-8.
10. Schoolcraft W, Sinton E, Schlenker T, Huynh D, Hamilton F, Meldrum DR. Lower pregnancy rate with premature luteinization during pituitary suppression with leuprolide acetate. Fertil Steril. 1991;55:563-6.
11. Papanikolaou EG, Pados G, Grimbizis G, Bili E, Kyriazi L, Polyzos NP, et al. GnRH-agonist versus GnRH-antagonist IVF cycles: Is the reproductive outcome affected by the incidence of progesterone elevation on the day of HCG triggering? A randomized prospective study. Hum Reprod. 2012;27:1822-8.
12. Kohler PO, Ross GT, Odell WD. Metabolic clearance and production rates of human luteinizing hormone in pre- and postmenopausal women. J Clin Invest. 1968;47:38-47.
13. Manau D, Fabregues F, Arroyo V, Jimenez W, Vanrell JA, Balasch J. Hemodynamic changes induced by urinary human chorionic gonadotropin and recombinant luteinizing hormone used for inducing final follicular maturation and luteinization. Fertil Steril. 2002;78:1261-7.
14. Turkgeldi E, Turkgeldi L, Seyhan A, Ata B. Gonadotropin-releasing hormone agonist triggering of oocyte maturation in assisted reproductive technology cycles. J Turk Soc Obstet Gynecol. 2015:12:96-101.
15. Baerwald AR, Adams GP, Pierson RA. Ovarian antral folliculogenesis during the human menstrual cycle: a review. Hum Reprod Update. 2012;18:73-91.
16. Hatirnaz S, Hatirnaz E, Ata B. Live birth following early follicular phase oocyte collection and vitrified-warmed embryo transfer 8 days later. Reprod Biomed Online. 2015;31:819-22.

CHAPTER 3

Endocrinology of Luteal Phase in Unstimulated Cycle

Rashmika Gandhi, Sunita Tandulwadkar

FOLLICULAR LUTEINIZATION

The onset of luteinization in granulosa-thecal cells is triggered by luteinizing hormone (LH) derived from the pituitary. This activation initiates a signal transduction pathway that relies on protein kinase A (PKA), along with a potential pathway connecting the LH receptor (LHr) to alterations in intracellular Ca2þ and diacylglycerol (IP3) generated through the activation of phospholipase C. The synthesis of estradiol shows a progressive increase originating from the dominant follicle, ultimately leading to the LH surge. Normal women exhibit a slight elevation in progesterone levels before the LH surge, indicative of the rising amplitude and frequency of LH pulses preceding the surge. In humans, a 24- to 36-hour LH surge is adequate to trigger the resumption of oocyte meiosis, disconnection of gap junctions between granulosa cells and the oocyte's plasma membrane, luteinization of granulosa cells, ovulation, and the initial phase of corpus luteum (CL) development. The LH surge also inhibits cell proliferation, likely influenced by changes in cyclins and other genes.[1-3] The surge-associated LH signaling enhances steroid biosynthesis, triggering the resumption of meiosis, ovulation, and subsequent luteinization in both theca and granulosa cells. In the latter stages of follicular maturation, LH, acting through the LHr on preovulatory granulosa cells, assumes the role traditionally played by FSH. Following the LH surge, plasma concentrations of progesterone (P) and 17a-hydroxyprogesterone (17aOHP) increase, marking the onset of luteinization in both granulosa and theca cells. The rapid elevation of P levels after the LH surge suggests that the necessary enzymes and proteins for P synthesis are either already present in the cells or are rapidly induced. The absence of the complete enzymatic machinery in human granulosa cells before the LH surge indicates that luteinization of thecal cells may serve as a potential immediate source for this rapid increase in P synthesis.[4] At this time, several morphologic and molecular changes take place in the granulosa cells.

CLASSIC PROGESTERONE RECEPTORS AND OVARIAN FUNCTION

The physiological effects of P are predominantly mediated through interaction with progesterone receptors (PR). Two classic isoforms of PR exist, namely PR-A and PR-B, with PR-A playing a crucial role in normal ovarian and uterine function, while PR-B is essential for mammary development.[5] LH serves as the primary signal for the rupture of preovulatory ovarian follicles and induces a transient expression of PR mRNA.

ENDOCRINE AUTOCRINE/PARACRINE REGULATION OF THE CORPUS LUTEUM

Regulation of the corpus luteum involves both endocrine and autocrine/paracrine mechanisms. The CL comprises steroidogenic cells (theca and granulosa lutein) and nonsteroidogenic cells (endothelial, immune, and fibroblast), all crucial for steroid synthesis and secretion.[6] Pituitary-derived LH plays a key role in this process, utilizing the cyclic adenosine monophosphate (cAMP) second messenger signaling system to regulate genes essential for hormone synthesis and luteal development. In conception cycles, trophoblastic human chorionic gonadotropin (hCG) production prevents CL regression. While LH is essential for primate CL development and maintenance, luteal regression occurs in the menstrual cycle due to reduced responsiveness of the aging CL to LH. Elevated hCG concentrations in fertile cycles overcome this regression.[7] Additionally, various molecules, including growth factors, hormones, nitric oxide, cytokines, insulin-like growth factor 1 (IGF-1), and IGF-binding proteins, modulate the in vitro effects of LH/hCG on human luteal cell steroidogenesis.[8]

STEROID BIOSYNTHESIS BY THECA AND LUTEINIZED GRANULOSA CELLS

The human CL is characterized by diverse cell types with distinct morphologic, endocrine, and biochemical phenotypes.[9] Throughout the luteal phase, these cells undergo changes in number, morphology, function, and secretory capabilities. Approximately 30% of CL cells are steroidogenic, with small luteal cells believed to originate from the theca-interna and large luteal cells from the granulosa cell lineage. Granulosa-lutein cells, responsible for both P and estradiol (E2) production, exhibit a greater basal P production and express aromatase for E2 synthesis. Theca-lutein cells, on the other hand, demonstrate a substantial increase in steroid production in response to hCG stimulation and express 17a-hydroxylase/17/20 lyase activity (P450c17). These cells produce androgen precursors, which are then aromatized by granulosa-lutein cells, and serve as the site for 17a-hydroxyprogesterone (17a-OHP) synthesis.

NONSTEROIDOGENIC LUTEAL CELLS

During the transition from the ovulatory follicle to a fully functional CL, there is a pronounced phase of proliferation among vascular endothelial cells, leading to the development of a robust capillary network. Endothelial cells constitute approximately 30–40% of mature CL cells. The luteal vasculature is crucial for transporting gonadotropins, plasma lipoproteins (a source of cholesterol for progesterone production), and facilitating the removal of secretory products, primarily steroid hormones, from luteal cells. The regulation of luteal vasculature is pivotal for controlling luteal function. Vascular endothelial growth factor (VEGF) mRNA and protein are localized in the granulosa-lutein cells of the CL. Inhibiting VEGF in vivo during the luteal phase in nonhuman primates hinders luteal angiogenesis and suppresses progesterone secretion.[10] In the past decade, an angiogenic factor known as endocrine gland-vascular endothelial growth factor (EG-VEGF), exhibiting a certain degree of specificity to the ovary, has been identified in human granulosa-lutein cells. Unlike VEGF mRNA, the mRNA levels of EG-VEGF increase in the mid and late CL stages. The presence of EG-VEGF is believed to empower the CL to respond to hCG, particularly in the early stages of pregnancy.[11] The significance of vasculature to CL function is evident in the modified parameters of blood flow observed in conditions such as luteinized unruptured follicle (LUF) and luteal phase defects.[12] Immune cells, including macrophages and T lymphocytes, are found within luteal tissue. Macrophages and endothelial cells form close connections with other luteal cells, enabling the regulation of luteal cells through paracrine mechanisms. The capability of macrophages to release interleukin (IL)-1b and tumor necrosis factor-α (TNF-α) is noteworthy, as both cytokines can influence luteal steroidogenesis. In vitro studies suggest that these cytokines reduce the LH/hCG-stimulated progesterone production in cultured human granulosa-lutein cells.[13] IL-1 and TNF-α are primarily secreted by activated luteal monocytes, macrophages, as well as T and B cells. The midluteal and late luteal phases of the corpus luteum are characterized by the presence of activated macrophages.[13] In normal physiological conditions, these cytokines likely contribute to functional and structural luteolysis, facilitating the initiation of a new menstrual cycle. However, the unregulated activation of these mechanisms could lead to dysfunction in the corpus luteum.

CHOLESTEROL TRANSPORT TO AND WITHIN LUTEAL STEROIDOGENIC CELLS

Obtaining the cholesterol precursor is the initial hurdle for steroid-producing cells, including luteal cells. While luteal steroidogenic cells have the capacity to synthesize cholesterol de novo, this pathway is of minor significance, as indicated by the low levels of 3-hydroxy-3-methyl-glutaryl-CoA (HMG-CoA) reductase, the key enzyme in this cholesterol pathway.[14] Steroidogenic luteal cells in humans acquire cholesterol carried by lipoproteins, particularly low-density lipoprotein (LDL), through endocytosis, maintaining reserves of esterified cholesterol. Additionally, high-density lipoproteins (HDL) may contribute cholesterol precursors for steroidogenesis via the SR-B1 receptors, facilitating the selective uptake of HDL cholesterol esters. Upon gonadotropin stimulation, cholesterol from various sources, including intracellular cholesterol esters stored in lipid droplets (which are hydrolyzed), is transported to the inner membrane of the mitochondria to serve as a substrate for pregnenolone (P5) production. The movement of cholesterol from the outer mitochondrial membrane to the inner membrane, where the cytochrome P450scc complex is situated, is believed to be the rate-limiting step in P synthesis. This sterol translocation in response to tropic hormones, including LH and hCG, is reliant on the essential role of steroidogenic acute regulatory (StAR) protein.[15,16]

LUTEAL PROGESTERONE SYNTHESIS

In primate ovarian physiology, three pivotal endocrine events support progesterone secretion:
1. *LH surge:* This surge serves as the signal for follicular rupture and the luteinization of theca and granulosa cells.
2. *LH pulses during luteal phase:* LH pulses during the luteal phase are crucial for the development and function of the CL.
3. *hCG secretion in early pregnancy:* hCG secretion by the embryo's trophoblast sustains CL function in early pregnancy.[17]

The biosynthesis of progesterone requires only two enzymatic steps: (1) The conversion of cholesterol to pregnenolone (P5), catalyzed by P450scc located on the inner mitochondrial membrane, and (2) its subsequent conversion to progesterone, catalyzed by 3β-HSD present in the smooth endoplasmic reticulum. Before the LH surge, StAR is virtually absent from human granulosa cells, rendering them unable to synthesize progesterone from cholesterol precursors.[18] On the contrary, StAR is present in high levels in the periovulatory human theca cells. These cells have the capability to synthesize androgens from cholesterol.[19] Therefore, the abrupt elevation in progesterone levels during the LH surge implies that the luteinizing theca cells might be the origin of progesterone. Moreover, the restricted vascular network of the human periovulatory granulosa cells could impede their access to cholesterol (low-density lipoprotein) through the vasculature. The formation of an insufficient vascular network in the corpus luteum is hypothesized to have substantial implications for steroid secretion in the later stages of the luteal phase. The expression of StAR transcripts and proteins is most prominent in the early and midluteal phases of the corpus luteum.

LUTEAL ESTRADIOL BIOSYNTHESIS

Small luteal cells are believed to be the primary source of luteal androgens,[20] while large luteal cells are considered the main site for luteal estrogen synthesis.[21] This suggests the preservation of the two-cell model of estrogen biosynthesis, initially proposed for follicular estrogen synthesis, in the primate corpus luteum. The enzyme P450c17, responsible for androgen synthesis, is in cells near the periphery of the gland along the vascular tract.[22] Although the two-cell system for estrogen production persists after luteinization of the follicle, the role of FSH in stimulating androgen aromatization is not conserved.[23] LH and IGF-1 appear to substitute for FSH, sustaining estradiol production by luteal cells in culture.[24]

A new model of follicular wave dynamics in the monovular mammalian ovary has been proposed, distinguishing between major and minor waves. Major waves lead to the development of the ovulatory follicle, while minor waves involve follicles that express P450arom and reach a diameter smaller than 5 mm. This raises the possibility that serum estradiol levels during the luteal phase may partly stem from luteal-phase follicle waves rather than exclusively from luteal tissue. The role of luteal estradiol secretion remains uncertain, as it was initially hypothesized to be involved in luteolysis in primates, where the luteolytic process is independent of uterine prostaglandin. However, the recent discovery of both types of estrogen receptors in the human corpus luteum supports a local role of estradiol in luteal function.[25]

LUTEOLYSIS

In a nonfertile cycle, the CL of primates undergoes a process of regression known as luteolysis. This process involves the loss of both functional and structural integrity of the gland.[26] The functional regression of the corpus luteum during luteolysis is characterized by a decrease in P production, while the structural regression occurs subsequently and is associated with various forms of cell death. The molecular events underlying luteal regression and how they are prevented by exposure to hCG remain unclear. A key feature of functional luteal regression is the reduced production of P, accompanied by a decline in the expression of the *StAR* gene and protein. This decrease in StAR expression precedes a decline in the expression of other steroidogenic enzymes, highlighting the critical role of StAR in luteal P production. Administration of hCG during the late human luteal phase restores StAR levels to those found in the midluteal phase corpus luteum, as well as plasma P and E2 levels. Various molecules, including prostaglandin F2-α (PGF2-α), TNF-α, interleukin-1β (IL-1β), endothelin, monocyte chemoattractant (MCP-1), estrogens, and reactive oxygen species, have been implicated in the luteolytic process.[27] The available data suggest that apoptosis is a characteristic feature of human luteal regression. Luteal cells showing a positive apoptotic signal and the number of luteal cells positive for inducible nitric oxide synthase (iNOS) increase within the human corpus luteum during luteal regression.[28] However, the percentages of luteal cells with apoptotic signals are relatively low, ranging from 5 to 7%, raising uncertainty about apoptosis being the sole mechanism responsible for luteal cell death. Other forms of cell death, including autophagy and necrosis, also seem to play a role in luteal regression.[29,30] The unscheduled activation of these mechanisms may contribute to luteal phase defects.

CORPUS LUTEUM RESCUE IN A FERTILE CYCLE

During the conception cycle, the trophoblast's production of hCG prevents the regression of the CL. Compelling evidence supporting the rescue role of hCG is demonstrated by the administration of a β-hCG vaccine to women, which inactivates endogenous hCG and leads to a decline in P levels and the onset of menstruation.[31] The hormonal profiles of conception and nonconception cycles differ during the early luteal phase. Conception cycles exhibit significantly higher levels of LH and E2 on days 4 and 5 after the LH peak in urine. However, serum levels of FSH, P, and relaxin are not significantly different during this period. These variations may indicate changes in signaling within the hypothalamic-pituitary-ovarian axis that commence in the periovulatory period of nonconception cycles.[32] Serum hCG becomes detectable around the time of implantation (day 8 after ovulation) and progressively increases up to the first 12 weeks of pregnancy. Vaginal ultrasound measurements show a rapid increase in CL volume during early human pregnancy, without a simultaneous rise in 17a-hydroxyprogesterone (17aOHP), P, or E2. However, the serum level of 17aOHP during the first 6 weeks of pregnancy is considered a reliable marker of luteal steroidogenesis because this steroid is not synthesized by the trophoblast, which lacks expression of P450c17. A positive correlation is observed between CL volume and serum concentrations of relaxin and hCG, suggesting that the growth of the CL in early pregnancy is mainly derived from the proliferation of nonsteroid-secreting cells.[33] Limited data are available on the molecular changes underlying the functional and structural alterations in the CL during pregnancy. Administration of exponentially increasing doses of LH or hCG extends the lifespan of the CL. Moreover, hCG administration during the late luteal phase restores the abundance of StAR mRNA and protein levels to those found in midluteal phase CL, along with an increase in plasma P levels. Additionally, hCG administration promotes the expansion of the vascular network in the theca and granulosa cell layers, with intense staining detected in the cytoplasm of steroidogenic cells.

The molecular changes underlying the functional and structural alterations in the CL during pregnancy are not extensively documented. However, studies have shown that the administration of exponentially increasing doses of LH or hCG can extend the lifespan of the CL.[7] Specifically, when hCG is administered during the late luteal phase, it restores the abundance of StAR mRNA and protein levels to those observed in the midluteal phase CL. This is accompanied by an increase in plasma P levels. Moreover, hCG administration induces the expansion of the vascular network within the theca and granulosa cell layers, and intense staining is detected in the cytoplasm of steroidogenic cells. These findings suggest that hCG plays a crucial role in maintaining the functional and structural integrity of the CL during pregnancy by influencing molecular factors such as StAR expression and vascular development.[13]

LABORATORY ASSESSMENT OF THE LUTEAL PHASE

The confirmation of ovulation has often relied on determining the P levels in the midluteal phase. There is variability in the cut-point values used to establish ovulation, ranging from 4 to 10 ng/mL in different settings. The considerable amplitude of pulsatile progesterone secretion during the late luteal phase, driven by large-amplitude LH pulses, poses a challenge to the accuracy of a single determination of this steroid. Alternatively, an increased daily excretion of pregnanediol, compared to the early menstrual cycle levels, is often considered as evidence that a woman has undergone ovulation. This method provides an alternative approach to assessing ovulation by looking at changes in pregnanediol excretion over time.

ULTRASONOGRAPHIC AND DOPPLER EVALUATION OF THE CORPUS LUTEUM

Ultrasonographic identification of the CL following ovulation is initially reported to occur in only 50–80% of natural menstrual cycles, as determined by transabdominal ultrasonography.[34] Two morphological types of CL can be observed after ovulation: those with and without a central fluid-filled cavity (CFFC). The majority of CLs contain a CFFC, and the incidence of CLs with a CFFC is highest immediately after ovulation, subsequently declining over time. The presence of a CFFC is associated with the leakage of blood into the follicular lumen following follicular rupture, and its ultrasonographic detection should be interpreted as a normal physiologic event during the menstrual cycle.[35]

A decrease in echogenicity during luteinization indicates increased vascularization of luteal tissue and a corresponding decrease in tissue density. In contrast, the increased echogenicity observed during luteolysis could be attributed to decreased vascularization and the replacement of luteal tissue with fibrous connective tissue.

ULTRASONOGRAPHIC AND DOPPLER EVALUATION OF THE LUTEAL PHASE ENDOMETRIUM

There is currently no reliable diagnostic method to evaluate endometrial receptivity, although various techniques have been proposed, including histologic assessment of endometrial biopsy,[36] evaluation of endometrial protein expression,[37] and ultrasound examination of the endometrium.[38]

Different ultrasound parameters have been suggested to assess endometrial receptivity, such as endometrial thickness, endometrial echogenic pattern, and endometrial volume.[39-41]

Endometrial Thickness and Pattern

Ultrasonographically, the endometrium appears as a thin, simple, hyperechogenic single stripe immediately after menses.

The stratum functionalis and basalis layers offer distinct views compared to the endometrial development during the mid-late follicular phase. In the periovulatory period, a pronounced triple-line echo-textural pattern, reflecting the separation between the stratum basalis and functionalis layers, is observed in association with rising estrogen (E2) levels. This triple-line pattern disappears after ovulation. A more homogeneous and hyperechogenic endometrium is observed as endometrial glands expand under the influence of luteal progesterone (P) production in the secretory phase.[42]

Endometrial Blood Flow

Doppler study of uterine arteries reflects blood flow to both the endometrium and myometrium. Blood flow to the endometrium originates from the radial artery, which divides after passing through the myometrial-endometrial junction to form basal arteries supplying the basal portion of the endometrium and spiral arteries continuing up toward the endometrium. Blood flow in the uterine vessels, assessed by color Doppler ultrasound, is typically expressed as downstream impedance to flow.

■ CONCLUSION

In conclusion, the CL in humans is a crucial temporary endocrine gland that produces significant amounts of steroid hormones, particularly progesterone, influencing menstrual cyclicity, endometrial receptivity, and early pregnancy maintenance. Regulation of the CL involves intricate endocrine, autocrine, and paracrine mechanisms, with luteolysis marking the regression of the CL in nonfertile cycles. The CL's rescue in a fertile cycle, facilitated by trophoblastic hCG production during conception, prevents regression, and sustains P levels. Various molecular events, including StAR expression and vascular development, contribute to the dynamic changes in the CL during pregnancy. Understanding the intricate mechanisms of CL development, function, and regression is essential for comprehending reproductive cycle dynamics and addressing potential issues related to fertility and luteal phase defects.

■ KEY LEARNING POINTS

The human corpus luteum (CL), a temporary endocrine gland originating from the ovulated follicle, serves as a significant source of steroid hormones, producing up to 40 mg of progesterone (P) daily. Unlike other species, the CL in many primates, including humans, exhibits a distinctive secretion pattern involving substantial amounts of androgens and estradiol (E2) alongside P. This secretion profile plays a critical role in shaping menstrual cyclicity, influencing endometrial receptivity for successful implantation, and is vital for the maintenance of early pregnancy. Therefore, gaining insights into the inherent endocrine, autocrine/paracrine, and molecular mechanisms governing P production during follicular cell luteinization, CL development, function, and rescue is crucial for comprehending the dynamics of a fertile reproductive cycle.

■ REFERENCES

1. Robker RL, Richards JS. Hormone-induced proliferation and differentiation of granulose cells: a coordinated balance of the cell cycle regulators cyclin D2 and p27Kip1. Mol Endocrinol. 1998;12:924-40.
2. Jirawatnotai S, Moons DS, Stocco CO, Franks R, Hales DB, Gibori G, et al. The cyclin-dependent kinase inhibitors p27Kip1 and p21Cip1 cooperate to restrict proliferative life span in differentiating ovarian cells. J Biol Chem 2003;278:7021-7.

3. Filicori M, Cognigni GE, Gamberini E, Parmegiani L, Troilo E, Roset B. Efficacy of low-dose human chorionic gonadotropin alone to complete controlled ovarian stimulation. Fertil Steril. 2005;84:394-401.
4. Christenson LK, Devoto L. Cholesterol transport and steroidogenesis by the corpus luteum. Reprod Biol Endocrinol. 2003;10:1-90.
5. Kastner P, Krust A, Turcotte B, Stropp U, Tora L, Gronemeyer H, et al. Two distinct estrogen-regulated promoters generate transcripts encoding the two functionally different human progesterone receptor forms A and B. EMBO J. 1990;9:1603-14.
6. Retamales I, Carrasco I, Troncoso JL, Las Heras J, Devoto L, Vega M. Morpho-functional study of human luteal cell subpopulations. Hum Reprod. 1994;9:591-6.
7. Zeleznik AJ. In vivo responses of the primate corpus luteum to luteinizing hormone and chorionic gonadotropin. Proc Natl Acad Sci USA. 1998;95:11002-7.
8. Devoto L, Vega M, Kohen P, Castro A, Castro O, Christenson LK, et al. Endocrine and paracrine-autocrine regulation of the human corpus luteum during the mid-luteal phase. J Reprod Fertil Suppl. 2000;55:13-20.
9. Carrasco I, Troncoso JL, Devoto L, Vega M. Differential steroidogenic response of human luteal cell subpopulations. Hum Reprod. 1996;11:609-14.
10. Fraser HM, Dickson SE, Lunn SF, Wulff C, Morris KD, Carroll VA, et al. Suppression of luteal angiogenesis in the primate after neutralization of vascular endothelial growth factor. Endocrinology. 2000;141:95-100.
11. Fraser HM, Bell J, Wilson H, Taylor PD, Morgan K, Anderson RA, et al. Localization and quantification of cyclic changes in the expression of endocrine gland vascular endothelial growth factor in the human corpus luteum. J Clin Endocrinol Metab. 2005;90:427-34.
12. Kupesic S, Kurjak A, Vujisic S, Petrovic Z. Luteal phase defect: comparison between Doppler velocimetry, histological and hormonal markers. Ultrasound Obstet Gynecol. 1997;9:105-12.
13. Kohen P, Castro A, Caballero-Campo P, Castro O, Vega M, Makrigiannakis A, et al. Interleukin-1beta (IL-1beta) is a modulator of human luteal cell steroidogenesis: localization of the IL type I system in the corpus luteum. J Clin Endocrinol Metab. 1999;84:4239-45.
14. Gwynne JT, Strauss JF 3rd. The role of lipoproteins in steroidogenesis and cholesterol metabolism in steroidogenic glands. Endocr Rev. 1982;3:299-329.
15. Stocco DM, Clark BJ. Regulation of the acute production of steroids in steroidogenic cells. Endocr Rev 1996;17:221-44.
16. Strauss JF 3rd, Kallen CB, Christenson LK, Watari H, Devoto L, Arakane F, et al. The steroidogenic acute regulatory protein (StAR): a window into the complexities of intracellular cholesterol trafficking. Recent Prog Horm Res. 1999;54:369-94.
17. Stouffer RL. Progesterone as a mediator of gonadotrophin action in the corpus luteum: beyond steroidogenesis. Hum Reprod Update. 2003;9: 99-117.
18. Chaffin CL, Dissen GA, Stouffer RL. Hormonal regulation of steroidogenic enzyme expression in granulosa cells during the peri-ovulatory interval in monkeys. Mol Hum Reprod. 2000;6:11-8.
19. Kiriakidou M, McAllister JM, Sugawara T, Strauss JF 3rd. Expression of steroidogenic acute regulatory protein (StAR) in the human ovary. J Clin Endocrinol Metab. 1996;81:4122-8.
20. Sanders SL, Stouffer RL, Brannian JD. Androgen production by monkey luteal cell subpopulations at different stages of the menstrual cycle. J Clin Endocrinol Metab. 1996;81:591-6.
21. Ohara A, Mori T, Taii S, Ban C, Narimoto K. Functional differentiation in steroidogenesis of two types of luteal cells isolated from mature human corpora lutea of menstrual cycle. J Clin Endocrinol Metab. 1987;65:1192-200.
22. Sanders SL, Stouffer RL. Localization of steroidogenic enzymes in macaque luteal tissue during the menstrual cycle and simulated early pregnancy: immunohistochemical evidence supporting the two-cell model for estrogen production in the primate corpus luteum. Biol Reprod. 1997;6:1077-87.
23. Devoto L, Kohen P, Vega M, Castro O, Gonzalez RR, Retamales I, et al. Control

of human luteal steroidogenesis. Mol Cell Endocrinol. 2002;186:137-41.
24. Johnson MC, Devoto L, Retamales I, Kohen P, Troncoso JL, Aguilera G. Localization of insulin-like growth factor (IGF-I) and IGF-I receptor expression in human corpora lutea: role on estradiol secretion. Fertil Steril. 1996;65:489-94.
25. Hosokawa K, Ottander U, Wahlberg P, Ny T, Cajander S, Olofsson IJ. Dominant expression and distribution of oestrogen receptor beta over oestrogen receptor alpha in the human corpus luteum. Mol Hum Reprod. 2001;7:137-45.
26. Stocco C, Telleria C, Gibori G. The molecular control of corpus luteum formation, function and regression. Endocr Rev. 2007;28:117-49.
27. Devoto L, Vega M, Kohen P, Castro O, Carvallo P, Palomino A. Molecular regulation of progesterone secretion by the human corpus luteum throughout the menstrual cycle. J Reprod Immunol. 2002;55:11-20.
28. Vega M, Urrutia L, Iniguez G, Gabler F, Devoto L, Johnson MC. Nitric oxide induces apoptosis in the human corpus luteum in vitro. Mol Hum Reprod. 2000;6:681-7.
29. Fraser HM, Lunn SF, Harrison DJ, Kerr JB. Luteal regression in the primate: different forms of cell death during natural and gonadotropin-releasing hormone antagonist or prostaglandin analogue-induced luteolysis. Biol Reprod. 1999;61:1468-79.
30. Del Canto F, Sierralta W, Kohen P, Muñoz A, Strauss JF 3rd, Devoto L. Features of natural and GnRH antagonist-induced corpus luteum regression and effects of in vivo human chorionic gonadotropin. J Clin Endocrinol Metab. 2007;92:4436-43.
31. Pal R, Singh O. Absence of corpus luteum rescue by chorionic gonadotropin in women immunized with a contraceptive vaccine. Fertil Steril. 2001;76:332-6.
32. Chen J, Oiu O, Lohstroh PN, Overstreet JW, Lasley BL. Hormonal characteristics in the early luteal phase of conceptive and nonconceptive menstrual cycles. J Soc Gynecol Investig. 2003;10:27-31.
33. Glock JL, Nakajima ST, Stewart DR, Badger GJ, Brumsted JR. The relationship of corpus luteum volume to relaxin, estradiol, progesterone, 17-hydroxyprogesterone and human chorionic gonadotropin levels in early normal pregnancy [published correction appears in Early Pregnancy 1996;2:76]. Early Pregnancy. 1995;3:206-11.
34. Queenan JT, O'Brien GD, Bains LM, Simpson J, Collins WP, Campbell S. Ultrasound scanning of ovaries to detect ovulation in women. Fertil Steril. 1980;34:99-105.
35. Baerwald AR, Adams GP, Pierson RA. Form and function of the corpus luteum during the human menstrual cycle. Ultrasound Obstet Gynecol. 2005;25:498-507.
36. Noyes RW, Hertig AT, Rock J. Dating the endometrial biopsy. Fertil Steril. 1950;1:3-25.
37. Gonzalez RR, Palomino A, Boric A, Vega M, Devoto L. A quantitative evaluation of alpha1, alpha4, alphaV and beta3 endometrial integrins of fertile and unexplained infertile women during the menstrual cycle. A flow cytometric appraisal. Hum Reprod. 1999;14:2485-92.
38. Ng EH, Chan CC, Tang OS, Yeung WS, Ho PC. Comparison of endometrial and subendometrial blood flow measured by three-dimensional power Doppler ultrasound between stimulated and natural cycles in the same patients. Hum Reprod. 2004;19:2385-90.
39. Ng EH, Chan CC, Tang OS, Yeung WS, Ho PC. Endometrial and subendometrial blood flow measured during early luteal phase by three-dimensional power Doppler ultrasound in excessive ovarian responders. Hum Reprod. 2004;19:924-31.
40. Coulam CB, Bustillo M, Soenksen DM, Britten S. Ultrasonographic predictors of implantation after assisted reproduction. Fertil Steril. 1994;62:1004-10.
41. Ueno J, Oehninger S, Brzyski RG, Acosta AA, Philput CB, Muasher SJ. Ultrasonographic appearance of the endometrium in natural and stimulated in-vitro fertilization cycles and its correlation with outcome Hum Reprod. 1991;6:901-4.
42. Baerwald AR, Pierson RA. Endometrial development in association with ovarian follicular waves during the menstrual cycle. Ultrasound Obstet Gynecol. 2004;24:453-60.

CHAPTER 4

Endocrinology of Luteal Phase in Stimulated Cycles

Madhuri Patil

■ INTRODUCTION

The human corpus luteum (CL) is a temporary endocrine gland that develops after ovulation from the ruptured follicle during the luteal phase and is a major source of steroid hormones **(Fig. 1)**. Normal luteal function is necessary for fertility and the maintenance of pregnancy. The human CL is composed of steroidogenic (theca and granulosa luteal cells) and nonsteroidogenic (endothelial, immune, and fibroblast) cells, both of which are critical for luteal steroid biosynthesis.[1]

The luteal phase is defined as the period between ovulation and either onset of menses 2 weeks later or the establishment of a pregnancy **(Fig. 1)**. The end of the luteal phase is due to luteolysis of the CL. Postovulation capillaries of the theca interna penetrate the basal membrane and the granulose layer becomes vascularized in response to secretion of angiogenic factors—vascular endothelial growth factor (VEGF), fibroblast growth factor, angiopoietins, and insulin-like growth factor.[2,3]

Capillary network extends throughout the fully differentiated CL tissue over the next few days due to intensive angiogenesis.[4] During luteinization, the granulosa cells are being reprogrammed to express a luteal phase-specific pattern of genes that encode enzymes, such as those required for cholesterol side-chain cleavage, P450 side-chain cleavage enzyme (P450scc), and the production of progesterone and 3β-hydroxysteroid dehydrogenase (3β-HSD).[5] The expression of P450scc in the CL

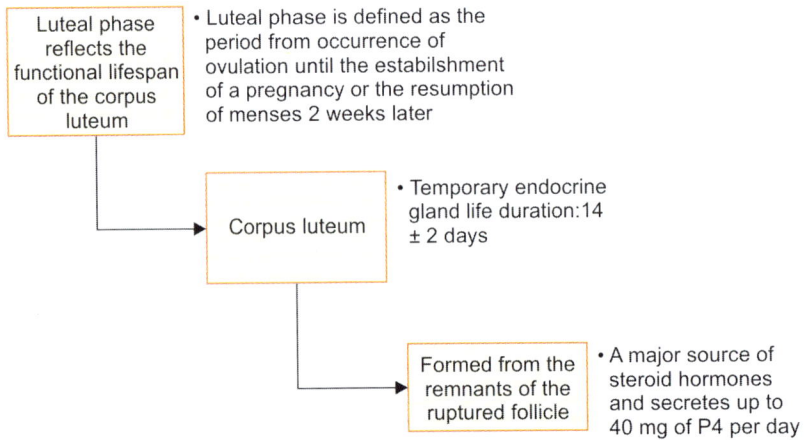

Fig. 1: Luteal phase in normal menstrual cycle. (P4: progesterone)

tissue in humans shows great variability in the late luteal phase, while 3β-HSD in vitro expression is reduced in late luteal phase and is "rescued" by human chorionic gonadotropin (hCG) given in vivo.[6]

Steroidogenic acute regulatory protein (StAR) is important for the transfer of cholesterol from the outer to the inner surface of the mitochondrial membrane.[7,8] The StAR protein is absent from the granulosa cells before the onset of the luteinizing hormone (LH) surge and this explains the inability of these cells to produce progesterone.[9] In vitro data have demonstrated that the expression of StAR protein increases in the human CL during the early and midluteal phase and declines in the late luteal phase.[10]

Increased vascularization allows large amounts of luteinizing hormone (LH) to enter the ovaries and the CL actively secretes progesterone, estrogen, and inhibin A, which are essential for secretory transformation of the endometrium, which enables the blastocyst to implant. LH is responsible for steroidogenic activity of the CL,[11] upregulation of growth factors VEGF-A, fibroblast growth factor 2 (FGF-2), and cytokines involved in implantation, and stimulation of LH receptors in the endometrium.[12,13]

During the luteal phase, a certain amplitude and frequency of LH is necessary to maintain an adequate steroid production by the CL.[14] Production of progesterone is initially from the theca-luteal cells, and later from the vascularized granulosa cells.[15] The amount of progesterone secreted daily from the CL is 25–50 mg. A midluteal progesterone value ≥10 ng/mL (≥32 nmol/L) or the sum of three random samples ≥30 ng/mL denotes a normal luteal function.[16,17]

Luteal progesterone rise plays critical role in implantation and development of normal pregnancy as it has the following functions:
- Downregulates estrogen receptors (ERs), thus indirectly suppressing the inhibitory effects of estradiol (E2) on integrins.
- Acts positively by increasing paracrine stromal factors—epidermal growth factor (EGF) and heparin-binding EGF (HB-EGF).
- Stimulates homeobox gene HOXA10—implicated in the regulation of β3 subunit expression.
- Transforms the endometrium into the secretory phase.
- Regulates the window of implantation (WOI).
- Increases endometrial vascularization.
- Acts as an immunomodulator.
- Reduces uterine contractions at the peri-implantation period.

If implantation occurs, the developing blastocyst secretes hCG, which is responsible for maintenance of the CL. Estrogen is also required in the luteal phase for implantation of the embryo and an optimal assisted reproductive technology (ART) outcome. Production of estrogen requires action of LH on the small luteal cells which produce androgens, which are then aromatized into estrogens in the large luteal cells under the influence of follicle-stimulating hormone (FSH).[18]

In the absence of conception luteolysis, an apoptotic process takes place, which results in reduction in secretion of progesterone due to reduced sensitivity to LH in the CL. Other mechanisms leading to luteolysis include upregulation of certain genes[19] which are favorable to prostaglandin F2-alpha (PGF2α) action,[20] and reduction in expression of N-cadherins in the late luteal phase, which are necessary to maintain cell-to-cell adhesion sites.[21] An in vitro data concluded that intraluteal substances, such as interleukin-1β, tumor necrosis factor α, and nitric oxide reduce the production of progesterone.[22]

LUTEAL PHASE IN STIMULATED CYCLES

Changes in the endocrine environment and CL dysfunction may be associated with different ovarian stimulation protocols especially those using gonadotropins. Thus, most ART cycles and those non-ART cycles where gonadotropins or gonadotropin-releasing hormone (GnRH) analogs have been used result in an abnormal luteal phase. One could also have an abnormal luteal phase in women stimulated with clomiphene citrate (CC). Luteal phase after ovarian stimulation is usually shorter and insufficient due to altered endocrinological parameters and thus associated with lower pregnancy rates.

The luteal phase defects (LPD) in stimulated cycles may be related to the multifollicular development, which alter the hormonal environment due to high concentration of E2 in the follicular phase and high estradiol and progesterone concentrations in the early luteal phase, especially when stimulation is performed with gonadotropins. These supraphysiological levels of steroids (both estrogen and progesterone) directly inhibit LH secretion via negative feedback actions at the hypothalamic–pituitary axis.[23] In the absence of adequate LH in the circulation, normal steroidogenic activity of the CL cannot be maintained.[24] Moreover, low levels of LH can also decrease inhibin levels and cause premature luteolysis.[25] Endogenous LH and or exogenous LH activity due to administration of hCG plays a crucial role in upregulation of growth factors[26,27] and cytokines, e.g., leukemia inhibitory factor (LIF), important for implantation.[28]

Luteal phase defect was documented in all ovulation–induction cycles using recombinant FSH plus a GnRH antagonist, whether recombinant hCG or recombinant LH or a GnRH agonist was given to induce final oocyte maturation.[29] When hCG with longer half-life is given for trigger, it can support the corpus luteal function only in the early luteal phase but not in the mid- and late-luteal phase, which is crucial for the implantation.[29]

The morphology, molecular phenotypes, and endocrine features of granulosa and theca cells of the preovulatory follicle is changed after midcycle LH surge following GnRH agonist trigger or hCG administration during a stimulated cycle. This marks the beginning of granulosa and theca cell luteinization due to increase in plasma concentration of progesterone and 17α-hydroxyprogesterone (17α-OHP). This is a result of an increase in expression of LH receptors, progesterone receptors, and the binding of activating transcription factors to the promoter of the StAR gene. GnRH agonist trigger or hCG administration also induces cytochrome P450scc, cyclo-oxygenase-2, and members of the matrix metalloproteinase (MMP) family, which are critical determinants of progesterone synthesis, oocyte maturation, and follicular rupture, respectively.[30]

Abnormal luteal function after ovarian stimulation with different protocols may be related to:

- Continuation of downregulation in long-GnRH agonist protocol which may prevent pituitary recovery[31,32]
- Induction of multiple follicle development in CC or gonadotrophin cycles which influences the duration of the luteal phase either directly or indirectly.[33,34]

- Removal of large quantities of granulosa cells at oocyte retrieval may decrease the most important source of progesterone synthesis by the CL, thus disrupting the luteal phase.[35,36]
- Supraphysiological levels of steroids due to multifollicular development with higher number of corpora lutea[37] during the early luteal phase could directly inhibit LH secretion from the pituitary via negative feedback actions at the hypothalamic–pituitary axis.[23]

Thus, stimulated cycles benefit with luteal phase support using either progesterone through different routes, hCG, and GnRH agonist or addition of E2. There is no difference in the outcome when different routes of administration of progesterone or addition of E2 were compared.[38-40] Both progesterone and hCG also have similar outcome; hCG may increase the risk of the ovarian hyperstimulation syndrome (OHSS).[41]

Luteal Phase in Clomiphene Citrate Cycles (Flowchart 1)

Clomiphene citrate initiates a series of endocrine events by displacing estrogen from the hypothalamus. Along with the central action, it also exhibits its antiestrogenic properties at the periphery. In addition, it also results in downregulation of cytosolic estrogen[42,43] and progesterone receptor concentrations,[42] which can alter the estrogen progesterone ratio. LPD after ovulation induction with CC has been observed in about 50% of CC initiated cycles.[44] The exact mechanism of endometrial abnormalities in CC cycles is not known. It may be related to direct CC action on the endometrium or due to hormonal imbalance induced by multiple follicular development. One must also remember that with long half-life (5 days), it remains active in the reproductive tract for a longer period of time following its discontinuation.

Luteal Phase in Assisted Reproductive Technology Cycles

Here we need to discuss the effect of gonadotropins used for stimulation, GnRH analogs used for pituitary downregulation, and hCG or GnRH agonist used as ovulation trigger.

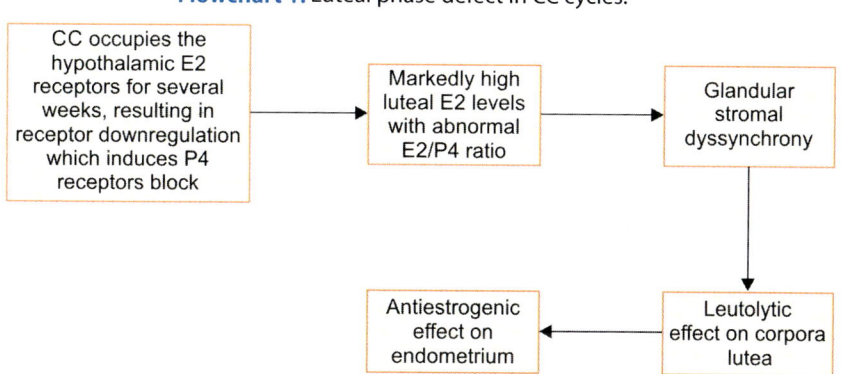

Flowchart 1: Luteal phase defect in CC cycles.

(CC: clomiphene citrate; E2: estradiol; P4: progesterone)

Luteal Phase Defect in Assisted Reproductive Technology Cycles

Effect on the luteal phase in ART cycles is related to decrease in LH levels due to:
- Supraphysiological concentrations of E2 in the late follicular and early luteal phase due to multifollicular development which result in deficient LH in the luteal phase
- Supraphysiologic progesterone levels that are in the early-to-midluteal phase have a negative effect on the pituitary gland, suppressing the LH release.
- Suppression of LH levels because of the use of GnRH agonist or antagonist to prevent premature LH surge.
- hCG given for trigger via short loop can suppress LH
- In ART cycles, oocyte retrieval results in removal of granulosa cells, which might diminish the most important source of progesterone synthesis by the corpora lutea, leading to a defect of the luteal phase.

EFFECT OF GONADOTROPIN-RELEASING HORMONE AGONIST USED FOR DOWNREGULATION ON LUTEAL PHASE

After stopping GnRH agonist in the downregulated patient, the recovery of LH and FSH levels takes at least 2–3 weeks.[32] In all ART cycles, GnRH agonist is stopped 2 days before the oocyte retrieval and therefore LH levels are low in the luteal phase. This is associated with a short luteal phase and reduced pregnancy rates,[45] unless the luteal phase support is provided with progesterone or hCG.[46] The luteal phase in ART cycles using GnRH agonist without luteal support is characterized by very high progesterone and E2 concentrations during the early luteal phase,[47] which is due to the effect of hCG bolus injection given to induce final oocyte maturation during the late follicular phase. Subsequently, premature luteolysis occurred during the midluteal phase due to low LH levels. Decrease in progesterone concentrations in the midluteal phase strongly correlates with the decrease in serum hCG levels.[47]

EFFECT OF GONADOTROPIN-RELEASING HORMONE ANTAGONIST ON LUTEAL PHASE

Initially, it was thought that luteal phase support may not be required in GnRH antagonist cycles as it has a rapid recovery of pituitary function.[48,49] Ragni et al. found no deleterious effects of GnRH antagonist administration on luteal phase hormonal profiles and duration of luteal phase in gonadotrophin-stimulated cycles both with and without GnRH antagonist therapy for IUI.[50] However, other studies using GnRH antagonist cotreatment in in vitro fertilization (IVF) noted premature luteolysis, resulting in a significant reduction in the luteal phase length which could then compromise the chances for pregnancy.[29] Stimulation with recombinant FSH (rFSH) and GnRH antagonist without progesterone supplementation results in dysregulation of 192 genes within the endometrium, resulting in implantation failure.[51] This luteal phase deficiency is seen whether r-hCG, r-LH, or GnRH agonist is used to trigger final oocyte maturation.[29]

Insufficient luteal phase is principally related to supraphysiological steroid levels in the late follicular and early luteal phase due to multifollicular development, resulting in subsequent multiple corpora lutea. Thus, for the rapid recovery of pituitary function,[48] luteal phase supplementation in GnRH antagonist protocols remains mandatory in IVF.[52]

A study by Ferraretti et al. looked at the luteal phase in IVF cycles stimulated using mild stimulation protocol. The study concluded that when IVF was done using CC, gonadotropins, and GnRH antagonist in good-prognosis (defined as ≤38 years old with normal ovarian reserve and normo-ovulatory cycles, body mass index < 29 kg/m², no previous cycles, no severe endometriosis, no history of recurrent miscarriage, no endocrine/autoimmune diseases, and no surgical semen extraction from the partner) patients, luteal phase support may not be necessary.[53] The hormonal (LH and progesterone) profiles of the luteal phase and its length were normal, with an implantation rate of 30% and live birth rate of 40%.[53] Despite their finding, they proposed that a larger, prospective controlled trial is needed to investigate whether luteal support is mandatory or not with mild stimulation.[53]

EFFECT OF HUMAN CHORIONIC GONADOTROPHIN USED FOR TRIGGER ON LUTEAL PHASE

Human chorionic gonadotropin administered for the final oocyte maturation in stimulated IVF cycles could potentially cause a LPD by suppressing LH production via a short-loop feedback mechanism.[54] However, the luteal phase in normal, unstimulated cycles in normo-ovulatory women, administration of hCG did not downregulate LH secretion.[55]

Due to its long half-life, HCG administered for final oocyte maturation covers the luteal phase for a maximum of 8 days.[56] Clearance of the exogenous hCG from the circulation is complete after 8 days and the maintenance of the nonsupported corpora lutea becomes dependent on endogenous LH production. In an unstimulated or natural cycle, LH will thereafter stimulate the corpora lutea. But in an stimulated cycle due to the suppressed LH levels as a result of supraphysiological steroid levels, there is no stimulus of the corpora lutea resulting in early luteolysis. Apart from this, the hCG bolus itself has a negative feedback effect on the pituitary LH synthesis and release.[29,57]

EFFECT OF HUMAN CHORIONIC GONADOTROPHIN AGONIST USED FOR TRIGGER ON LUTEAL PHASE

The spontaneous LH surge of the natural menstrual cycle is characterized by a short ascending phase of 14 hours, a peak plateau of 20 hours, and a descending phase of 20 hours.[58] The GnRH agonist-induced LH surge has a short ascending phase of <4 hours[58] and a descending phase of 20 hours without a peak plateau. Thus, GnRH agonist trigger is associated with an extremely short duration of the endogenous LH surge.[59] The duration of LH surge is more critical to normal luteal function than its amplitude.[60-62] Too short a duration of LH surge prevents the granulosa cells from completing luteinization, leading to a CL with impaired secretory function and a shortened lifespan.[63] The median LH levels 4 days post-trigger were also significantly low (2 IU/L) for early luteal phase, which results in low progesterone production throughout the luteal phase.[64] A short luteal phase then results in a low progesterone and estrogen concentration throughout the luteal phase as compared to hCG trigger.[58,65-71] These low progesterone levels after GnRH agonist triggers are very low for optimal embryo implantation, thus associated with absence of pregnancy.[72]

Moreover, the LPD that occurs following agonist-triggered ovulation is a patient-dependent response and thus could be variable from one patient to the other.[63]

Luteal phase deficiency following GnRH agonist trigger for ovulation is mainly due to lack of LH activity[73] which may be due to following mechanisms:

- LH activity is compromised after GnRH agonist triggering due to the shorter duration of the endogenous LH surge and a potential weaker activation of the LH/hCG receptor which result in a significant reduction in LH activity throughout the early/midluteal phase, leading to premature luteolysis and implantation failure.[71]
- Absent or reduced endogenous LH support of the early CL due to persistent pituitary desensitization.[74]
- Direct inhibitory effect of the agonist itself on the CL, which is endowed with GnRH receptors.[75]
- Dramatic decrease of supraphysiological concentrations of steroids after GnRH agonist administration.[76]

Human chorionic gonadotrophin supplementation on the day of oocyte retrieval extends the LH effect of the agonist and can restore a normal luteal phase[70] with optimal implantation and pregnancy rate, though may be responsible for occurrence of OHSS. The hCG produced by the implanting embryo is detectable in maternal serum as early as the 8th day after ovulation, which results in normal production of progesterone and estrogen by the CL thereafter.[77] Thus, after the end of the LH surge, continued luteal LH support is necessary in the early-to-midluteal phase to prevent early luteolysis and, subsequently, shortening of the luteal phase to sustain an early pregnancy.

■ CONCLUSION

Luteal phase defect can occur in natural ovulatory cycles and stimulated cycles resulting in infertility. LPD in stimulated cycles can be a result of suppression of LH secretion from the pituitary by supraphysiological steroid levels, GnRH analogs (agonists or antagonists) used to prevent premature ovulation during ovarian stimulation, and/or by the inhibitory action of the ovulation trigger (HCG or GnRH agonist), which is responsible for the maintenance of the CL activity for endometrial receptivity until its role is taken over by embryo-derived hCG. LPD can cause implantation failure and miscarriage through inappropriate endometrial preparation for implantation, embryo expulsion through uterine contractions after embryo transfer, or immune rejection due to a failure of progesterone-induced reprogramming of uterine T cells and natural killer (NK) cells. LPD caused by insufficient progesterone secretion by the CL can be easily corrected, either by hormonal stimulation of the CL or by a direct supplementation of exogenous progesterone.

■ KEY LEARNING POINTS

- Diagnosis of luteal phase defect remains controversial.
- A defective luteal phase in a natural cycle is defined as presence of serum mid-luteal progesterone levels of less than 10 ng/mL or lag of more than two days in endometrial histological development compared to the expected day of the cycle.
- Luteal phase of all stimulated cycles are abnormal.
- Luteal phase defect in a stimulated cycle may be due to:
  - Multifollicular development achieved during ovarian stimulation, alter hormonal environment completely.

- Multiple corpora lutea result in supraphysiologic levels of steroids in early luteal phase which directly inhibit the LH release via negative feedback actions at the hypothalamicpituary axis level.
- Prolonged pituitary recovery that follows the GnRH agonist co-treatment, to prevent spontaneous LH surge.
- Luteolysis may be initiated prematurely in antagonist co-treated cycles, resulting in a significant reduction in the luteal phase length.
- hCG administered for the final oocyte maturation in stimulated cycles could suppress the LH production via a short-loop feedback mechanism resulting in LPD.
- Removal of large quantities of granulosa cells during the oocyte retrieval (OR), which might diminish the most important source of progesterone synthesis by the corpora lutea.

- LPD in stimulated cycles can cause implantation failure and miscarriage through inappropriate endometrial preparation for implantation.

■ REFERENCES

1. Retamales I, Carrasco I, Troncoso JL, Las Heras J, Devoto L, Vega M. Morpho-functional study of human luteal cell subpopulations. Hum Reprod. 1994;9(4):591-6.
2. Anasti JN, Kalantaridou SN, Kimzey LM, George M, Nelson LM. Human follicle fluid vascular endothelial growth factor concentrations are correlated with luteinization in spontaneously developing follicles. Hum Reprod. 1998;13(5):1144-7.
3. Fraser HM, Wulff C. Angiogenesis in the corpus luteum. Reprod Biol Endocrinol. 2003;1(1):1-8.
4. Fraser HM, Lunn SF. Regulation and manipulation of angiogenesis in the primate corpus luteum. Reproduction. 2001;121(3):355-62.
5. McNatty KP, Fidler AE, Juengel JL, Quirke LD, Smith PR, Heath DA, et al. Growth and paracrine factors regulating follicular formation and cellular function. Mol Cell Endocrinol. 2000;163(1-2):11-20.
6. Duncan WC, Cowen GM, Illingworth PJ. Steroidogenic enzyme expression in human corpora lutea in the presence and absence of exogenous human chorionic gonadotrophin (HCG). Mol Hum Reprod. 1999;5(4):291-8.
7. Miller WL. Steroidogenic acute regulatory protein (StAR), a novel mitochondrial cholesterol transporter. Biochim Biophys Acta. 2007;1771(6):663-76.
8. Miller WL. StAR search—what we know about how the steroidogenic acute regulatory protein mediates mitochondrial cholesterol import. Mol Endocrinol. 2007;21(3):589-601.
9. Kiriakidou MA, Mcallister JM, Sugawara T, Strauss 3rd JF. Expression of steroidogenic acute regulatory protein (StAR) in the human ovary. J Clin Endocrinol Metab. 1996;81(11):4122-8.
10. Devoto L, Kohen P, Gonzalez RR, Castro O, Retamales I, Vega M, et al. Expression of steroidogenic acute regulatory protein in the human corpus luteum throughout the luteal phase. J Clin Endocrinol Metab. 2001;86(11):5633-9.
11. Stouffer RL. Progesterone as a mediator of gonadotrophin action in the corpus luteum: beyond steroidogenesis. Hum Reprod Update. 2003;9(2):99-117.
12. Tesarik J, Hazout A, Mendoza C. Luteinizing hormone affects uterine receptivity independently of ovarian function. Reprod Biomed Online. 2003;7(1):59-64.
13. Galvão AM, Skarzynski D, Ferreira-Dias G. Luteolysis and the auto-, paracrine role of cytokines from tumor necrosis factor α and transforming growth factor β superfamilies. Vitam Horm. 2018;107:287-315.
14. Filicori M, Butler JP, Crowley WF Jr. Neuroendocrine regulation of the corpus luteum in the human. Evidence for pulsatile progesterone secretion. J Clin Invest. 1984;73:1638-47.

15. Christenson LK, Devoto L. Cholesterol transport and steroidogenesis by the corpus luteum. Reprod Biol Endocrinol. 2003;1(1):1-9.
16. Lenton EA, Landgren BM, Sexton L. Normal variation in the length of the luteal phase of the menstrual cycle: identification of the short luteal phase. Br J Obstet Gynaecol. 1984;91(7):685-9.
17. Jordan J, Craig K, Clifton DK, Soules MR. Luteal phase defect: the sensitivity and specificity of diagnostic methods in common clinical use. Fertil Steril. 1994;62(1):54-62.
18. Sanders SL, Stouffer RL. Localization of steroidogenic enzymes in macaque luteal tissue during the menstrual cycle and simulated early pregnancy: immunohistochemical evidence supporting the two-cell model for estrogen production in the primate corpus luteum. Biol Reprod. 1997;56:1077-87.
19. Xu J, Stouffer RL, Searles RP, Hennebold JD. Discovery of LH-regulated genes in the primate corpus luteum. Mol Hum Reprod. 2004;11(3):151-9.
20. Priyanka S, Jayaram P, Sridaran R, Medhamurthy R. Genome-wide gene expression analysis reveals a dynamic interplay between luteotropic and luteolytic factors in the regulation of corpus luteum function in the bonnet monkey (Macaca radiata). Endocrinology. 2009;150(3): 1473-84.
21. Makrigiannakis A, Coukos G, Blaschuk O, Coutifaris C. Follicular atresia and luteolysis evidence of a role for N-Cadherin. Ann N Y Acad Sci. 2000;900(1):46-55.
22. Devoto L, Kohen P, Vega M, Castro O, González RR, Retamales I, et al. Control of human luteal steroidogenesis. Mol Cell Endocrinol. 2002;186(2);137-41.
23. Fauser BC, Devroey P. Reproductive biology and IVF: ovarian stimulation and luteal phase consequences. Trends Endocrinol Metab. 2003;14(5):236-42.
24. Casper RF, Yen SS. Induction of luteolysis in the human with a long-acting analog of luteinizing hormone-releasing factor. Science. 1979;205:408-10.
25. Duffy DM, Stewart DR, Stouffer RL. Titrating luteinizing hormone replacement to sustain the structure and function of the corpus luteum after gonadotropin-releasing hormone antagonist treatment in rhesus monkeys. J Clin Endocrinol Metab. 1999;84(1):342-9.
26. Sugino N, Kashida S, Takiguchi S, Karube A, Kato H. Expression of vascular endothelial growth factor and its receptors in the human corpus luteum during the menstrual cycle and in early pregnancy. J Clin Endocrinol Metab. 2000;85:3919-24.
27. Wang XF, Xing FQ, Chen SL. Interleukin-1beta expression on ovarian granulosa cells and its clinical implication in women undergoing in vitro fertilization. Di Yi Jun Yi Da Xue Xue Bao. 2002;22:934-6.
28. Licht P, Russu V, Lehmeyer S, Wildt L. Molecular aspects of direct LH/hCG effects on human endometrium—lessons from intrauterine microdialysis in the human female in vivo. Reprod Biol. 2001;1:10-9.
29. Beckers NG, Macklon NS, Eijkemans MJ, Ludwig M, Felberbaum RE, Diedrich K, et al. Nonsupplemented luteal phase characteristics after the administration of recombinant human chorionic gonadotropin, recombinant luteinizing hormone, or gonadotropin-releasing hormone (GnRH) agonist to induce final oocyte maturation in in vitro fertilization patients after ovarian stimulation with recombinant follicle-stimulating hormone and GnRH antagonist cotreatment. J Clin Endocrinol Metab. 2003;88(9):4186-92.
30. Richards JS. Genetics of ovulation. Semin Reprod Med. 2007;25(4):235-42.
31. Smitz J, Erard P, Camus M, Devroey P, Tournaye H, Wisanto A, et al. Pituitary gonadotrophin secretory capacity during the luteal phase in superovulation using GnRH-agonists and HMG in a desensitization or flare-up protocol. Hum Reprod. 1992;7(9):1225-9.
32. Donderwinkel PF, Schoot DC, Pache TD, De Jong FH, Hop WC, Fauser BC. Endocrinology: Luteal function following ovulation induction in polycystic ovary syndrome patients using exogenous gonadotrophins in combination

with a gonadotrophin-releasing hormone agonist. Hum Reprod. 1993;8(12):2027-32.
33. Messinis IE, Templeton AA. Disparate effects of endogenous and exogenous oestradiol on luteal phase function in women. Reproduction. 1987;79(2):549-54.
34. Hohmann FP, Laven JS, De Jong FH, Eijkemans MJ, Fauser BC. Low-dose exogenous FSH initiated during the early, mid or late follicular phase can induce multiple dominant follicle development. Hum Reprod. 2001;16(5):846-54.
35. Garcia J, Jones GS, Acosta AA, Wright Jr GL. Corpus luteum function after follicle aspiration for oocyte retrieval. Fertil Steril. 1981;36(5):565-72.
36. Vargyas J, Kletzky O, Marrs RP. The effect of laparoscopic follicular aspiration on ovarian steroidogenesis during the early preimplantation period. Fertil Steril. 1986;45(2):221-5.
37. Smitz J, Devroey P, Van Steirteghem AC. Endocrinology in luteal phase and implantation. Brit Med Bull. 1990;46(3):709-19.
38. Gelbaya TA, Kyrgiou M, Tsoumpou I, Nardo LG. The use of estradiol for luteal phase support in in vitro fertilization/intracytoplasmic sperm injection cycles: a systematic review and meta-analysis. Fertil Steril. 2008;90(6):2116-25.
39. Kolibianakis EM, Venetis CA, Papanikolaou EG, Diedrich K, Tarlatzis BC, Griesinger G. Estrogen addition to progesterone for luteal phase support in cycles stimulated with GnRH analogues and gonadotrophins for IVF: a systematic review and meta-analysis. Hum Reprod. 2008;23(6):1346-54.
40. Zarutskie PW, Phillips JA. A meta-analysis of the route of administration of luteal phase support in assisted reproductive technology: vaginal versus intramuscular progesterone. Fertil Steril. 2009;92(1):163-9.
41. Pritts EA, Atwood AK. Luteal phase support in infertility treatment: a meta-analysis of the randomized trials. Hum Reprod. 2002;17(9):2287-99.
42. Aksel S, Saracoglu OF, Yeoman RR, Wiebe RH. Effects of clomiphene citrate on cytosolic estradiol and progesterone receptor concentrations in secretory endometrium. Am J Obstet Gynecol. 1986;155(6):1219-23.
43. Nakamura Y, Ono M, Yoshida Y, Sugino N, Ueda K, Kato H. Effects of clomiphene citrate on the endometrial thickness and echogenic pattern of the endometrium. Fertil Steril. 1997;67(2):256-60.
44. Cook CL, Schroeder JA, Yussman MA, Sanfilippo JS. Induction of luteal phase defect with clomiphene citrate. Am J Obstet Gynecol. 1984;149(6):613-6.
45. Smitz J, Ron-El R, Tarlatzis BC. The use of gonadotrophin releasing hormone agonists for in vitro fertilization and other assisted procreation techniques: experience from three centres. Hum Reprod. 1992;7(suppl_1):49-66.
46. Soliman S, Daya MS, Collins J, Hughes EG. The role of luteal phase support in infertility treatment: a meta-analysis of randomized trials. Fertil Steril. 1994;61(6):1068-76.
47. Beckers NG, Laven JS, Eijkemans MJ, Fauser BC. Follicular and luteal phase characteristics following early cessation of gonadotrophin-releasing hormone agonist during ovarian stimulation for in-vitro fertilization. Hum Reprod. 2000;15(1):43-9.
48. Dal Prato L, Borini A. Use of antagonists in ovarian stimulation protocols. Reprod Biomed Online. 2005;10(3):330-8.
49. Elter K, Nelson LR. Use of third generation gonadotropin-releasing hormone antagonists in in vitro fertilization-embryo transfer: a review. Obstet Gynecol Surv. 2001;56(9):576-88.
50. Ragni G, Vegetti W, Baroni E, Colombo M, Arnoldi M, Lombroso G, et al. Comparison of luteal phase profile in gonadotrophin stimulated cycles with or without a gonadotrophin-releasing hormone antagonist. Hum Reprod. 2001;16(11):2258-62.
51. Macklon NS, Van Der Gaast MH, Hamilton A, Fauser BC, Giudice LC. The impact of ovarian stimulation with recombinant FSH in combination with GnRH antagonist on the

endometrial transcriptome in the window of implantation. Reprod Sci. 2008;15:357-65.
52. Tarlatzis BC, Kolibianakis EM. GnRH agonists vs antagonists. Best Pract Res Clin Obstet Gynaecol. 2007;21(1):57-65.
53. Ferraretti AP, Devroey P, Magli MC, Gianaroli L. No need for luteal phase support in IVF cycles after mild stimulation: proof-of-concept study. Reprod Biomed Online. 2017;34(2):162-5.
54. Miyake A, Aono T, Kinugasa T, Tanizawa O, Kurachi K. Suppression of serum levels of luteinizing hormone by short-and long-loop negative feedback in ovariectomized women. J Endocrinol. 1979;80(3):353-6.
55. Tavaniotou A, Devroey P. Effect of human chorionic gonadotropin on luteal luteinizing hormone concentrations in natural cycles. Fertil Steril. 2003;80(3):654-5.
56. Fatemi HM, Popovic-Todorovic B, Papanikolaou E, Donoso P, Devroey P. An update of luteal phase support in stimulated IVF cycles. Hum Reprod Update. 2007;13(6):581-90.
57. Smitz J, Platteau P. Influence of human chorionic gonadotrophin during ovarian stimulation: an overview. Reprod Biol Endocrinol. 2020;18(1):1-7.
58. Itskovitz J, Boldes R, Levron J, Erlik Y, Kahana L, Brandes JM. Induction of preovulatory luteinizing hormone surge and prevention of ovarian hyperstimulation syndrome by gonadotropin-releasing hormone agonist. Fertil Steril. 1991;56:213-20.
59. Fauser BC, de Jong D, Olivennes F, Wramsby H, Tay C, Itskovitz-Eldor J, et al. Endocrine profiles after triggering of final oocyte maturation with GnRH agonist after cotreatment with the GnRH antagonist ganirelix during ovarian hyperstimulation for in vitro fertilization. J Clin Endocrinol Metab. 2002;87(2):709-15.
60. Zelinski-Wooten MB, Lanzendorf SE, Wolf DP, Chandrasekher YA, Stouffer RL. Titrating luteinizing hormone surge requirements for ovulatory changes in primate follicles. I. Oocyte maturation and corpus luteum function. J Clin Endocrinol Metab. 1991;73(3):577-83.
61. Hoff JD, Quigley ME, Yen SS. Hormonal dynamics at midcycle: a reevaluation. J Clin Endocrinol Metab. 1983;57(4):792-6.
62. Cohlen BJ, te Velde ER, Scheffer G, van Kooij RJ, de Brouwer CP, van Zonneveld P. The pattern of the luteinizing hormone surge in spontaneous cycles is related to the probability of conception. Fertil Steril. 1993;60(3):413-7.
63. Emperaire JC, Parneix I, Ruffie A. Luteal phase defects following agonist-triggered ovulation: a patient-dependent response. Reprod Biomed Online. 2004;9:22-7.
64. Chandrasekher YA, Hutchison JS, Zelinski-Wooten MB, Hess DL, Wolf DP, Stouffer RL. Initiation of periovulatory events in primate follicles using recombinant and native human luteinizing hormone to mimic the midcycle gonadotropin surge. J Clin Endocrinol Metab. 1994;79(1):298-306.
65. Segal S, Casper RF. Gonadotropin-releasing hormone agonist versus human chorionic gonadotropin for triggering follicular maturation in in vitro fertilization. Fertil Steril. 1992;57(6):1254-8.
66. Khoury CA, Itskovitz-Eldor JO, Bar-Ami S. Induction of maturation of cumulus-oocyte complex by gonadotropin-releasing hormone analog is associated with lower progesterone secretion. J Clin Endocrinol Metab. 1994;79(4):1001-6.
67. Scott RT, Bailey SA, Kost ER, Neal GS, Hofmann GE, Illions EH. Comparison of leuprolide acetate and human chorionic gonadotropin for the induction of ovulation in clomiphene citrate-stimulated cycles. Fertil Steril. 1994;61(5):872-9.
68. Humaidan P, Bungum L, Bungum M, Yding AC. Rescue of corpus luteum function with peri-ovulatory HCG supplementation in IVF/ICSI GnRH antagonist cycles in which ovulation was triggered with a GnRH agonist: a pilot study. Reprod Biomed Online. 2006;13:173-8.
69. Humaidan P. Luteal phase rescue in high-risk OHSS patients by GnRHa triggering in combination with low-dose HCG: a pilot study. Reprod Biomed Online. 2009;18:630-4.

70. Humaidan P, Ejdrup BH, Westergaard LG, Yding AC. 1,500 IU human chorionic gonadotropin administered at oocyte retrieval rescues the luteal phase when gonadotropin-releasing hormone agonist is used for ovulation induction: a prospective, randomized, controlled study. Fertil Steril. 2010;93:847-54.
71. Humaidan P, Kol S, Papanikolaou EG. GnRH agonist for triggering of final oocyte maturation: time for a change of practice? Hum Reprod Update. 2011;17:510-24.
72. Andersen CY, Andersen KV. Improving the luteal phase after ovarian stimulation: reviewing new options. Reprod Biomed Online. 2014;28(5):552-9.
73. Humaidan P, Papanikolaou EG, Kyrou D, Alsbjerg B, Polyzos NP, Devroey P, et al. The luteal phase after GnRH-agonist triggering of ovulation: present and future perspectives. Reprod Biomed Online. 2012;24:134-41.
74. Kol S, Lewit N, ltskovitz-Eldor J. Ovarian hyperstimulation syndrome after using gonadotrophin-releasing hormone analogue as a trigger of ovulation: causes and implications. Hum Reprod. 1996;11(6):1143-4.
75. Minaretzis DE, Jakubowski MO, Mortola JF, Pavlou SN. Gonadotropin-releasing hormone receptor gene expression in human ovary and granulosa-lutein cells. J Clin Endocrinol Metab. 1995;80(2):430-4.
76. Kol S. Luteolysis induced by a gonadotropin-releasing hormone agonist is the key to prevention of ovarian hyperstimulation syndrome. Fertil Steril. 2004;81(1):1-5.
77. Bonduelle ML, Dodd R, Liebaers I, Van SA, Williamson R, Akhurst R. Chorionic gonadotrophin-beta mRNA, a trophoblast marker, is expressed in human 8-cell embryos derived from tripronucleate zygotes. Hum Reprod. 1988;3:909-14.

CHAPTER 5

Endocrinology of Ovulation and Its Clinical Application

Tejas Gundewar

ENDOCRINOLOGY OF OVULATION

Ovulation is a physiologic process defined by the rupture of dominant follicle and release of the oocyte from the ovary into the fallopian tube. Normal functioning hypothalamic–pituitary–ovarian axis coupled with the orchestrated release of hormones like gonadotropin-releasing hormone (GnRH), follicle-stimulating hormone (FSH), luteinizing hormone (LH), estradiol (E2), and progesterone is essential for ovulation to occur.

In the human ovary, an orderly sequence of events in the follicular phase of the menstrual cycle results in the selection of a single follicle (dominant follicle) from within a group of immature follicles, which is eventually ready for ovulation. This process, which occurs over the space of 10–14 days, features a series of sequential actions of hormones and autocrine-paracrine peptides on the follicle, leading the follicle destined to ovulate through a period of initial growth from a primordial follicle through the stages of the preantral, antral, and preovulatory follicle.

DEVELOPMENT OF PREOVULATORY FOLLICLE

The primordial germ cells originate in the endoderm of the yolk sac, allantois, and hindgut of the embryo and migrate to the genital ridge by 6–8 weeks. They undergo rapid mitotic multiplication to reach a total of 6–7 million in both ovaries by 16–20 weeks. The number then starts decreasing, with the sharpest fall prior to birth reaching 2 million and 300,000 at puberty. Out of these, 400 ovulate during women's reproductive years.

The primordial follicle consists of an oocyte arrested in the diplotene stage of meiotic prophase, surrounded by a single layer of spindle-shaped granulosa cells. With multiplication of the cuboidal granulosa cells, the primordial follicle becomes a primary follicle. Once growth is accelerated, the follicle progresses to the preantral stage as the oocyte enlarges and is surrounded by a membrane, the zona pellucida. The granulosa cells undergo a multilayer proliferation and have the ability to synthesize all three classes of steroids, however, significantly more estrogens than either androgens or progestins. The aromatase enzyme system acts to convert androgens to estrogens and is a factor limiting ovarian estrogen production. Initial follicular development occurs independent of hormone influence. FSH stimulation propels follicles to the preantral stage. FSH-induced aromatization of androgen in the granulosa results in the production of estrogen. Together, FSH and estrogen increase the FSH-receptor content of the follicle. The success of a follicle depends upon its ability to convert an androgen-dominated microenvironment to an estrogen-dominated microenvironment.[1,2]

Under the synergistic influence of estrogen and FSH, there is an increase in the production of follicular fluid that accumulates in the intercellular spaces of the granulosa, eventually coalescing to form a cavity, as the follicle makes its gradual transition to the antral stage. The accumulation of follicular fluid, which is rich in hormones, growth factors, and cytokines, provides the milieu that is required for the orderly maturation and development of the oocyte and its surrounding cells. The granulosa cells surrounding the oocyte are now designated the cumulus oophorus. In the presence of FSH, estrogen becomes the dominant substance in the follicular fluid. Conversely, in the absence of FSH, androgens predominate.[3,4] LH is not normally present in follicular fluid until the midcycle. If LH is prematurely elevated in the plasma and antral fluid, mitotic activity in the granulosa decreases, degenerative changes ensue, and intrafollicular androgen levels rise.

The successful conversion to an estrogen-dominant follicle marks the "selection" of a follicle destined to ovulate.[5] This selection process is, to a significant degree, the result of two estrogen actions: (1) A local interaction between estrogen and FSH within the follicle and (2) the effect of estrogen on the pituitary secretion of FSH. While estrogen exerts a positive influence on FSH action within the maturing follicle, its negative feedback relationship with FSH at the hypothalamic–pituitary level serves to withdraw gonadotropin support from the other less-developed follicles. The fall in FSH leads to a decline in FSH-dependent aromatase activity, limiting estrogen production in the less mature follicles. The dominant follicle, therefore, must escape the consequences of declining FSH induced by its own accelerating estrogen production.

■ OVULATION

Estrogen levels sufficient to achieve and maintain peripheral threshold concentrations of E2 are required to induce the LH surge. LH initiates luteinization and progesterone production in the granulosa layer. The preovulatory rise in progesterone facilitates the positive feedback action of estrogen at the level of pituitary, which results in the LH surge. Preovulatory rise in progesterone may also be required to induce the midcycle FSH peak.

Ovulation occurs approximately 10–12 hours after the LH peak and 24–36 hours after peak E2 levels are attained.[6,7] The onset of the LH surge appears to be the most reliable indicator of impending ovulation, occurring 34–36 hours prior to follicle rupture.[7] Usually, the LH surge lasts 48–50 hours. The details are depicted in **Figure 1**.

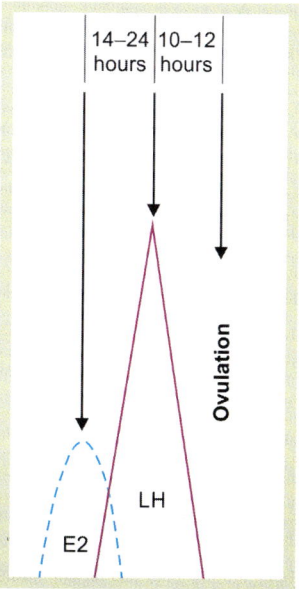

Fig. 1: Timeline of hormonal interplay prior to ovulation. (E2: estradiol; LH: luteinizing hormone)

The LH surge initiates the resumption of meiosis in the oocyte (meiosis is not completed until after the sperm has entered and the second polar body is released), luteinization of granulosa cells and progesterone production, expansion of the cumulus, and the synthesis of prostaglandins and other eicosanoids essential for follicle rupture.

An LH-induced increase in cyclic adenosine monophosphate (AMP) occurs within the follicle just prior to ovulation. Cyclic AMP is transferred from the granulosa cells to the oocyte via the gap junction network, and thus a reduction in cyclic AMP occurs when LH causes a breakdown of the gap junctions. This results in a decrease in the local inhibitory action of oocyte maturation inhibitor (OMI) and luteinization inhibitor (LI), which originates from granulosa cells.

With the LH surge, levels of progesterone in the follicle continue to rise up until the time of ovulation. The progressive rise in progesterone may act to terminate the LH surge as a negative feedback effect is exerted at higher concentrations. In addition to its central effects, progesterone increases the distensibility of the follicle wall, which is necessary to accommodate the rapid increase in follicular fluid volume occurring just prior to ovulation, unaccompanied by any significant change in intrafollicular pressure. FSH, LH, and progesterone stimulate the activity of proteolytic enzymes. The escape of the ovum is associated with degenerative changes of the collagen in the follicular wall so that just prior to ovulation, the follicular wall becomes thin and stretched.

The granulosa and theca cells produce plasminogen activator in response to the gonadotropin surge. Plasminogen is activated by either of two plasminogen activators: Tissue-type plasminogen activator and urokinase-type plasminogen activator. Plasminogen activators produced by granulosa cells activate plasminogen in the follicular fluid to produce plasmin. Plasmin, in turn, generates active collagenase to disrupt the follicular wall. Thus, before and after ovulation, the inhibitor activity is high, while just at ovulation, activator activity dominates and the inhibitors are at a nadir. Plasminogen activator synthesis in granulosa cells is expressed only at a precise preovulatory stage in response to LH. The inhibitor system, which is very active in the theca and interstitial cells, prevents inappropriate activation of plasminogen and disruption of growing follicles.

Physical migration of the preovulatory follicle to the surface of the ovary is an important step in which the exposed surface of the follicle is now prone to rupture because it is now separated from the cells rich in the plasminogen inhibitor system. Ovulation is the result of proteolytic digestion of the follicular apex, a site called the stigma. The matrix metalloproteinase (MMP) enzymes and their endogenous inhibitors, tissue inhibitors of metalloproteinases (TIMPs), are increased in response to LH and progesterone and are also involved in this event.

Prostaglandins E2 and F2α and other eicosanoids [especially hydroxyeicosatetraenoic acids (HETEs)] increase markedly in the preovulatory follicular fluid in response to the LH surge, reaching a peak concentration at ovulation. Prostaglandins act to free proteolytic enzymes within the follicular wall and contract smooth muscle cells, thereby aiding the extrusion of the oocyte cumulus cell mass from the ruptured follicle.[8-10] This ovulatory role of prostaglandins is so well demonstrated that infertility patients should be advised to avoid the use of drugs that inhibit prostaglandin synthesis.[11-13] A large number of leukocytes enter the follicle prior to ovulation. Neutrophils are a prominent feature in the theca compartment of both healthy and atretic antral follicles. The accumulation of leukocytes is mediated by chemotactic mechanisms of the interleukin system.

Estradiol levels plunge as LH reaches its peak. This may be a consequence of LH-mediated downregulation of its own receptors on the periovulatory follicle. Theca tissue derived from healthy antral follicles exhibits marked suppression of steroidogenesis when exposed to high levels of LH, whereas exposure over a low range stimulates steroid production. The low-midcycle levels of progesterone exert an inhibitory action on further granulosa cell multiplication, and the drop in estrogen may also reflect this local follicular role for progesterone. Finally, estrogen can exert an inhibitory effect on P450c17, a direct action on the gene that is not receptor-mediated.

The FSH peak, partially and perhaps totally dependent on the preovulatory rise of progesterone, has several functions. An adequate FSH peak ensures an adequate complement of LH receptors on the granulosa layer. Plasminogen activator production is sensitive to FSH as well as LH. Expansion and dispersion of the cumulus cells allow the oocyte cumulus cell mass to become free-floating in the antral fluid just before follicle rupture. It should be noted that a shortened or inadequate luteal phase is observed in cycles when FSH levels are low or selectively suppressed at any point during the follicular phase.

■ CLINICAL APPLICATION

Detection of Ovulation

The ability to identify the precise time of ovulation is important for women who want to plan conception or practice contraception. Urinary LH kits and ultrasound are the most commonly used methods for detecting ovulation. **Table 1** details all the methods available.

TABLE 1: Methods for detecting ovulation.

Name of test	Cost	Accuracy	Accessibility	Detects before ovulation
Urinary LH kits	Low	High	Easily available	Yes
Computerized monitor (urinary LH + E1-3-G)	Moderate	High	Easily available	Yes
Ultrasound	High	High	Less (needs to be performed by a physician)	Yes
Serum progesterone	Moderate	High	Less (needs to be done in a laboratory)	No
Urinary PDG	Moderate	High	Less (needs to be done in a laboratory)	No
Basal body temperature	Low	Low	High	No
Cervical mucus	No cost	Moderate	High	Yes
Salivary ferning	Low	Moderate	High	Yes

(E1-3-G: Estrone-3-glucuronide; LH: luteinizing hormone; PDG: pregnanediol 3-glucuronide)

Triggering of Ovulation

Therapeutic triggering of ovulation is an important step in patients undergoing infertility treatment. The basic issue regarding the precise dose that is both necessary and sufficient to trigger adequate ovulation has really never been resolved. More out of habit than from solid scientific evidence, the typical urinary human chorionic gonadotropin (hCG) dosing level has become:

- Approximately 5,000 IU for a monofollicular stimulation
- Approximately 5,000–10,000 IU in controlled ovarian hyperstimulation (COH).

Recombinant hCG 250 µg is commonly used in COH programs. Gonadotropin-releasing agonist (triptorelin acetate or leuprolide acetate) is also used if ovulation is not triggered with hCG.

CONCLUSION

A rightful interplay of hormones from hypothalamopituitary-ovarian axis brings about the process of ovulation. Ovulation is quintessential for fertility and hence its detection or artificial triggering carries paramount importance in fertility practice. Continuing research to develop patient friendly yet highly specific methods for detecting ovulation can simplify fertility practice. Similarly, more research is required for developing safe and effective medicines for triggering ovulation.

KEY LEARNING POINTS

- Initial follicle development is hormone independent and FSH stimulation propels the follicle to pre-antral stage.
- Estrogen-dominant follicle marks the "selection" of a follicle destined to ovulate.
- When estradiol secretion peaks, it induces the LH surge which causes luteinization of granulosa cells and progesterone production.
- Ovulation occurs approximately 10–12 hours after the LH peak and 24–36 hours after peak E2 levels are attained.
- Urinary LH kits and ultrasound are the most commonly used methods to detect ovulation.
- hCG injections (5,000 or 10,000 IU) are most commonly used for triggering ovulation in clinical practice. Use of recombinant hCG injections and agonist for triggering ovulation is on the rise.

REFERENCES

1. Chabab A, Hedon B, Arnal F, Diafouka F, Bressot N, Flandre O, et al. Follicular steroids in relation to oocyte development and human ovarian stimulation protocols. Hum Reprod. 1986;1(7):449-54.
2. Greisen S, Ledet T, Ovesen P. Effects of androstenedione, insulin and luteinizing hormone on steroidogenesis in human granulosa luteal cells. Hum Reprod. 2001;16(10):2061-5.
3. McNatty KP, Smith DM, Makris A, Osathanondh R, Ryan KJ. The microenvironment of the human antral follicle: interrelationships among the steroid levels in antral fluid, the population of granulosa cells, and the status of the oocyte in vivo and in vitro. J Clin Endocrinol Metab. 1979;49(6):851-60.
4. McNatty KP, Makris A, DeGrazia C, Osathanondh R, Ryan KJ. Steroidogenesis by recombined follicular cells from the human ovary in vitro. J Clin Endocrinol Metab. 1980;51(6):1286-92.
5. Goodman AL, Hodgen GD. The ovarian triad of the primate menstrual cycle. Recent Prog Horm Res. 1983;39:1-73.
6. Pauerstein CJ, Eddy CA, Croxatto HD, Hess R, Siler-Khodr TM, Croxatto HB. Temporal relationships of estrogen, progesterone, and luteinizing hormone levels to ovulation in women and infrahuman primates. Am J Obstet Gynecol. 1978;130(8):876-86.

7. Temporal relationships between ovulation and defined changes in the concentration of plasma estradiol-17β, luteinizing hormone, follicle stimulating hormone, and progesterone. I. Probit analysis. World Health Organization, Task Force on Methods for the Determination of the Fertile Period, Special Programme of Research, Development and Research Training in Human Reproduction. Am J Obstet Gynecol. 1980;138(4):138:383.
8. Markosyan N, Duffy DM. Prostaglandin E2 acts via multiple receptors to regulate plasminogen-dependent proteolysis in the primate periovulatory follicle. Endocrinology. 2009;150(1):435-44.
9. Espey LL, Tanaka N, Adams RF, Okamura H. Ovarian hydroxyeicosatetraenoic acids compared with prostanoids and steroids during ovulation in rats. Am J Physiol. 1991; 260:E163.
10. Miyazaki T, Katz E, Dharmarajan AM, Wallach EE, Atlas SJ. Do prostaglandins lead to ovulation in the rabbit by stimulating proteolytic enzyme activity? Fertil Steril. 1991;55(6):1183-8.
11. Pall M, Fridén BE, Brännström M. Induction of delayed follicular rupture in the human by the selective COX-2 inhibitor rofecoxib: a randomized double-blind study. Hum Reprod. 2001;16(7):1323-8.
12. Priddy AR, Killick SR, Elstein M, Morris J, Sullivan M, Patel L, et al. The effect of prostaglandin synthetase inhibitors on human preovulatory follicular fluid prostaglandin, thromboxane, and leukotriene concentrations. J Clin Endocrinol Metab. 1990;71(1):235-42.
13. Smith G, Roberts R, Hall C, Nuki G. Reversible ovulatory failure associated with the development of luteinized unruptured follicles in women with inflammatory arthritis taking non-steroidal anti-inflammatory drugs. Br J Rheumatol. 1996; 35(5):458-62.

SECTION 2

Investigations and Counseling

6. **Evaluation of Female Partner**
   Nikita Banerjee

7. **Evaluation of Male Partner to Optimize Intrauterine Insemination Success**
   Sunil Jindal, Anshu Jindal

8. **Selection and Counseling of Couple for Intrauterine Insemination**
   Surveen Ghumman, Pinkee Saxena

CHAPTER 6

Evaluation of Female Partner

Nikita Banerjee

INTRODUCTION

Infertility is defined as the failure to achieve pregnancy after 12 months of regular unprotected sexual intercourse. In approximately 85% of infertility cases, an identifiable cause can be ascertained in one of both the partners. The remaining 15% have unexplained infertility.[1] We, therefore, have an opportunity to identify and treat the cause leading to infertility in majority of cases. The most common causes of infertility include ovulatory disorders, tubal factor infertility, and male factor infertility. In this chapter, evaluation of female partner has been addressed.

Any couple trying to conceive for >12 months without unprotected intercourse should be evaluated for infertility. Earlier evaluation can be considered for:[2]

- Women who are >35 years of age trying for >6 months and considering the age-related decline in fertility, immediate attention should be given to those who are >40 years of age. Early evaluation can also be done for special circumstances such as amenorrhea, oligomenorrhea, those who have history of premature menopause in first-degree relatives, known or suspected uterine, tubal, and peritoneal disease such as stage III or IV endometriosis
- Known or suspected male factor
- Sexual dysfunction
- Genetic or acquired conditions that predispose to infertility (chemotherapy, radiation exposure, and *FMR1* premutation).

HISTORY AND PHYSICAL EXAMINATION

The initial assessment in the evaluation of female partner requires patient and sufficient time of thorough history taking and physical examination.

Fertility History

- Length/duration of unprotected sexual intercourse. The couple may be married for certain length of time but may not be cohabiting for sufficient length of time
- Coital frequency
- Sexual discomfort such as dyspareunia, erectile dysfunction, ejaculatory disorder, and vaginismus
- Prior fertility treatment—use of ovulation induction drugs, history of intrauterine insemination (IUI) or any form of assisted reproductive techniques. All previous documents related to previous fertility treatment should be read carefully.

Gynecological History

- Menstrual history:
  - Age at menarche
  - Cycle interval, duration, and amount of bleeding

- Presence of dysmenorrhea, intermenstrual bleeding, and molimina
- Obstetric history:
  - Previous pregnancies along with outcomes
  - Ectopic pregnancy, biochemical pregnancy, pregnancy of unknown location, termination, clinical miscarriage, stillbirth, and live birth
  - Nature of conception—spontaneous or with fertility treatment
  - History of surgical procedure—surgical evaluation for pregnancy loss or surgical treatment for ectopic pregnancy
  - Obstetric complications in previous pregnancies—hypertension, gestational diabetes, preterm delivery, fatal growth restriction, and placental disease.

Medical History

- Medical disorders such as endocrine, autoimmune, genetic, psychiatric, and malignant disorders.
- Prior surgical procedures. Take note of case history and surgical findings.
- History of diagnosis and treatment of tuberculosis.
- Current use of drugs ensuring that the patient takes the medication that is safe during pregnancy.
- Prompt identification and review of any potential teratogenic medication before the start of fertility treatment.
- Review antihypertensive, oral hypoglycemic medication and psychiatric medication. Shift to safer choice after discussion with the multidisciplinary team.
- History of drug allergy.

Family History

- Consanguineous marriage
- Inherited disorders, birth defects, and developmental delay
- Infertility
- Early menopause (<40 years)
- Multiple spontaneous abortions
- Hereditary cancer disorders.

Social History

- Use of alcohol, tobacco, or recreational drugs
- History of psychological, physical, or sexual trauma.

EXAMINATION OF FEMALE PARTNER

In case of infertility, apart from the general physical examination, a targeted examination should be performed to look for conditions that may affect fertility treatment or can have an impact on pregnancy.

- *Body mass index (BMI):* Extremes of weight can have negative impact on fertility and pregnancy.
- *Hirsutism:* Evaluate for androgen excess.
- *Acne:* Evaluate for androgen excess.
- *Acanthosis nigricans:* Evaluate for insulin resistance and polycystic ovary syndrome (PCOS).
- *Midline neck swelling:* Evaluate for thyroid disorders.
- Blood pressure assessment.
- Breast examination to look for galactorrhea or breast lump.
- *Abdominal examination:* Look for previous surgical scars. Abdominal palpation for lump.
- *Per speculum examination:* Vaginal and cervical abnormalities, discharge, and cervical polyp.

- *Bimanual pelvic vaginal examination:* tenderness, rectovaginal modularity, and uterine and ovarian masses.

DIAGNOSTIC EVALUATION

After a meticulous history-taking and examination, diagnostic evaluation should be done to look for common causes. Evaluation of infertility in female partner should be conducted in systematic, swift, and cost-effective manner with emphasis on least invasive methods to start with.

Ovulatory Factor

Ovulatory dysfunction accounts for approximately 40% of infertility in women.[3] It can present itself clinically as irregular cycles, oligomenorrhea, and amenorrhea, but regular cycles do not confirm ovulation. First step in a patient with secondary amenorrhea is to test for pregnancy. Once pregnancy is excluded, other causes of ovulatory dysfunction should be addressed. Common causes of ovulatory dysfunction include PCOS, thyroid disorder, hyperprolactinemia, obesity, extreme weight gain or weight loss, strenuous exercise, and perimenopausal status **(Table 1)**.

The World Health Organization (WHO) categorizes ovulation disorders into three groups:

1. *Group I ovulation disorders* (hypogonadotropic hypogonadal anovulation) are caused by the hypothalamic pituitary failure. This category includes conditions such as hypothalamic amenorrhea and hypogonadotropic hypogonadism. Typically, women present with amenorrhea (primary or secondary) which is characterized by low gonadotropins and estrogen deficiency. Approximately, 10% of women with ovulation disorders have a group I ovulation disorder.
2. *Group II ovulation disorders* (normogonadotropic and normoestrogenic anovulation) are defined as dysfunctions of the hypothalamic-pituitary-ovarian axis. This category includes conditions such as polycystic ovary syndrome and hyperprolactinemic amenorrhea. Around 85% of women with ovulation disorders have a group II ovulation disorder.

TABLE 1: Common causes, presentation, and assessment of ovulatory dysfunction.

Clinical condition	Clinical presentation	Evaluation and diagnosis
PCOS	Irregular cycles, oligomenorrhea, and amenorrhea	Ultrasound assessment
Thyroid disorder	Irregular cycles, oligomenorrhea, amenorrhea, and scanty menstruation	Serum TSH
Prolactin disorder	Oligomenorrhea, amenorrhea, scanty menstruation, and galactorrhea	Serum prolactin, Serum TSH. Hyperprolactinemia secondary to hypothyroidism
Obesity	Irregular cycles, amenorrhea, association with PCOS	Increased leptin, insulin resistance
Luteinized unruptured follicle syndrome	Anovulation despite regular periods, association with pelvic inflammatory disease, endometriosis, hyperprolactinemia, and PCOS	• Ultrasonographic evidence of dominant follicle failing to rupture after LH surge • Low midluteal serum progesterone

(LH: luteinizing hormone; PCOS: polycystic ovary syndrome; TSH: thyroid-stimulating hormone)

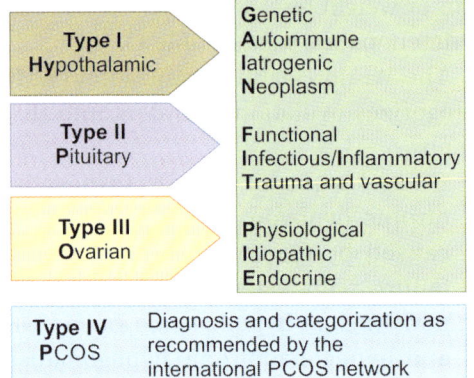

Fig. 1: The International Federation of Gynecology and Obstetrics (FIGO) Ovulatory Disorders Classification (HyPO-P). (PCOS: polycystic ovary syndrome)

3. *Group III ovulation disorders* (hypergonadotropic and hypoestrogenic anovulation) are caused by ovarian failure. Around 5% of women with ovulation disorders have a group III ovulation disorder.

The proposed International Federation of Gynecology and Obstetrics (FIGO) classification now includes ovulatory disorders categorized into four groups as follows: (1) *Type I:* Hypothalamic; (2) *Type II:* Pituitary; (3) *Type III:* Ovarian; and (4) *Type IV:* PCOS **(Fig. 1)**.

Ovulation Prediction Tests

- *Basal body temperature (BBT):* Serial, daily BBT testing is an inexpensive, often unreliable, method of predicting ovarian function. Ovulatory cycles are generally associated with biphasic BBT recordings unlike anovulatory cycles that typically result in monophasic patterns. Theoretically, the period of highest fertility spans the 7 days before the midcycle rise in BBT. Given the tedious nature of the testing and its lack of accuracy, this test is not routinely recommended today.
- *Urinary luteinizing hormone (LH) kits* can identify the midcycle LH surge that precedes ovulation within 1–2 days. Patients with PCOS may have a tonic elevation in basal LH levels, leading to false-positive results with urinary LH levels. Self-testing may result in false negative and false positive results and is often difficult to interpret by the patient.
- *Ultrasound monitoring:* This is a useful and commonly used tool to identify and time the ovulation. Serial growth and eventual rupture of dominant follicle with other associated signs of ovulation like presence of fluid in pelvis, luteal changes in the appearance of endometrium gives accurate assessment of ovulation.
- *Endometrial biopsy:* Historically, endometrial biopsy was used to look for the evidence of secretory changes in the histopathological examination of endometrial tissue obtained in the luteal phase. Due to its invasive nature and presence of other noninvasive better investigative modalities, use of endometrial biopsy is now obsolete for the purpose of identification of ovulation.
- *Serum luteal progesterone:* Serum progesterone can be measured 1 week before the expected onset of next menstrual cycle rather than one specific (day 21) day. A progesterone concentration >3 ng/mL provides presumptive and sufficient evidence of recent ovulation.[4] Serum progesterone levels can fluctuate sevenfold over a few hours, a single progesterone value may be used to confirm ovulation, but not to assess the quality of the luteal phase.

Ovarian Reserve Testing

The concept of ovarian reserve describes reproductive potential as a function of the number of oocytes. Women with decreased or diminished ovarian reserve may have regular menses while the response to ovarian stimulation is reduced relative to those in women of comparable age. Female age is the single most important predictor of fecundity. The goal of using ovarian reserve testing is to identify women who may be poor responders to gonadotropin stimulation in efforts to individualize treatment and discuss realistic expectations of response to treatment.[5]

Poor ovarian reserve testing does not necessarily imply an inability to conceive or subfertility. Ovarian reserve testing can be done using ultrasound assessment of astral follicle count or biochemical assessment of anti-Müllerian hormone and basal follicle-stimulating hormone (FSH) and estradiol levels. As the follicle pool diminishes in size, inhibition of pituitary FSH secretion by estrogen is lost and early follicular phase serum FSH rises. Basal FSH and estradiol should be measured together in the early follicular phase between menstrual cycle days 2–4. Anti-Müllerian hormone can be measured at any point in the menstrual cycle.

Antral follicles are 2–10 mm size range of well-defined anechoic cysts with smooth margins and absence of internal septations or nodularity measured and counted in each ovary **(Figs. 2A and B)**.

POSEIDON group (*Patient-Oriented Strategies Encompassing Individualize D Oocyte Number*) was recently established to focus specifically on the diagnosis and management of low prognosis patients.[6]

Four subgroups have been suggested based on quantitative and qualitative parameters **(Box 1)**, namely:
- Age and the expected aneuploidy rate
- Ovarian biomarkers [i.e., antral follicle count (AFC) and anti-Müllerian hormone (AMH)], and
- Ovarian response—provided a previous stimulation cycle was performed.

Tubal Factor Infertility

Tubal pathology accounts for 30–40% of all infertility cases.[7] Although the obvious causes include blocked tubes or presence of hydrosalpinx. However, mere latency of tube does not confirm adequate tubal

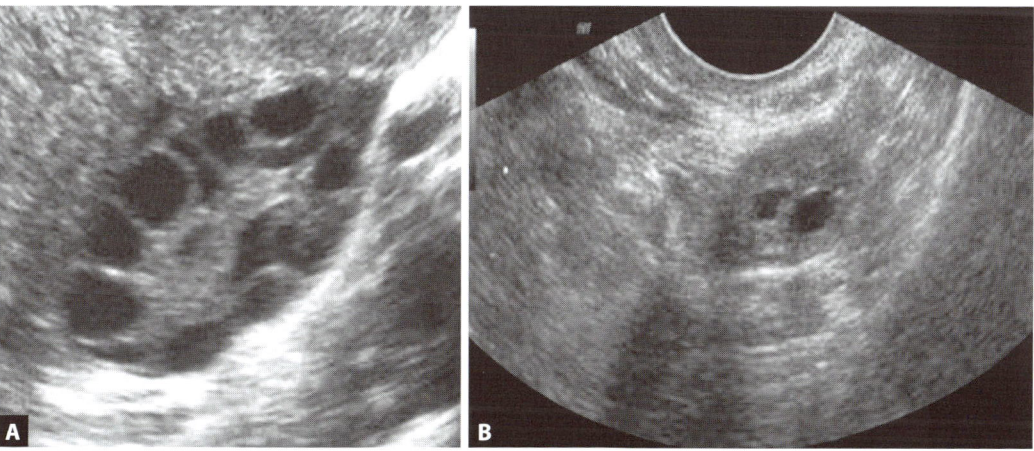

Figs. 2A and B: Ultrasound picture of astral follicles. (A) Ovary with good antral follicle count; (B) Ovary with low antral follicle count.

> **BOX 1:** Four groups of "low prognosis patients" in assisted reproductive technology according to the POSEIDON's stratification based on oocyte quantity and quality.
>
> *POSEIDON Group 1*
> Young patients <35 years with adequate ovarian reserve parameters (AFC ≥5; AMH ≥1.2 ng/mL) and with an unexpected poor or suboptimal ovarian response:*
> - Subgroup 1a: <4 oocytes
> - Subgroup 1b: 4–9 oocytes retrieved
>
> *POSEIDON Group 2*
> Older patients ≥35 years with adequate ovarian reserve parameters (AFC >5; AMH >1.2 ng/mL) and with an unexpected poor or suboptimal ovarian response.
>
> *POSEIDON Group 3*
> Young patients <35 years with poor ovarian reserve prestimulation parameters (AFC <5; AMH <1.2 ng/mL)
>
> *POSEIDON Group 4*
> Older patients ≥35 years with poor ovarian reserve prestimulation parameters (AFC <5; AMH <1.2 ng/mL)
>
> *After standard ovarian stimulation
> (AFC: antral follicle count; AMH: anti-Müllerian hormone)

function. There are various ways to test for tubal patency. Hysterosalpingography (HSG) is the most commonly used diagnostic modality. The HSG can document proximal or distal tubal occlusion. It may suggest the presence of fimbrial phimosis or peritubal adhesions when the escape of contrast is delayed or becomes loculated, respectively. It can also identify presence of hydrosalpinx. HSG may cause corneal spasm which may be falsely interpreted as corneal block. This can be avoided by performing HSG under anesthesia.

Sonohysterography can also be used to demonstrate tubal patency where tubal patency can be observed by the appearance of fluid in the cul-de-sac with the saline infusion. This test does not differentiate between unilateral or bilateral patency.

Uterine Abnormalities

Uterine abnormalities occur in 16.2% of women presenting for infertility evaluation, most commonly polyps (13%), submucous fibroids (2.8%), and adhesions (0.3%).

Ultrasonography is the best imaging modality and can simultaneously identify uterine anatomical abnormalities along with adnexal pathology. Leiomyoma, adenomyosis, and endometrial polyps are usual findings in infertile women.

Hysterosalpingography can aid in the identification of Müllerin anomalies such as arcuate, septate and bicornuate uterus which may further require assessment through three-dimensional (3D) ultrasound, MRI or laparoscopy and hysteroscopy. Laparoscopy, however, is not recommended as a routine method for assessing tubal patency. Acquired anomalies such as endometrial polyp, submucous myoma, and uterine synechiae can also be identified.

Sonosalpingography involves transvaginal ultrasonography after the introduction of saline into the uterine cavity. It better defines the size and shape of the uterine cavity and can be a valuable tool for the detection of intrauterine pathologies (endometrial polyps, submucous myomas, and synechiae).

Hysteroscopy is the definitive method for the diagnosis and treatment of intrauterine pathologies.

Peritoneal Factors

Peritoneal factors, such as endometriosis and pelvic or adnexal adhesions, may cause or contribute to infertility. History and examination can raise suspicion but are not enough to make diagnosis. Transvaginal sonography may reveal endometrioma. Laparoscopy with direct visualization is a reliable method for specific diagnosis of peritoneal factors such as peritoneal adhesions and altered tubo-ovarian anatomy. the impact of minimal and mild endometriosis on fertility is relatively small.[8] However, laparoscopy is not recommended for the routine evaluation of an infertile woman without a suspected pelvic pathology **(Box 2)**.

Flowchart 1 shows the systematic evaluation of female partner.

BOX 2: Infertility tests that should not be routinely ordered, unless specifically indicated.

- Laparoscopy
- Advanced sperm function testing and DNA fragmentation test
- Postcoital test
- Thrombophilia testing
- Immunologic testing
- TORCH test
- Endometrial biopsy
- Karyotype
- Hormonal test like FSH, LH, estradiol, and progesterone

(FSH: follicle-stimulating hormone; LH: luteinizing hormone; TORCH: toxoplasmosis, rubella, cytomegalovirus, and herpes simplex virus)

Unexplained Infertility

The Practice Committee of the American Society for Reproductive Medicine (ASRM) has published guidelines for a standard infertility evaluation.[9] It includes a semen analysis, assessment of ovulation, a hysterosalpingogram, and, if indicated, tests for ovarian reserve and laparoscopy. When the results of a standard infertility evaluation are normal, a provisional diagnosis of unexplained infertility is made. Although estimates vary, the likelihood of such diagnosis (unexplained infertility) is approximately 15–30%.[10] Majority of cases where females are diagnosed as unexplained are actually caused by following three conditions **(Flowchart 1)**:

1. Premature ovarian aging
2. Tubal disease and endometriosis
3. *Immunological infertility:* Role of antithyroid antibodies and antisperm antibodies has been studied in causation of infertility.

SUMMARY AND RECOMMENDATIONS

- Infertility evaluation is to be offered to couples who have not been able to conceive after 12 months of unprotected and frequent intercourse.
- Earlier evaluation (e.g., after 6 months) is indicated in some couples, such as those in whom the female partner is over 35 years of age or has a history of oligo-/amenorrhea, known or suspected tubal disease or endometriosis, a history of chemotherapy or radiation therapy, and those in whom the male partner is known to be subfertile.
- The history and physical examination are directed at identifying signs and symptoms suggestive of the etiology of the infertility.

Flowchart 1: Algorithm for systematic evaluation of female partner.

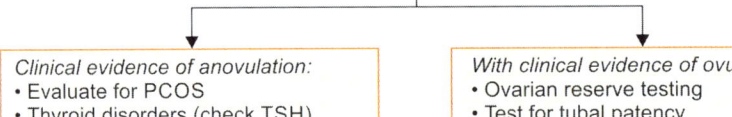

(AFC: antral follicle count; AMH: anti-Müllerian hormone; ATT: antitubercular treatment; PCOS: polycystic ovary syndrome; TSH: thyroid-stimulating hormone)

Noteworthy Mentions in the Evaluation of Female Infertility

- Chlamydia antibodies—Chlamydia trachomatis immunoglobulin G (IgG) antibody testing is a simple, inexpensive, and noninvasive test with some evidence supporting its use as a method for predicting the presence of tubal disease.
- Test of endometrial receptivity—endometrial receptivity array is a tissue test which evaluates the receptivity of the endometrial lining to determine the optimal timing for pregnancy, or the "window of implantation". This is usually done in patient undergoing assisted reproduction and those with history of recurrent implantation failures.
- Immunological causes:
  - *Antisperm antibodies (ASA):* ASA affect fertility potential through various pre-/postfertilization processes, such as sperm agglutination and motility, cervix mucous penetration, capacitation, acrosome reaction, zona pellucida (ZP) binding and penetration, oolemma binding, sperm-oocyte fusion, and embryo implantation.[11] It has been shown that

the ASA present in cervical mucus are of an agglutinating character.[12] Role of seminal fluid (SF) in female immune infertility—some seminal constituents, such as cathepsin D, are able to degrade proteins vaginally exposed that may be involved in antibody formation related to immune infertility.[13] SF has already been considered to be linked to the immunoglobulin E (IgE)-mediated rare reaction to semen. It has been suggested that female patients experiencing any allergic symptoms after/during the first-time intercourse might be sensitive to other antigens/allergens that cross-react with SF.
- Autoimmune aspects in female infertility—antiphospholipid, antinuclear, antithyroid, antiannexin V, antiprothrombin, antilaminin, anti-ZP antibody formation, the high level of natural killer (NK) cells are considered as the risk factors but not as those pathognomonic.[14] Peritoneal endometriosis is characterized by retrograde menstruation causing secondary inflammation. Factors typical for such a condition are high level of autoantibodies, presence of T-lymphocytes in peritoneal fluid, and elevated level of NK cells.[15]
- *Disordered uterine microbiome as a cause of female infertility:* Lactobacillus dominant (>90%) endometrial microbiome improves fertility potential and recurrent infections may shift the flora to lactobacillus nondominant. This may lead to infertility and recurrent implantation failure.[16]

Following test can be performed on endometrial tissue:
- EMMA: Endometrial microbiome metagenomic analysis
- ALICE: Analysis of infectious chronic endometritis.

These tests should not be used in routine practice and should be utilized only under special circumstances and for research purposes.

CONCLUSION

The basic infertility evaluation of all couples consists of:[17]
- Semen analysis.
- Assessment of ovulatory status by history or laboratory testing.
- Determination of tubal patency and presence or absence of abnormalities of the uterine cavity, usually by hysterosalpingogram.
- Ovarian reserve is assessed in women over 35 years of age and younger women with risk factors for premature ovarian failure. Antral follicle count and anti-Müllerian hormone (AMH) levels are utilized for ovarian reserve testing. Basal (day 3) FSH and estradiol may aid in further assessment.
- Thyroid dysfunction should be identified using serum thyroid-stimulating hormone (TSH).
- Serum prolactin wherever there is clinical evidence of hyperprolactinemia (amenorrhea, scanty menstruation, and/or galactorrhea).
- Diagnostic laparoscopy is indicated for women with suspected endometriosis or pelvic adhesions.

KEY LEARNING POINTS

- To identify common causes of female infertility.
- To evaluate common causes of female infertility.

- Systematic approach to the evaluation of female partner.
- Future research.

REFERENCES

1. American College of Obstetricians and Gynecologists Committee on Gynecologic Practice and Practice Committee. Female age-related fertility decline: committee opinion No. 589. Fertil Steril. 2014;101(3): 633-4.
2. Infertility workup for the women's health specialist: ACOG committee opinion number 781. Obstet Gynecol. 2019;133(6):1294-5.
3. Mosher WD, Pratt WF. Fecundity and infertility in the United States: incidence and trends. Fertil Steril. 1991;56:192-3.
4. Wathen NC, Perry L, Lilford RJ, Chard T. Interpretation of single progesterone measurement in diagnosis of anovulation and defective luteal phase: observations on analysis of the normal range. Br Med J (Clin Res Ed). 1984;288:7-9.
5. Practice Committee of the American Society for Reproductive Medicine. Testing and interpreting measures of ovarian reserve: a committee opinion. Fertil Steril. 2020; 114:115-7.
6. Roque M, Haahr T, Esteves SC, Humaidan P. The POSEIDON stratification—moving from poor ovarian response to low prognosis. JBRA Assist Reprod. 2021;25(2):282-92.
7. Dun EC, Nezhat CH. Tubal factor infertility: diagnosis and management in the era of assisted reproductive technology. Obstet Gynecol Clin North Am. 2012;39:551-566.
8. Marcoux S, Maheux R, Berube S. Laparoscopic surgery in infertile women with minimal or mild endometriosis. Canadian Collaborative Group on Endometriosis. N Engl J Med. 1997;337:217-22.
9. The Practice Committee of the American Society for Reproductive Medicine. Optimal evaluation of the infertile female. Fertil Steril. 2006;86(5 suppl):S264-7.
10. The Practice Committee of the American Society for Reproductive Medicine. Effectiveness and treatment for unexplained infertility. Fertil Steril. 2006;86(5 suppl):S111-4.
11. Brazdova A, Zidkova J, Peltre G, Ulcova-Gallova Z. IgG, IgA and IgE reactivities to sperm antigens in infertile women. Jordan J Biol Sci. 2012;5(2):85-9.
12. Ulcova-Gallova Z. Immunological and physicochemical properties of cervical ovulatory mucus. J Reprod Immunol. 2010; 86(2):115-21.
13. Pardesi SR, Dandekar SP, Jamdar SN, Harikuma P. Identification and purification of an aspartic proteinase from human semen. Indian J Clin Biochem. 2004;19(2):84-90.
14. Gleicher N, Barad D. Unexplained infertility: does it really exist? Hum Reprod. 2006;21(8):1951-5.
15. Nisolle M, Paindaveine B, Bourdon A, Berlière M, Casanas-Roux F, Donnez J. Histologic study of peritoneal endometriosis in infertile women. Fertil Steril. 1990;53(6):984-8.
16. Toson B, Simon C, Moreno I. The endometrial microbiome and its impact on human conception. Int J Mol Sci. 2022;23(1):485.
17. Akhter N, Jebunnaher S. Evaluation of female infertility. J med. 2012;13(2):200-9.

CHAPTER 7

Evaluation of Male Partner to Optimize Intrauterine Insemination Success

Sunil Jindal, Anshu Jindal

INTRODUCTION

In the ever-evolving landscape of assisted reproductive technologies (ARTs), intrauterine insemination (IUI) has emerged as a widely embraced and efficacious method for addressing infertility. While historical emphasis often leaned toward the female partner, recent breakthroughs underscore the pivotal role played by the male partner in achieving favorable outcomes. As an andrologist and IVF specialist, this chapter endeavors to offer gynecologists a comprehensive manual for assessing and refining the male partner, thereby optimizing the IUI results.

SIGNIFICANCE OF MALE FACTOR IN INFERTILITY

Infertility is a shared challenge affecting both male and female partners, with approximately 50% of cases attributed solely to male factors or a combination of male and female factors. Recognizing the gravity of male factor infertility is the initial stride toward augmenting IUI success rates.[1]

Male contribution to reproductive success is multifaceted, extending beyond numerical considerations. Qualitative aspects such as sperm morphology, motility, and deoxyribonucleic acid (DNA) integrity play pivotal roles in determining fertility. Recent research underscores the impact of sperm DNA fragmentation as a significant factor in male infertility, influencing not only natural conception but also ARTs.

Moreover, the male reproductive system is susceptible to environmental influences like endocrine-disrupting chemicals and lifestyle choices such as smoking and excessive alcohol intake. These elements can compromise spermatogenesis, emphasizing the need for tailored interventions.

HOLISTIC APPROACH TO EVALUATING MALE PARTNERS

A systematic approach to assessing male partners is imperative for identifying potential barriers to fertility. This involves an in-depth medical history, a comprehensive physical examination, and targeted diagnostic tests.[2]

Medical History

A meticulous medical history forms the foundation of male infertility evaluation. Beyond general health inquiries, specific attention is devoted to reproductive history, sexual function, and lifestyle factors. Occupational exposures, history of sexually transmitted infections, and previous surgeries impacting fertility are carefully documented. This thorough assessment aids in pinpointing potential etiological factors and guides subsequent diagnostic steps.

Physical Examination

A thorough physical examination zeroes in on male reproductive anatomy and associated structures. Detecting varicoceles, linked with impaired sperm quality, is pivotal. Assessment of secondary sexual characteristics offers insights into hormonal function, and an evaluation of anatomical abnormalities ensures a comprehensive understanding of potential obstacles to fertility.[1]

Diagnostic Tests

Advanced diagnostic tests complement the clinical evaluation. A good semen analysis by WHO guidelines in a lab trained to do the procedure is first priority. It may be repeated in case the need be. Computer-assisted semen analysis (CASA) provides detailed insights into sperm parameters, including concentration, motility, and morphology. Genetic testing, hormonal assessments, and specialized sperm functional tests refine the understanding of the male partner's reproductive health.[3] This integrated approach ensures a comprehensive grasp of individual needs, facilitating targeted interventions.

UNDERSTANDING SEMEN ANALYSIS

Semen analysis remains pivotal in evaluating male fertility. Grasping the parameters of sperm count, motility, and morphology provides valuable insights into reproductive potential and aids in predicting IUI success.

Semen analysis remains fundamental, with the World Health Organization (WHO) offering critical insights. WHO guidelines establish standardized methodologies for evaluating semen parameters. Understanding and interpreting these parameters within the WHO framework are crucial for predicting IUI success and informing tailored treatment strategies.[4]

A good semen analysis even if done manually by WHO criteria in a lab where training is adequate is of prime importance. Computer-assisted semen analysis is recommended for a nuanced evaluation, allowing a deeper understanding of potential fertility challenges. This approach ensures an evidence-based prediction of IUI success and facilitates informed decision-making.

BALANCING HORMONES FOR OPTIMAL FERTILITY

Hormonal imbalances can significantly impact male fertility. A comprehensive hormonal evaluation, including testosterone, follicle-stimulating hormone (FSH), and luteinizing hormone (LH), aids in identifying underlying endocrine disorders and guides appropriate management strategies.[5] Hormonal assessment is pivotal in elucidating the endocrine milieu crucial for male fertility. Practical solutions involve a comprehensive approach to identifying and addressing hormonal imbalances contributing to infertility.

Testosterone, the principal male sex hormone, is a focal point in hormonal assessment. Low testosterone levels can adversely impact sperm production. Interventions may include testosterone replacement therapy under careful medical supervision.

Follicle-stimulating hormone and LH are essential regulators of spermatogenesis. Elevated FSH levels may indicate testicular dysfunction, while low levels of LH can suggest a disruption in the hypothalamic–pituitary–gonadal axis. Tailoring treatment to normalize FSH and LH levels can involve hormonal therapies and lifestyle modifications.

In cases of hormonal imbalance, clinicians may consider selective estrogen receptor modulators (SERMs) to manage elevated estrogen levels, thereby restoring hormonal equilibrium. Lifestyle modifications such as weight management and stress reduction contribute to hormonal optimization.

Regular monitoring and adjustment of hormonal therapies, coupled with lifestyle interventions, offer practical solutions for optimizing hormonal balance. This tailored approach ensures that hormonal imbalances are comprehensively addressed, fostering an environment conducive to improved male reproductive health.

Navigating Genetic and Chromosomal Landscape

Genetic abnormalities can contribute to male factor infertility. Genetic testing, including karyotyping and screening for specific gene mutations, aids in identifying hereditary factors that may impact IUI success.[6]

Practical evaluation of genetic tests involves a targeted approach to identify genetic anomalies impacting reproductive potential. Key genetic tests include karyotyping and Y-chromosome microdeletion analysis, offering insights for tailored interventions.[7]

Karyotyping assesses the chromosomal structure and detects numerical and structural abnormalities. In cases like Klinefelter syndrome, genetic counseling addresses potential hereditary implications and guides family planning decisions.

Y-chromosome microdeletion analysis identifies specific microdeletions (AZFa, AZFb, AZFc) associated with spermatogenic failure. Genetic counseling is integral to understanding implications, risks, and available reproductive options. In cases of identified genetic abnormalities, options like preimplantation genetic testing (PGT) or donor sperm may be considered, emphasizing a personalized and informed approach to infertility management.[8]

ADDRESSING VARICOCELES FOR IMPROVED OUTCOMES

Varicoceles, characterized by enlarged veins in the scrotum, are a treatable cause of male infertility. Evaluating and managing varicoceles can significantly improve sperm parameters and enhance the success of IUI.

Practical evaluation involves a comprehensive approach encompassing diagnostic assessments and tailored management strategies to optimize male fertility.

Diagnostic assessments: Accurate diagnosis typically involves scrotal ultrasound to assess varicocele size and characteristics. Evaluation of sperm parameters through semen analysis is crucial, guiding clinicians in determining clinical significance and the need for intervention.

Management strategies: Varicocele management aims to improve sperm quality and alleviate associated symptoms. Surgical intervention, specifically varicocelectomy, is common. Practical application involves preoperative assessment, considering factors such as varicocele severity, symptoms, and fertility goals. Microsurgical techniques offer improved outcomes. Postoperative care includes monitoring sperm parameters to assess varicocele repair impact on fertility potential. In cases where surgery is not feasible, ARTs like IUI or in vitro fertilization (IVF) may be considered.[9] Practical decision-making involves collaborative discussions with the couple to determine the most suitable course of action based on individual circumstances.

UNRAVELING IMMUNE FACTORS AND INFLAMMATION

Inflammation and immune dysregulation may impact sperm function. Assessing inflammatory markers and immune factors provides a holistic understanding of male reproductive health in the context of IUI.

Practical evaluation involves a nuanced understanding of the immune system's impact on sperm function and fertility outcomes.

Immune factors: Investigating immune factors such as antisperm antibodies is controversial in cases of unexplained infertility. These antibodies can impair sperm motility and function. Practical evaluation includes specific tests to detect antisperm antibodies, guiding clinicians in determining the appropriate course of intervention.

Inflammatory markers: Chronic inflammation in the male reproductive tract can adversely affect sperm production and function. Practical yet controversial evaluation involves assessing inflammatory markers such as interleukins and tumor necrosis factor-alpha (TNF-α). Elevated levels of these markers may indicate localized inflammation, impacting sperm quality. Targeted interventions may include anti-inflammatory therapies or lifestyle modifications to mitigate inflammation.[10]

Understanding the interplay between immune factors and fertility requires a comprehensive approach. Practical solutions involve tailored treatment plans based on the specific immune profile of the individual. In cases where inflammation is identified, anti-inflammatory agents, antioxidants, or lifestyle modifications may be recommended to create an environment conducive to optimal sperm function.

IMPACT OF LIFESTYLE AND ENVIRONMENT

Practical evaluation of lifestyle and environmental factors in male infertility involves recognizing the significant impact of daily choices and external exposures on reproductive health.

Lifestyle choices and environmental exposures can influence male fertility. Evaluating and modifying factors such as smoking, alcohol consumption, and exposure to toxins contribute to optimizing reproductive health for IUI success.

Smoking and alcohol consumption: Cigarette smoking and excessive alcohol intake have been linked to reduced sperm quality. Practical assessment includes obtaining detailed information about the frequency and intensity of these habits. Interventions may include smoking cessation programs and moderate alcohol consumption to mitigate their adverse effects on sperm parameters.[11]

Weight management: Obesity and under-weight conditions are associated with altered reproductive hormone levels and impaired sperm production. Practical evaluation involves assessing body mass index (BMI) and guiding individuals toward achieving a healthy weight through diet and exercise. Weight optimization contributes to the restoration of hormonal balance and improves fertility potential.

Toxin exposure: Occupational and environmental exposures to toxins, such as pesticides and heavy metals, can adversely affect male fertility. Practical evaluation entails identifying potential sources of exposure and implementing protective measures, such as personal protective equipment or lifestyle adjustments, to minimize risks.

Understanding the interconnectedness of lifestyle and environmental factors with male fertility requires a holistic approach. Practical solutions involve personalized counseling, lifestyle modifications, and targeted interventions to create an environment conducive to optimal reproductive health.

PROVIDING SUPPORT BEYOND MEDICINE

The practical integration of counseling and emotional support in male infertility recognizes the profound impact of psychological factors on the journey to parenthood. Acknowledging the emotional toll of infertility and providing structured support are vital components of a holistic approach.

Psychological assessment: Practical evaluation involves conducting a psychological assessment to identify the emotional and mental well-being of the male partner. Questionnaires and interviews may be utilized to gauge stress levels, anxiety, and coping mechanisms. Understanding the emotional landscape allows healthcare professionals to tailor support strategies accordingly.[12]

Educational counseling: Providing educational counseling is crucial for empowering individuals with knowledge about infertility, available treatments, and coping strategies. Practical solutions include structured sessions that address concerns, clarify misconceptions, and set realistic expectations. Educational counseling fosters informed decision-making and enhances the resilience of individuals navigating the challenges of infertility.

Couple-based support: Recognizing infertility as a shared experience, practical solutions involve including the partner in counseling sessions. Couples benefit from open communication, shared coping mechanisms, and mutual understanding. Couple-based support fosters a collaborative approach to overcoming challenges, strengthening the emotional bond between partners.

Peer support groups: Facilitating access to peer support groups offers practical avenues for individuals to connect with others facing similar challenges. Sharing experiences, coping strategies, and success stories within a supportive community can alleviate feelings of isolation and provide valuable emotional support.

Emotional well-being is integral to the overall success of infertility treatments. Practical integration of counseling and emotional support ensures that individuals and couples receive personalized guidance, fostering resilience and a positive mindset throughout the infertility journey.

SEAMLESS INTEGRATION INTO INTRAUTERINE INSEMINATION PROTOCOLS

The successful integration of male partner evaluation into IUI protocols is essential for optimizing overall reproductive outcomes. This process involves incorporating comprehensive male fertility assessments seamlessly into the broader framework of IUI treatment.

Joint consultations: Practical integration begins with joint consultations involving both the male and the female partners. This collaborative approach ensures that both individuals actively participate in discussions about medical history, diagnostic assessments, and treatment plans. Joint consultations foster a shared understanding of the fertility journey and encourage mutual support.

Simultaneous evaluation: Conducting simultaneous evaluations of both partners streamlines the diagnostic process. This approach enables healthcare professionals to identify any concurrent fertility challenges in real time, facilitating the development of targeted treatment strategies. Practical solutions include synchronized appointments for male and female evaluations, minimizing delays in initiating IUI protocols.

Tailored treatment plans: The integration of male evaluation data informs the development of personalized treatment plans. Practical solutions involve tailoring IUI protocols based on male fertility parameters, such as sperm count, motility, and morphology. Specific interventions, such as optimizing sperm preparation techniques or adjusting the timing of the IUI procedure, can be implemented to enhance the chances of success.

Education and empowerment: Educational components within IUI protocols should encompass both partners. Practical integration involves providing detailed information about the male partner's role, the significance of male factor evaluation, and the potential impact on IUI success. This education empowers couples, fostering a proactive approach to their fertility journey.

Ongoing monitoring and adjustment: Practical integration extends to continuous monitoring and adjustment throughout the IUI cycle. Regular assessments of sperm parameters during the treatment cycle allow for real-time adjustments to optimize conditions for conception. This dynamic approach ensures that the IUI protocol remains adaptive to the unique needs of each couple.

By seamlessly integrating male partner evaluation into IUI protocols, healthcare professionals create a comprehensive and patient-centric approach that maximizes the chances of successful outcomes.

CONCLUSION AND KEY LEARNING POINTS

- *Importance of male factor in infertility:* Understanding the critical role of the male partner in infertility and acknowledging the impact of male-factor infertility on reproductive outcomes.
- *Comprehensive male partner evaluation:* Outlining a systematic approach to evaluate male partners undergoing IUI, including medical history, physical examination, and advanced diagnostic tests.
- *Semen analysis:* Interpreting the significance of semen analysis parameters and their relevance in predicting IUI success, with a focus on sperm count, motility, and morphology.
- *Hormonal assessment:* Exploring the role of hormonal evaluation in assessing male fertility, including the measurement of testosterone, FSH, and LH.
- *Genetic and chromosomal assessment:* Highlighting the importance of genetic testing to identify potential genetic abnormalities affecting male fertility and their implications for IUI success.
- *Varicocele assessment and management:* Discussing the impact of varicoceles on male fertility and the role of evaluation and management in optimizing IUI outcomes.
- *Immune factors and inflammatory markers:* Examining the influence of immune factors and inflammatory markers on male fertility and their significance in the context of IUI.
- *Lifestyle and environmental factors:* Exploring the impact of lifestyle choices and environmental factors on male

fertility, with recommendations for optimizing reproductive health.

- *Counseling and emotional support:* Recognizing the psychological aspects of male infertility and the importance of counseling and emotional support for couples undergoing IUI.
- *Integrating male evaluation into IUI protocols:* Providing guidelines for gynecologists to seamlessly integrate comprehensive male partner evaluation into the overall IUI treatment protocol.

REFERENCES

1. Agarwal A, Mulgund A, Hamada A, Chyatte MR. A unique view on male infertility around the globe. Reprod Biol Endocrinol. 2015;13:37.
2. Esteves SC, Miyaoka R, Agarwal A. An update on the clinical assessment of the infertile male. [corrected]. Clinics (Sao Paulo). 2011; 66(4):691-700.
3. Esteves SC, Agarwal A. Novel concepts in male infertility. Int Braz J Urol. 2011;37(1):5-15.
4. World Health Organization. (2021). WHO laboratory manual for the examination and processing of human semen. [online] Available from: https://www.who.int/publications/i/item/9789240030787 [Last accessed January, 2024].
5. Practice Committee of the American Society for Reproductive Medicine. Diagnostic evaluation of the infertile male: a committee opinion. Fertil Steril. 2015;103(3):e18-25.
6. Krausz C, Riera-Escamilla A. Genetics of male infertility. Nat Rev Urol. 2018;15(6):369-84.
7. Foresta C, Moro E, Ferlin A. Y chromosome microdeletions and alterations of spermatogenesis. Endocr Rev. 2001;22(2): 226-39.
8. Lo Giacco D, Chianese C, Sánchez-Curbelo J, Bassas L, Ruiz P, Rajmil O, et al. Clinical relevance of Y-linked CNV screening in male infertility: new insights based on the 8-year experience of a diagnostic genetic laboratory. Eur J Hum Genet. 2014;22(6):754-6.
9. Esteves SC, Oliveira FV, Bertolla RP. Clinical outcome of intracytoplasmic sperm injection in infertile men with treated and untreated clinical varicocele. J Urol. 2010; 184(4):1442-6.
10. Fraczek M, Kurpisz M. Inflammatory mediators exert toxic effects of oxidative stress on human spermatozoa. J Androl. 2007;28(2):325-33.
11. Ricci E, Al Beitawi S, Cipriani S, Candiani M, Chiaffarino F, Viganò P, et al. Semen quality and alcohol intake: a systematic review and meta-analysis. Reprod Biomed Online. 2017;34(1):38-47.
12. Gameiro S, Boivin J, Dancet E, de Klerk C, Emery M, Lewis-Jones C, et al. ESHRE guideline: routine psychosocial care in infertility and medically assisted reproduction and guide for fertility staff. Hum Reprod. 2015;30(11):2476-85.

CHAPTER 8

Selection and Counseling of Couple for Intrauterine Insemination

Surveen Ghumman, Pinkee Saxena

INTRODUCTION

Artificial intrauterine insemination (IUI) is often favored as method of choice both by the clinicians and the infertile couples. The success of IUI depends on varied factors like proper patient selection, infertility diagnosis, stimulation protocol used, semen preparation, and the procedure itself. Appropriate patient selection is one of the most important factors which determine success of the IUI program.

Detailed history, examination, and investigations of the couple are required to arrive at a correct diagnosis. The cause of infertility must be established, which is essential to decide if IUI is appropriate therapy. Equally important is to rule out any contraindications that may give poor results **(Box 1)**.

Patients must be counseled on success rates, other options, and risks of IUI.

SELECTION FOR INTRAUTERINE INSEMINATION

Various factors need to be kept in mind while selecting couples for IUI.

Age

Maternal age is an important factor that predicts the success of IUI. Studies have shown that as the chronological age increases, the success rates of IUI decrease especially after 35 years. Success of IUI cycles is 13.7–17% in <40 years old and 4.1–7% in >40 years old. In older women between 38 and 42 years

---

BOX 1: Indications and contraindications of intrauterine insemination (IUI).

Indications for IUI:
- Male factor infertility:
  - Subnormal sperm parameters
  - Nonliquefying or highly viscous semen
  - Retrograde ejaculation
  - Impotence or ejaculatory dysfunction
  - Hypospadias
  - Hypospermia
- Female factor infertility:
  - Vaginismus
  - Cervical factor
  - Ovulatory dysfunction
  - Mild endometriosis
  - Unexplained
- Immunological infertility
- Unexplained infertility
- HIV, HbsAg-positive
- Donor insemination: Azoospermia of primary testicular origin

Contraindications for IUI:
- Bilateral tubal block
- Very severe oligoasthenospermia
- Genital tract infection—cervicitis, endometritis
- Unexplained genital tract bleeding
- Ovarian failure
- Uterine pathology—Intrauterine adhesions, large submucous fibroid or polyp
- Multiple infertility etiologies

(HbsAg: hepatitis B surface antigen; HIV: human immunodeficiency virus; IUI: intrauterine insemination)

of age, the Forty and Over Treatment Trial (FORT-T) trial (n = 154) observed an increased clinical pregnancy rates per cycle (24.7 vs. 7.3%) and live birth rates per cycle (15.3 vs. 5.1%) in the in vitro fertilization (IVF) group than in IUI group. Many clinicians hence do not recommend IUI in women >38 years of age.[1]

Studies have shown that increased paternal age >35 years may have a negative impact on pregnancy, though controversial. In addition, increased parental body mass index (BMI) may also negatively affect fertility.[2]

Duration of Infertility

The duration of infertility is yet another important factor that predicts the chance of successful pregnancy. A study has reported pregnancy rates of 14.2% when the duration of infertility was below 6 years and 6.1% when it was >6 years. Others have reported >80% of pregnancies in patients where the duration of infertility was <4 years. A reasonable threshold for duration of infertility by most clinicians to switch over to IVF rather than IUI is 4–5 years.[3]

Number of Failed Intrauterine Insemination Cycles

Best results are observed in initial cycles. Cycle fecundity has been reported to be relatively constant for the first three to six cycles.

Number of treatment cycle	Pregnancy/cycle (%)
1	51/283 (18.0)
2	26/228 (11.4)
3	15/160 (9.4)
4	7/73 (9.6)
5	3/67 (4.5)[3]

Usually 3–4 IUI treatment cycles give optimal results. Most pregnancies occur within the first four IUI cycles, after which IVF should be considered.[2]

Cause of Infertility

Various causes of infertility have varied impact on the success rate of IUI **(Table 1)**.

- *Cervical factors:* The best results of IUI were obtained in women with infertility due to cervical factors. Women with an isolated cervical factor infertility had a clinical pregnancy rate per couple of 55.6%.[4]
- *Unexplained infertility:* IUI for unexplained infertility had gone into disrepute since the National Institute for Health and Care Excellence (NICE) guidelines 2013 on it. Many studies were done to study the role of it in various settings. A large randomized controlled trial (RCT) was done to assess the role of intrauterine insemination in a natural cycle and expectant management in infertile couple with unexplained infertility. It was observed that there was no significant difference in the live-birth rate between IUI cycles (23%) and expectant management (16%).[5] A systematic review done to assess the role of ovulation induction with IUI and

TABLE 1: Causes of infertility and impact on success rate.

Infertility etiology	Pregnancy rate/cycles
Unexplained	22.6%
Mild male factor	18.8%
Ovarian dysfunction	12.4%
Endometriosis	6.5%
Tubal factor	7.6%
Combined factors	9.7%

expectant management in unexplained infertility showed that IUI with ovulation induction has better results over expectant management, particularly in patients with poor prognosis. The odds ratio (OR) for cumulative live birth rate was 4.48 [95% confidence interval (CI): 2.00–10.01; 1 RCT, 201 patients] in patients with poor prognosis and 0.82 (95% CI: 0.45–1.49; 1 RCT, 253 patients) in patients with moderate prognosis.[6] Ovulation induction or IUI alone is not effective when compared to expectant management or IUI in a natural cycle. However, IUI in combination with ovulation induction is as effective as IVF without added risk and extra cost of IVF. The European Society of Human Reproduction and Embryology (ESHRE) recommends IUI with ovarian stimulation as a first-line treatment in patients with unexplained infertility, for three to six cycles.[7] Also, low-dose regimen is suggested for ovarian stimulation to decrease the multiple pregnancy rate without compromising on the live birth rate. Parameters like increased age, duration of infertility, previous treatments, and previous pregnancy can help to decide if patients will benefit from IVF over IUI on case-to-case basis.

- *Anovulation:* This is the most common cause of infertility. The majority of patients with anovulation will conceive using simpler treatments. IUI has good results in these patients. A pregnancy rate per couple of 47.4% was obtained for an IUI carried out in cases of anovulation.[4]
- *Endometriosis:* Endometriosis is the most difficult cases to treat. IUI with ovulation induction can be tried in mild endometriosis. In mild endometriosis (I–II), cycle specific pregnancy rate was lower with endometriosis when compared to women with unexplained infertility (5.2–6.5% and 14%, respectively.[3] Prado-Perez et al. have observed that pregnancy rate with IUI decreased from 22.7% in those with stage I and II endometriosis to 5.6% in those with stages III–IV endometriosis.[8]

A study done to evaluate the efficacy of IUI and IVF in women with endometriosis showed higher pregnancy rates for IVF compared to IUI irrespective of age or stage of endometriosis. The IUI pregnancy rate per cycle was 11% with a cumulative pregnancy rate of 41% after six cycles, while the IVF pregnancy rate per cycle was 47% with cumulative pregnancy rate of 73%.[9] In endometriosis, the toxins released from the implants can affect the quality of oocyte and its fertilization. IUI is done for mild endometriosis in a young ovulating woman with normal anatomy and no male factor. However, in presence of other factors like pelvic adhesions, male factor, advanced age, diminished ovarian reserve, stage III & IV endometriosis, long duration of infertility and previous failed treatments IVF is preferred.

Male Factor

- *Ejaculatory dysfunction:* The quality of semen is generally poor in men who are continent for long periods. The motility is low despite high-sperm density. The success of treatment depends on sperm quality.
- *Hypospadias:* Deposition of semen occurs outside the vagina or much away from the os. However, hypospadias is usually repaired in infancy.
- *Hypospermia:* Need for IUI in such cases exists because IUI is done for low semen volume seen in hypospermia.

- The very small volume of ejaculate may be deposited away from the cervix in the vagina, but away from cervix.
- The small volume of semen deposited in the vagina may be inadequate to change the acidic ph of vagina to alkaline. This acidic pH kills the sperms present in the semen.
- *Tubal factor:* IUI can be done for unilateral tubal blockage. Presence of pelvic adhesions however decreases the success rate of IUI.

Semen Parameters

Sperm parameters which can influence the outcome of IUI includes total sperm count, total inseminating motile count, sperm motility, abnormal forms and DNA fragmentation index (DFI).

Highly viscous semen: Increased viscosity impedes the escape of sperms from the ejaculate into the cervical canal before it's destruction by vaginal acidity.

IUI is performed in these cases after treating semen by:
- Enzymatic digestion of mucus by plasmin or chymotrypsin
- Mechanical methods—Semen is drawn in a hypodermic needle of 18-G (gauge) or pipette and then pushed or forced through it to decrease its viscosity.

Recommendation regarding the ideal sperm count for IUI is varied. A study observed clinical pregnancy rate of 44.3% when total motile sperm (TMS) count was >5 million and 28.5% when the TMS was lower than 5 million. Also, the count of inseminated spermatozoa >1 million was associated with higher pregnancy rate (14 vs. 6.4% per cycle; $p = 0.10$). The lowest count of inseminated spermatozoa that resulted in pregnancy was 45,000.[4] Studies have demonstrated cutoffs value for TMC of 5–10 million sperm and 1 million for post-wash total sperm count. The pregnancy rate per couple diminished from 40.7 to 21.4%, if teratospermia exceeds than 70% of abnormal forms. Intracytoplasmic sperm injection (ICSI) is usually suggested if the percentage of abnormal forms is >70%.[4]

DFI has a negative effect on sperm motility, however, not much difference was seen in the pregnancy outcome. Miscarriages are reported for increased DFI. A study[10] found decreased pregnancy, and delivery rates when the DFI >30% compared to couples with DFI ≤30%. Since not much difference is seen in pregnancy outcomes by levels of DFI routine testing for DFI is not required for couples undergoing IUI.

Couples with mild male factor fertility problems can be offered up to six cycles of IUI because this increases the chance of pregnancy. Usually, when IUI is done for male factor infertility, ovulation induction is not performed as it increases the chances of unwanted multiple pregnancies. Also, single IUI and not double IUI is recommended in such patients.

In a meta-analysis of 2014,[11] cutoff values for IUI for male factor infertility suggested were:
- Inseminating motile count after washing: Between 0.8 and 5 million
- Sperm morphology using strict criteria: >4% normal
- Total motile sperm count in native sperm sample: 5–10 million
- Total motility in native sperm sample: Threshold value of 30%.

IUI is a reasonable first-line therapy for patients with normal sperm morphology of >4%, provided other parameters are normal. Less than 4% normal sperms or inseminate motile count of <1 million should be considered for fertilization by ICSI.

Donor Intrauterine Insemination

In case of azoospermia donor IUI is an option. Donor IUI may also be considered where there is a genetic disease in the father and the couple does not want to do IVF and preimplantation genetic testing (PGT).

Human Immunodeficiency Virus Positive Partners

In order to avoid infection IUI is recommended in these cases as sperm washing helps in decreasing chance of virus being attached to sperm and transmission to partner or vertical transmission to baby.

■ COUNSELING

Counseling is an important before any infertility procedure. The couples must be informed the probable reason for infertility and explained in detail about the available options. The pros and cons of any procedure suggested and its success rate in achieving live pregnancy must be told. In cases where both IUI and IVF can be done couples must be told about the cost involved, complications like ovarian hyperstimulation syndrome (OHSS), multiple pregnancy, and success rates. All options must be discussed. Diagnostic tests required before procedure must be explained. A step-wise explanation is given of the IUI cycle which includes the drugs to be taken, time duration, monitoring by ultrasound, any injection required, how and when semen would be collected and prepared, and the IUI procedure. Legal issues must be discussed specially in donor sperm IUI. Required consent forms must be signed.

■ CONCLUSION

The proper selection of infertile couple for IUI is imperative for the success of the procedure. IUI would only be successful in a certain sect of patients. Counseling on success rates and other available options is also a vital part of treatment plan.

■ KEY LEARNING POINTS

- IUI is an inexpensive and non invasive treatment modality for infertile couple.
- Couple should be counselled on the success rates, risk of IUI and other options available.
- Proper selection of couples is imperative for success of this procedure.
- Age, duration of infertility, previous failed treatment, cause of infertility, male factors especially the semen parameters are few important factors to be assessed and evaluated while planning an IUI for a couple.

■ REFERENCES

1. Goldman MB, Thornton KL, Ryley D, Alper MM, Fung JL, Hornstein MD, et al. A randomized clinical trial to determine optimal infertility treatment in older couples: the Forty and Over Treatment Trial (FORT-T). Fertil Steril. 2014;101:1574-81.e1-2.
2. Starosta A, Gordon CE, Hornstein MD. Predictive factors for intrauterine insemination outcomes: a review. Fertil Res Pract. 2020;6(1):23.
3. Nuojua-Huttunen S, Tomas C, Bloigu R, Tuomivaara L, Martikainen H. Intrauterine insemination treatment in subfertility: an analysis of factors affecting outcome. Hum Reprod. 1999;14(3):698-703.
4. Merviel P, Heraud MH, Grenier N, Lourdel E, Sanguinet P, Copin H. Predictive factors for pregnancy after intrauterine insemination (IUI): an analysis of 1038 cycles and a review of the literature. Fertil Steril. 2010;93(1):79-88.
5. Bhattacharya S, Harrild K, Mollison J, Wordsworth S, Tay C, Harrold A, et al. Clomifene citrate or unstimulated intrauterine insemination compared with

expectant management for unexplained infertility: pragmatic randomised controlled trial. BMJ (Clin Res). 2008;337:a716.
6. Ayeleke RO, Asseler JD, Cohlen BJ, Veltman-Verhulst SM. Intra-uterine insemination for unexplained subfertility. Cochrane Database Syst Rev. 2020;3:Cd001838.
7. Guideline Group on Unexplained Infertility; Romualdi D, Ata B, Bhattacharya S, Bosch E, Costello M, et al. Evidence-based guideline: unexplained infertility. Hum Reprod. 2023; 38(10):1881-90.
8. Prado-Perez J, Navarro-Maritnez C, Lopez-Rivadeneira E, Sanon-Julien Flores E. The impact of endometriosis on the rate of pregnancy of patients submitted to intrauterine insemination. Fertil Steril. 2002;77:51.
9. Dmowski WP, Pry M, Ding J, Rana N. Cycle-specific and cumulative fecundity in patients with endometriosis who are undergoing controlled ovarian hyperstimulation-intrauterine insemination or in vitro fertilization-embryo transfer. Fertil Steril. 2002;78:750-6.
10. Bungum M, Humaidan P, Axmon A, Spano M, Bungum L, Erenpreiss J, et al. Sperm DNA integrity assessment in prediction of assisted reproduction technology outcome. Hum Reprod. 2007;22:174-9.
11. Ombelet W, Dhont N, Thijssen A, Bosmans E, Kruger T. Semen quality and prediction of IUI success in male subfertility: a systematic review. Reprod Biomed Online. 2014;28(3):300-9.

SECTION 3: Ultrasonography in Intrauterine Insemination

9. Monitoring of Intrauterine Insemination Cycles and Dopplers in Intrauterine Insemination
   Sonal Panchal, Chaitanya Nagori

CHAPTER 9

Monitoring of Intrauterine Insemination Cycles and Dopplers in Intrauterine Insemination

Sonal Panchal, Chaitanya Nagori

INTRODUCTION

Intrauterine insemination (IUI) is considered as one of the primary treatments for subfertility. Though patients undergoing IUI are commonly stimulated with oral ovulogens, like clomiphene citrate and letrozole, gonadotropins are preferred and claimed to have better results. Literature documents much better pregnancy rates with IUI when it is combined with superovulation, which means stimulating the ovary to produce follicles with gonadotropins. In unexplained infertility, superovulation with IUI has a higher pregnancy rate than only superovulation.[1] Superovulation with IUI should be offered as the first line of treatment in male immunological infertility.[2] The absolute pregnancy rate was 8.4% for monofollicular and 15% for multifollicular growth and is statistically significant in the presence of two, three, or four follicles (LOE 1a) in a meta-analysis.[3]

The success of IUI is grossly dependent on the time of the trigger, and therefore, optimal assessment of the follicular maturity is essential. Therefore, whatever the agent used for ovarian stimulation, the follicle growth needs to be monitored to decide the follicular maturity and plan the trigger for ovulation. This can be decided by ultrasound and Doppler because hormonal changes are closely related to morphological and vascular changes in the ovary and the endometrium. When gonadotropins are used, there is an additional risk of ovarian hyperstimulation syndrome (OHSS), which needs to be prevented by individualizing the gonadotrophin dose, and this also requires a close ultrasound assessment.

TECHNIQUE OF ULTRASOUND AND DOPPLER STUDY FOR FOLLICLE

- Transvaginal route is used for follicle monitoring always.
- Locate the uterus and manipulate the probe to image the uterus in the midsagittal plane.
- Endometrial thickness is measured from the outer margin of the anterior hyperechoic line of the endometrium to the outer margin of the posterior hyperechoic line of the endometrium, perpendicular to the central line of endometrium.
- For Doppler assessment of the endometrium, power Doppler is used with the color box size, just large enough to accommodate the endometrium.
- Pulsed wave Doppler is used to quantitatively assess the endometrial flow in intraendometrial vessels.
- Follow the transverse section of the uterus to locate the ovary along the adnexal soft-tissue band.

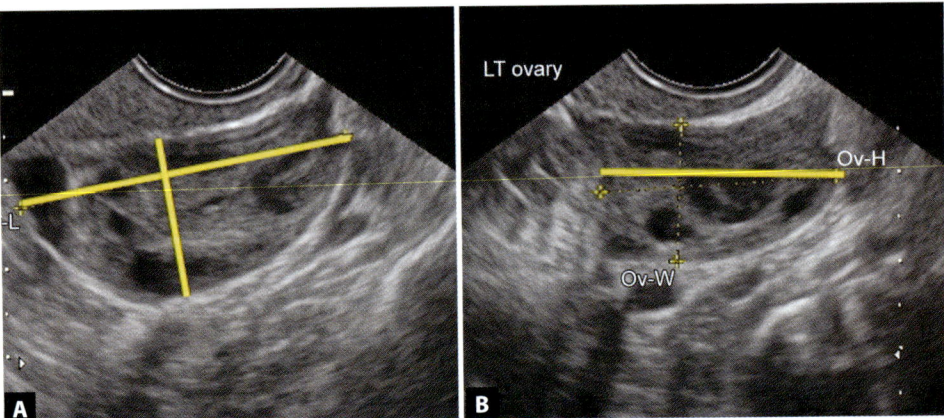

Figs. 1A and B: Measurement of three orthogonal diameters of ovary on B-mode ultrasound. (LT: left)

- Rotate the probe to find out the long plane of the ovary, and then the probe is spanned across this plane to find out the longest section. Measure the largest longitudinal diameter.
- This image is stored as one frame on a dual screen.
- Then the probe is rotated 90° with no other movements of the probe to get a true transverse section of the ovary.
- Anteroposterior (AP) diameter is the longest diameter perpendicular to the long diameter on long section (**Figs. 1A and B**).
- Transverse diameter is side-to-side diameter on transverse section.
- Ovarian volume is calculated by the equation (L × W × H × 0.523).
- Antral follicles are counted by eyeballing, when spanning across the ovary in any one plane, without rotation of the probe.
- After B-mode assessment, the color is switched on to assess the stromal vessels.
- The color box should be large enough to include the entire ovary only.
- The vessels that are in the middle of the stroma and not close to the follicles are stromal vessels (**Fig. 2**).

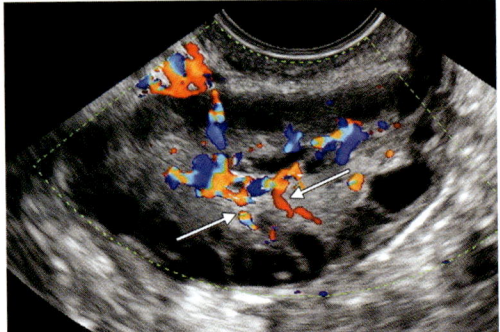

Fig. 2: Color Doppler image of the ovary showing stromal vessels.

- For color Doppler assessment, pulse repetition frequency (PRF) is set at 0.3–0.4. Optimum gains and wall filter are set at the lowest for both color and the power Doppler. Sample volume for spectral Doppler is usually 2 mm for follicular, corpus luteal, and endometrial scans. Angle correction is essential for these scans.
- For pulse Doppler, PRF is set at 0.9–1.3 but may be lowered if required and the wall filters are set at 30 Hz as stromal flows at baseline scan are low-velocity flows.
- The follicular size can be measured as mean diameter or volume. The mean

CHAPTER 9: Monitoring of Intrauterine Insemination Cycles and Dopplers in Intrauterine Insemination

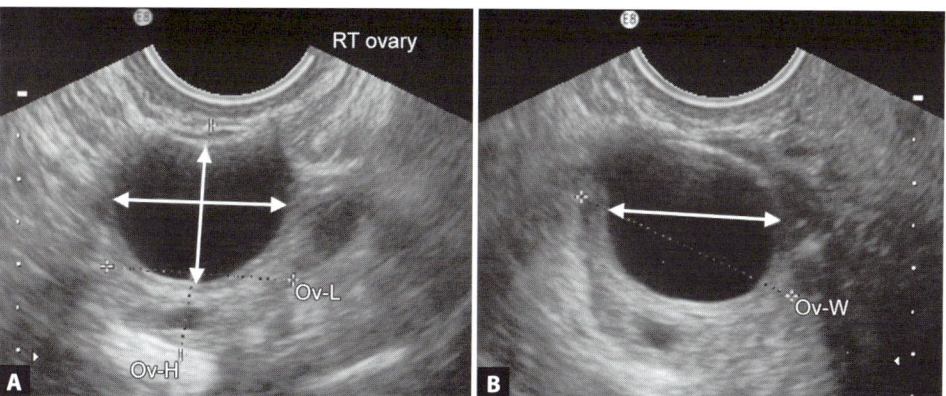

Figs. 3A and B: Measuring follicle size by three orthogonal diameters and mean of them when the follicle does not appear round on screen. (RT: right)

diameter of the follicle is measured by first rotating the probe and finding out the longest follicular diameter; on that same image, the AP diameter is measured as the longest diameter perpendicular to this diameter. The probe is then rotated 90° and side-to-side longest diameter is the transverse diameter **(Figs. 3A and B)**. The mean of these three orthogonal diameters is mean follicular diameter.

- For the preovulatory scan, blood vessels that overlap the follicular margin are to be considered as perifollicular and blood flow in these vessels is also assessed by spectral Doppler **(Fig. 4)**.
- Pick up the brightest vessels for spectral Doppler assessment. Take at least three measurements and select the combination of the lowest resistive index (RI) and highest peak systolic velocity (PSV) for decision-making.

MONITORING OVARIAN STIMULATION

Secondary antral follicles (2 mm) are the first follicular structures that may be visualized on ultrasound **(Figs. 5A and B)**. Follicular

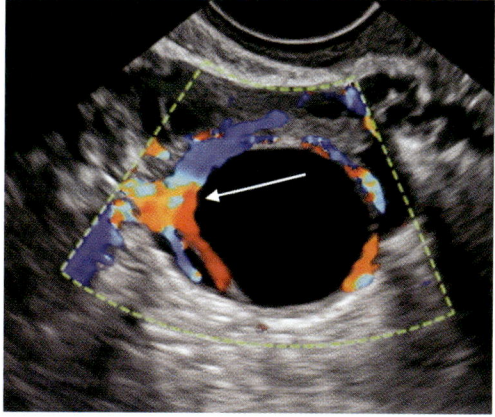

Fig. 4: Color Doppler image of the follicle showing perifollicular vessels.

dominance is selected by day 5 of the cycle and becomes evident on ultrasound as a follicle becomes >9 mm. Dominance indicates follicle-stimulating hormone (FSH) sensitivity and is confirmed by follicular vascularity as it reaches a size of 8–10 mm.

The scan is done on day 2 or 3 of the menstrual cycle, when estrogen and progesterone levels are at baseline, ovaries are silent, and have no active follicle or corpus luteum. This is done to assess ovarian reserve and response.

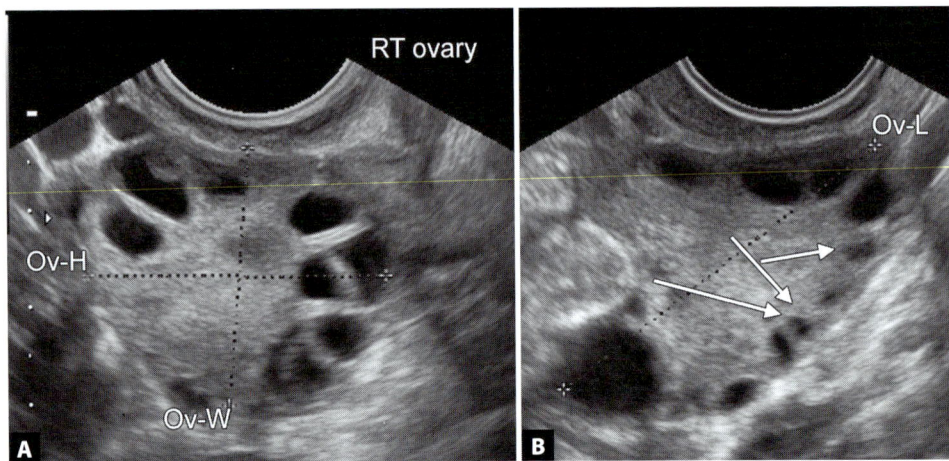

Figs. 5A and B: B-mode ultrasound of the ovary showing small secondary antral follicles. (RT: right)

Reserve indicates a likely number of follicles that may develop or a likely number of ova that may be retrieved at the end of ovarian stimulation, and this is decided by antral follicle count (AFC) and ovarian volume.

Response indicates approximate doses of gonadotropins that would be required to produce one or more mature follicles and that is decided by ovarian stromal flow parameters, RI and PSV.

It is important to mention here that the ovarian reserve assessment is not of much practical application in IUI cycles because the total follicles required for this mode of treatment is only two to three. Only three to four antral follicle counts also, therefore, may be adequate. However, ovarian reserve assessment is still done to predict the risk of OHSS.

The AFC and ovarian stromal flow parameters on the baseline scan are predictive of the ovarian response after pituitary downregulation.[4] According to a study by Popovic-Todorovic et al.,[5] the total number of antral follicles and ovarian stromal blood flow were the two most significant predictors of ovarian response, and ovarian volume was a highly significant predictor of the number of follicles and oocytes retrieved. Total AFC >21 could lead to the decision to adjust the gonadotropin dose in trying to prevent a hyper-response leading to OHSS[6] whereas a volume of >10 cc indicates polycystic ovary and risk of OHSS.

Measurement of ovarian stromal flow in the early follicular phase is related to subsequent ovarian response.[7] Ovarian stromal blood flow velocity is a true representative of baseline ovarian blood flow and predictive of ovarian responsiveness.[8] Those who had low stromal PSV in the early follicular phase were poor responders.[8,9] Ovarian stromal flow is less in obese and in patients with advanced age; this explains why these patients require higher doses for stimulation.[10]

Using age, body mass index (BMI), AFC, ovarian volume, stromal RI, and PSV as parameters to individualize the stimulation doses of gonadotropins, a scoring system has been devised. This method simplifies the dose calculation for individual patients and has proved to be an important guide for

CHAPTER 9: Monitoring of Intrauterine Insemination Cycles and Dopplers in Intrauterine Insemination

TABLE 1: Baseline score calculation.

Score	1	2	3	4	5
Age	>40	35.1–40	30.1–35	25.1–30	<25
BMI	>30	30–28.1	28–25.1	25–22.1	<22
AFC	<5	5–10	10–15	15–20	>20
Ovarian volume	<3	3.1–5	5.17	7.1–10	>10
Stromal RI	>0.75	0.75–0.66	0.65–0.56	0.55–0.45	<0.45
Stromal PSV	<3	3.1–5	5.1–7	7.1–10	>10

(AFC: antral follicle count; BMI: body mass index; PSV: peak systolic velocity; RI: resistance index)

TABLE 2: Dose calculation of rFSH for IUI and IVF cycles depending on the baseline score.

Score	IUI starting dose of rFSH	IVF starting dose of rFSH—fresh transfer	IVF starting dose of rFSH—frozen transfer
≥25	25 IU	75 IU	150 IU
21–24	37.5 IU	150 IU	225 IU
16–20	75 IU	225 IU	300 IU
11–15	112.5 IU	300 IU	375 IU
6–10	150 IU	375 IU	450 IU

(IUI: intrauterine insemination; IVF: in-vitro fertilization; rFSH: recombinant follicle stimulating hormone)

the safe use of gonadotropins for ovulation induction in assisted reproductive technology (ART) cycles[11,12] with zero severe OHSS rates **(Tables 1 and 2)**.

The final dose calculation is based on the factors given in **Table 1**.[8,9]

Once the stimulation is started, follow-up scan is done on the day of the last dose of oral ovulogen if it is an oral ovulogen cycle and on the day of the first dose of gonadotrophin (which is usually the 5th day of the cycle) if gonadotrophin is to be used for ovulation induction. If on this scan no dominant follicle is found, the patient is called after 5 days. If one of the follicles has reached dominance, the follow-up scan is done when the follicle is expected to reach 17–18 mm in diameter, based on the normal growth rate of dominant follicle of 2 mm a day. If the follicle is dominant, it will definitely respond to endogenous or exogenous FSH and grow.

But if no follicle was dominant on the above-said scan and the patient is called after 5 days and either follicle or endometrium is growing, it indicates that the patient is responding and the same dose is continued till the follicle matures. But if both the follicle and the endometrium are not growing, that means the patient is not responding and the dose needs to be increased. The schedule to dose rise is illustrated in **Flowchart 1** for IUI. Gonadotropins are to be continued till the day of trigger.

Individualizing the ovarian stimulation protocol by this method has resulted in zero moderate/severe OHSS and also zero cycle cancellation rate for poor response.

PREOVULATORY SCAN

Follicle

A follicle approximately reaches a size of 18–24 mm before ovulation in a natural cycle.[13]

Flowchart 1: Gonadotrophin dose modification chart for IUI.

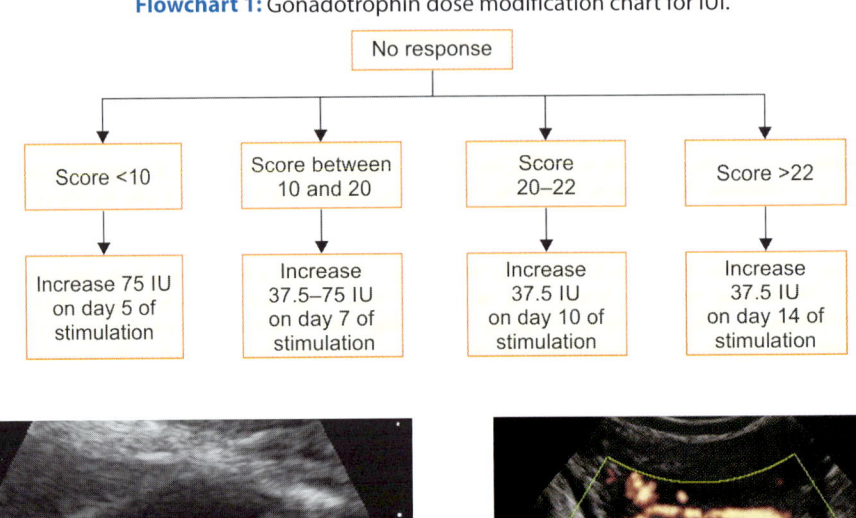

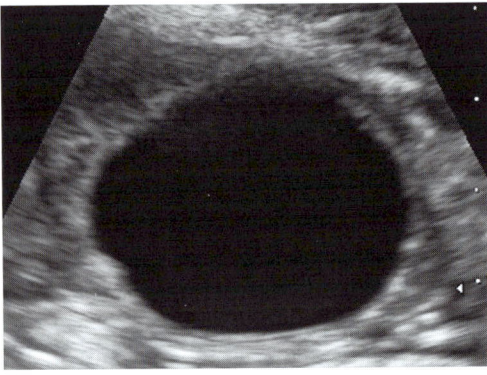

Fig. 6: B-mode ultrasound image of a mature follicle.

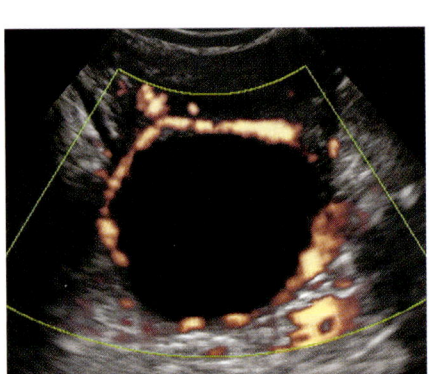

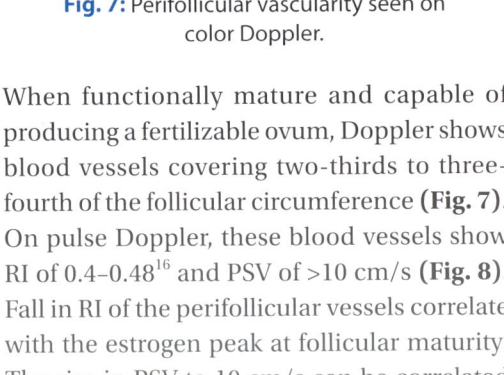

Fig. 7: Perifollicular vascularity seen on color Doppler.

A follicular size of 17–18 mm is considered optimum for a gonadotropin-stimulated cycle, whereas for clomiphene citrate (CC)-stimulated cycles, a minimum size of 18–20 mm is required.[14] A normal follicle scan has a regular round shape and no echogenicity in the lumen and shows a thin hypoechoic rim surrounding the follicle **(Fig. 6)**. Though the size of the follicle has been considered a parameter for follicular maturity, this only assesses the anatomical maturity and not the functional maturity that would correlate with the ovum yield.

Doppler

About 2 days before ovulation, when estrogen peaks, the RI of these vessels starts falling.[15]

When functionally mature and capable of producing a fertilizable ovum, Doppler shows blood vessels covering two-thirds to three-fourth of the follicular circumference **(Fig. 7)**. On pulse Doppler, these blood vessels show RI of 0.4–0.48[16] and PSV of >10 cm/s **(Fig. 8)**. Fall in RI of the perifollicular vessels correlate with the estrogen peak at follicular maturity. The rise in PSV to 10 cm/s can be correlated with the kick to LH surge.

Follicle flow correlates well with oocyte recovery rates and hence may be useful in determining the most appropriate time to administer trigger. Our data of >1,000 IUI cycles has shown that when the perifollicular RI >0.53 and PSV <9 cm/s, 12 hours before ovulation trigger, the conception rates were

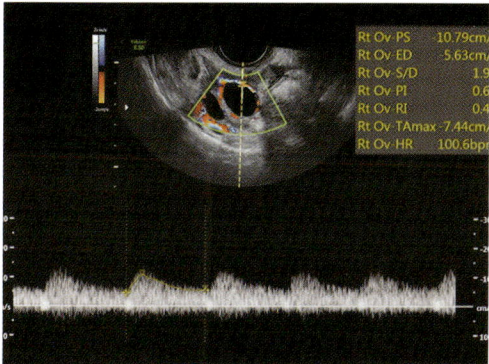

Fig. 8: Pulse Doppler image of the low-resistance perifollicular flow.

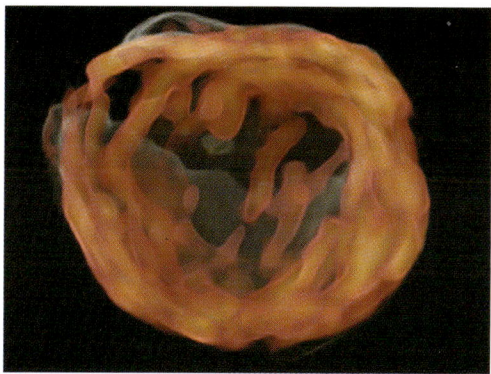

Fig. 9: Three-dimensional power Doppler image rendered in glass-body mode showing uniformly distributed perifollicular flow.

only 8.3% and 10%, respectively, as compared to 32.8% and 28.2%, and individually when perifollicular RI <0.50 and PSV >11 cm/s.[17] We have, therefore, always preferred to wait, with no extra medication, when the patient is on oral ovulogens or continue with the same dose of gonadotropin till we get desired perifollicular RI and PSV, though sometimes the follicular size may reach up to 22–24 mm. Oocytes from hypoxic follicles are associated with a high frequency of chromosomal abnormalities and catastrophic mosaics in embryo[18-20] and follicles with a more uniform perifollicular network contain oocytes capable of producing pregnancy[21] **(Fig. 9)**.

Three-dimensional power Doppler gives the most precise information about the vascularization and follicular blood flow.[22] We have found perifollicular vascularization index (VI) between 6 and 20 and perifollicular flow index (FI) >35 as most optimum for best conception rates[23] **(Fig. 10)**.

In response to LH surge, resulting preovulatory changes in the follicle are seen as appearance of a sonolucent halo surrounding the follicle and appearance of cumulus (a small solid projection from the follicle wall) 24–36 hours before ovulation **(Fig. 11)**.

At the start of the LH surge, the perifollicular PSV is 10 cm/s. LH surge leads to increased vascularity of the inner wall of the follicle and a coincident surge in blood velocity just prior to erruption.[24] PSV increases 29 hours before the time of follicular rupture.[25] A marked increase in the PSV around the follicle, in the presence of a relatively constant pulsatility index (PI), could be a sign of follicle maturity and impending ovulation.[20] In IUI cycles, these findings suggest the start of the surge, and therefore, ovulation may occur earlier than 36–42 hours, and thus, earlier or double IUI is recommended in these cases.

ENDOMETRIAL ASSESSMENT

B-mode Features of Endometrium with Good Receptivity

A minimum endometrial thickness is 6 mm but 8-10 mm is optimum, with preferably multilayered endometrium, to indicate anatomical endometrial maturity. Multilayered morphology of endometrium is named grade A, when it is a triple-line endometrium with echogenicity in the intervening area, which is not more than that of anterior myometrium **(Fig. 12)**.

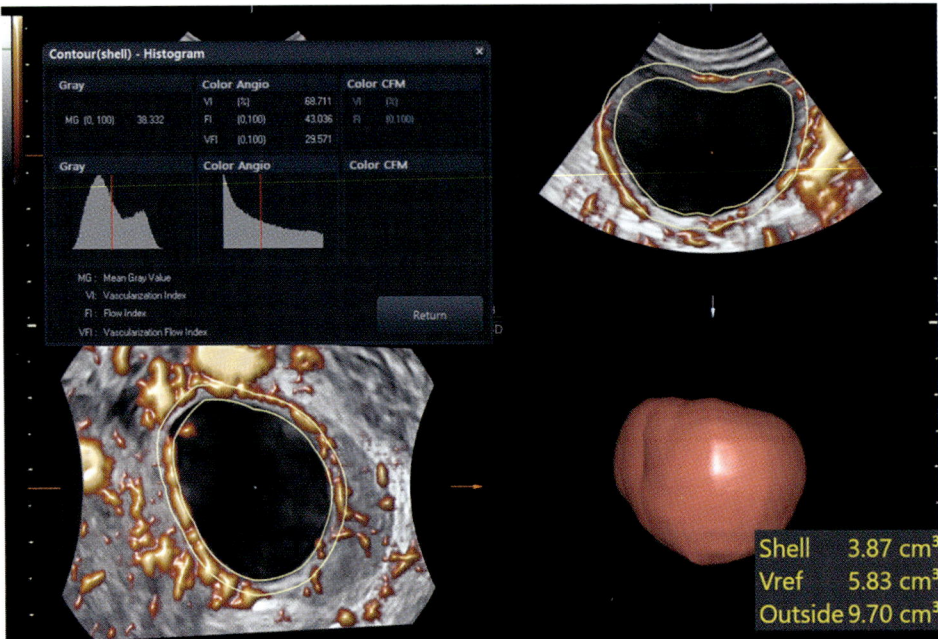

Fig. 10: 3D power Doppler ultrasound-acquired image of the follicle, processed by VOCAL and followed by volume histogram, shows VI, FI, and VFI values of the follicle. (3D: three-dimensional; FI: flow index; VFI: vascularization flow index; VI: vascularization index; VOCAL: virtual organ computer-aided analysis)

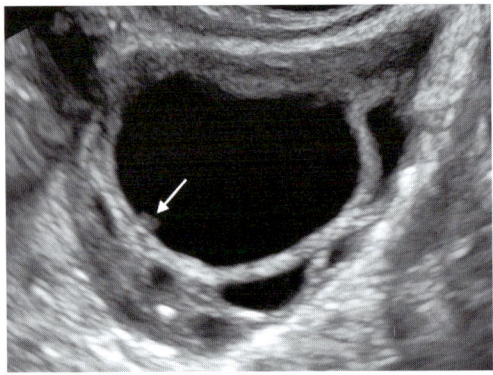

Fig. 11: B-mode ultrasound image of the follicle showing cumulus.

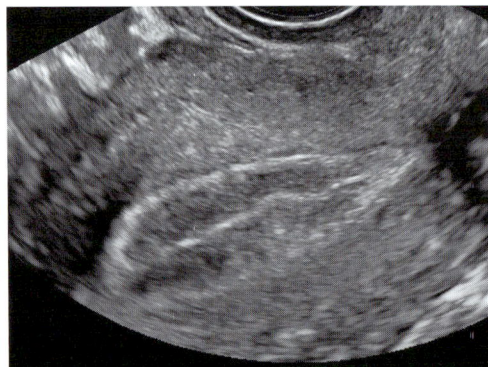

Fig. 12: B-mode ultrasound image of grade A endometrium.

It is termed grade B **(Fig. 13)** when it is multilayered with a hypoechoic/anechoic intervening area and grade C for homogenous isoechoic endometrium[26] **(Fig. 14)**. Changing endometrium morphology can be correlated with the rising estrogen level from grade B to grade A to grade C.

Doppler Features of Endometrium with Good Receptivity

Implantation rates are more correlated with the vascularity of the endometrium rather than the thickness and morphology of the endometrium. On Doppler, vascularity in

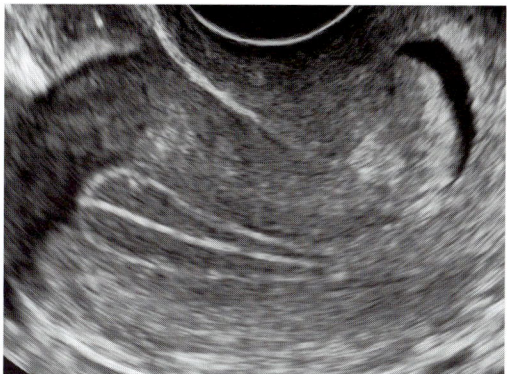

Fig. 13: B-mode ultrasound image of grade B endometrium.

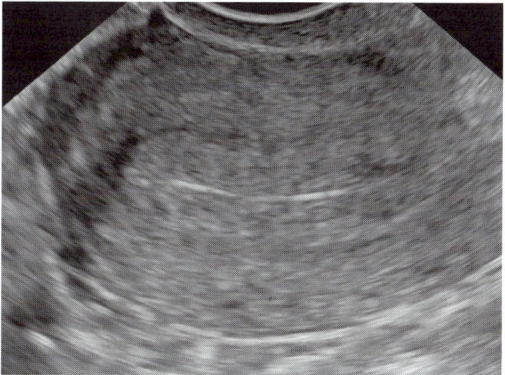

Fig. 14: B-mode ultrasound image of grade C endometrium.

endometrium is defined as vascularity in zones 3 and 4, which indicates functional maturity of the endometrium[27] **(Figs. 15A to D)**.

The zones of vascularity are defined according to Applebaum[27] as: Zone 1 when the vascularity on power Doppler is seen only at endometrial–myometrial junction, zone 2 when vessels penetrate through the hyperechogenic endometrial edge, zone 3 when they reach intervening hypoechogenic zone, and zone 4 when they reach the endometrial cavity and only cover at least 5 mm^2 area of that zone. Better conception rates and lower abortion rates are associated with vascularity in zones 3–4[28] **(Table 3)**.

These arteries should have an RI <0.6 and on pulse Doppler of the uterine artery, PI should be <3.2. Absence of flow in the endometrial and subendometrial zones on the day of trigger indicates total failure of implantation[29] **(Fig. 16)**.[30]

Endometrial volume assessment by three-dimensional ultrasound volume calculation correlates the cycle outcome with quantitative parameters rather than endometrial thickness. Pregnancy and implantation rates were significantly lower when endometrial volume <2 mL when measured by virtual organ computer-aided analysis (VOCAL).[31,32]

If these parameters are not reached, the cycle is not canceled, but stimulation is continued and trigger is delayed. Stimulation is continued till these parameters are achieved or LH surge is predicted by rising perifollicular RI and hyperechogenincity of the follicular wall.

This shows the fluffiness of the outer margin of the multilayered endometrium **(Fig. 17)**. However, hyperechogenicity of the endometrium may indicate deteriorating endometrial receptivity due to high preovulatory progesterone.

CONCLUSION

Ultrasound is the most cost-effective, accurate, and reliable tool for monitoring the follicles, understanding their behavior, and controlling their response to ovarian stimulation. Doppler adds to follow the hormonal changes and so to closely monitoring the cycle. Ultrasound with Doppler can be used as the only and a more relevant modality for monitoring ovarian stimulation cycles in patients undergoing infertility treatment **(Table 4)**.

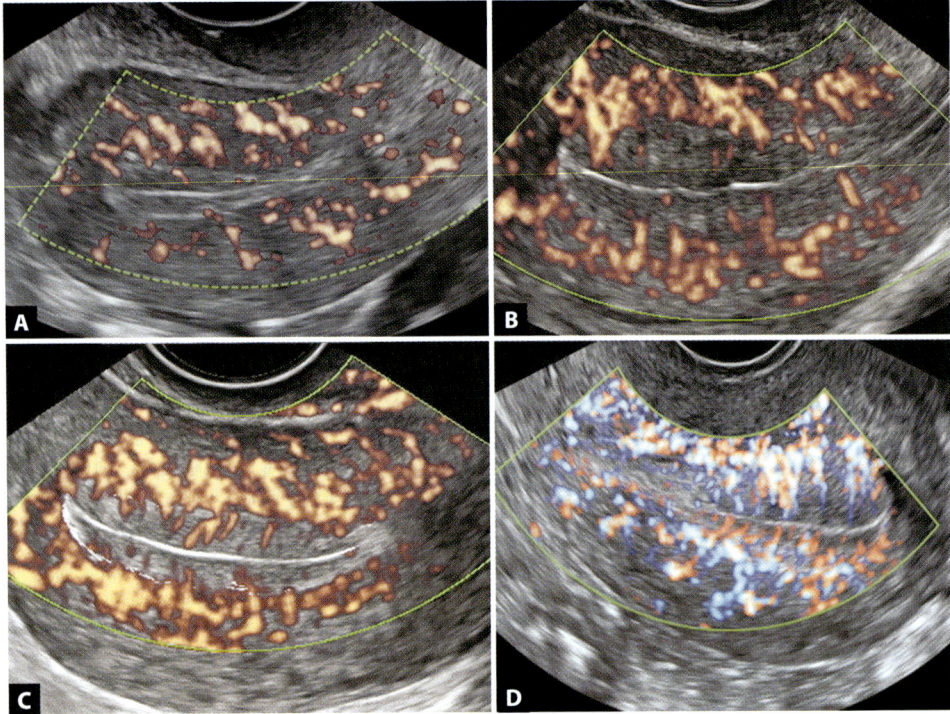

Figs. 15A to D: Power Doppler images of zones 1–4 of endometrium.

TABLE 3: Endometrial vascularity and its relation to implantation rates.[20]

Vascularity in % of patients	Zone 1 6.69%	Zone 2 20.73%	Zone 3 58%	Zone 4 14.47%
+ β-hCG	19%	21.87%	39.77%	70.14
Gestational sac	9.6%	14.58%	36.8%	68.65%
Abortions	50%	23.8%	5.6%	1.5%

(β-hCG: beta human chorionic gonadotropin)

TABLE 4: Ultrasound and Doppler features of mature follicle and endometrium.

Features	Follicle	Endometrium
Size/thickness	16–18 mm	8–10 mm
Morphology	Thin wall, no internal echoes, and halo	Grade A/B
Vascularity	Three-fourth circumference	Zones 3–4
RI	0.4–0.48	<0.5
PSV	>10 cm/s	–
Uterine artery PI	–	<3.2
Volume	3–7 cc	3–7 cc
3D morphology	Cumulus	Intact endometrial–myometrial junction
3D PD	More symmetrical the better	Higher the better

(3D: three-dimensional; PI: pulsatility index; PSV: peak systolic velocity; RI: resistance index; PD: power Doppler)

CHAPTER 9: Monitoring of Intrauterine Insemination Cycles and Dopplers in Intrauterine Insemination

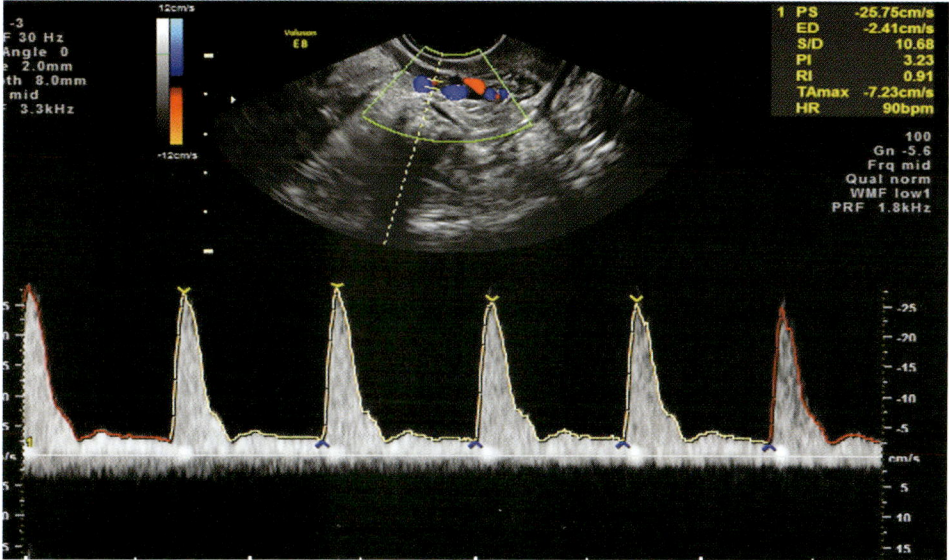

Fig. 16: Pulse Doppler image showing high-resistance uterine artery flow waveform.

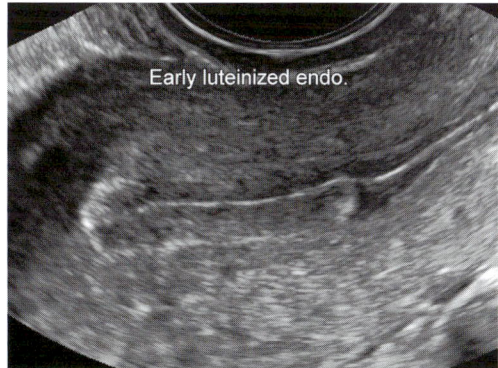

Fig. 17: Endometrium of the early luteal phase seen on B-mode ultrasound and fluffiness of the outer margins of the multilayered endometrium.

■ KEY LEARNING POINTS

- Results of IUI can be improved by gonadotrophin stimulation.
- Individualising the dose of gonadotrophin is a key to prevent ovarian hyper stimulation or poor response.
- Assessment of the follicle maturity and endometrial receptivity should be done with ultrasound and doppler for best results.
- Doppler and 3D ultrasound not only helps decide the time of trigger, it also helps in deciding the time of trigger and the trigger agent.

■ REFERENCES

1. Verhulst SM, Cohlen BJ, Hughes E, Te Velde E, Heineman MJ. Intrauterine insemination for unexplained subfertility. Cochrane Database Syst Rev. 2006;(4):CD001838.
2. Ombelet W, Vandeput H, Jansen M, Cox A, Vossen C, Pollet H, et al. Treatment of male infertility due to sperm surface antibodies: IUI or IVF? Hum Reprod. 1997;12(6):1165-70.
3. van Rumste MM, Custers IM, van der Veen F, van Wely M, Evers JL, Mol BW. The influence of number of follicles on pregnancy rates in intrauterine insemination with ovarian stimulation: a meta-analysis. Hum Reprod Update. 2008;14(6):563-70.
4. Kupesic S, Kurjak A. Predictors of IVF outcome by three-dimensional ultrasound. Hum Reprod. 2002;17(4):950-5.

5. Popovic-Todorovic B, Loft A, Lindhard A, Bangsbøll S, Andersson AM, Anderson AN. A prospective study of predictive factors of ovarian response in 'standard' IVF/ICSI patients treated with recombinant FSH. A suggestion for recombinant FSH dosage normogram. Hum Reprod. 2003;18(4):781-7.
6. Kwee J, Elting ME, Schats R, McDonnell J, Lambalk CB. Ovarian volume and antral follicle count for the prediction of low and hyper responders with in vitro fertilization. Reprod Biol Endocrinol. 2007;5:9.
7. Lass A, Skull J, McVeigh E, Margara R, Winston RM. Measurement of ovarian volume by transvaginal sonography before ovulation induction with human menopausal gonadotrophin for in-vitro fertilization can predict poor response. Hum Reprod. 1992;12:294-7.
8. Engmann L, Sladkevicius P, Agrawal R, Bekir JS, Campbell S, Tan SL. Value of ovarian stromal blood flow velocity measurement after pituitary suppression in the prediction of ovarian responsiveness and outcome of in vitro fertilization treatment. Fertil Steril. 1999;71(1):22-9.
9. Zaidi J, Barber J, Kyei-Mensah A, Bekir J, Campbell S, Tan SL. Relationship of ovarian stromal blood flow at baseline ultrasound to subsequent follicular response in an in vitro fertilization program. Obstet Gynecol. 1996;88:779-84
10. Lam PM, Johnson IR, Rainne-Fenning NJ. Three-dimensional ultrasound features of the polycystic ovary and the effect of different phenotypic expressions on these parameters. Hum Reprod. 2007 Dec;(12): 3116-23.
11. Panchal S, Nagori C. Ultrasound-based decision making on stimulation protocol for superovulated IUI cycles. IJIFM. 2016; 7(1):7-13.
12. Panchal S, Nagori C. Ultrasound Based decision making on stimulation protocol for IVF cycles. DSJUOG. 2016;10(3):330-7.
13. Hackelöer BJ, Fleming R, Robinson HP, dam AH, Coutts JR. Correlation of ultrasonic and endocrinological assessment of human follicular development. Am J Obstet Gynecol. 1979;135(1):122-8.
14. Luciano GN, Tarek AG. Ultrasonography and IVF. In: Rizk B (Ed). Ultrasonography in Reproductive Medicine and Infertility. Cambridge: Cambridge University Press; 2010. pp. 193-201.
15. Jokubkeine L, Sladkevicius P, Rovas L, Valentine L. Assessment of changes in volume and vascularity of ovaries during the normal menstrual cycle using three-dimensional power Doppler ultrasound. Hum Reprod. 2006;21(10):2661-8.
16. Nargund G, Doyle PE, Bourne TH, Parsons JH, Cheng WC, Campbell S, et al. Ultrasound derived indices of follicular blood flow before HCG administration and prediction of oocyte recovery and preimplantation embryo quality. Hum Reprod. 1996;11(11):2512-7.
17. Glock JL, Brumsted JR. Colour flow pulsed Doppler ultrasound in diagnosing luteal phase defect. Fertil Steril. 1995,64(3):500-4.
18. Nargund G, Doyle PE, Bourne TH, Parsons JH, Cheng WC, Campbell S, et al. Ultrasound-derived indices of follicular blood flow before HCG administration and prediction of oocyte recovery and preimplantation embryo quality. Hum Reprod. 1996;11(11):2512-7.
19. Nargund G, Bourne T, Doyle P, Parsons J, Cheng W, Campbell S, et al. Association between ultrasound indices of follicular blood flow, oocyte recovery and pre-implantation embryo quality. Hum Reprod. 1996;1(1)1:109-13.
20. Van Blerkom J, Antczak M, Schrader R. The developmental potential of human oocyte is related to the dissolved oxygen content of follicular fluid: association with vascular endothelial growth factor levels and perifollicular blood flow characteristics. Hum Reprod. 1997;12(5):1047-55.
21. Vlaisavljević V, Reljic M, Gavrić Lovrec V, Zazula D, Sergent N. Measurement of perifollicular blood flow of the dominant preovulatory follicle using three dimensional power doppler. Ultrasound Obstet Gynecol. 2003;22(5):520-6.

22. Mercé LT, Barco MJ, Kupesic S, Kurjak A. Two- and three-dimensional power Doppler ultrasound: from ovulation to implantation. In: Kurjak A, Chervenak F (Eds). Textbook of Perinatal Medicine, 2nd edition. London: CRC Press; 2005.
23. Panchal SY, Nagori CB. Can 3D PD be a better tool for assessing the pre-HCG follicle and endometrium? A randomized study of 500 cases. Presented at 16th World Congress on Ultrasound in Obstetrics and Gynecology, 2006, London. J Ultrasound Obstet Gynecol. 2006;28(4):504.
24. Bourne TH, Jurkovic D, Waterstone J, Campbell S, Collins WP. Intrafollicular blood flow during human ovulation. Ultrasound Obstet Gynecol. 1991;1(1):53-9.
25. Bourne TH, Athanasiou S, Bauer B. Ovulation and the periovulatory follicle. In: Bourne TH, Jauniaux E, Jurkovic D (Eds). Transvaginal Colour Doppler. Berlin: Springer-Verlag; 1995. pp. 119-30.
26. Smith B, Porter R, Ahuja K, Craft I. Ultrasonic assessment of endometrial changes in stimulated cycles in an in vitro fertilization and embryo transfer program. J In Vitro Fert Embryo Transf. 1984;1(4):233-8.
27. Applebaum M. The 'steel' and 'teflon' endometrium-ultrasound visualization of endometrial vascularity in IVF patients and outcome. Presented at The Third World Congress of Ultrasound in Obstetrics and Gynecology. Ultrasound Obstet Gynecol 1993;3(Suppl 2):10.
28. Nagori C, Panchal S. Endometrial vascularity: Its relation to implantation rates. Int J Infertility Fetal Med. 2012;3(2):48-50.
29. Zaidi J, Pittrof R, Shaker A, Kyei-Mensah A, Campbell S, Tan SL. Assessment of uterine artery blood flow on the day of human chorionic gonadotrophin administration by transvaginal color Doppler ultrasound in an in vitro fertilization program. Fertil Steril. 1996;65(2):377-81.
30. Steer CV, Campbell S, Tan SL, Crayford T, Mills C, Mason BA, et al. The use of transvaginal color flow imaging after in vitro fertilization to identify optimum uterine conditions before embryo transfer. Fertil Steril. 1992;57(2):372-6.
31. Raga F, Bonilla-Musoles F, Casan EM, Klein O, Bonilla F. Assessment of endometrial volume by three-dimensional ultrasound prior to embryo transfer: clues to endometrial receptivity. Hum Reprod. 1999;14(11):2851-4.
32. Kupesic S, Bekavac I, Bjelos D, Kurjak A. Assessment of endometrial receptivity by transvaginal color Doppler and three-dimensional power Doppler ultrasonography in patients undergoing in vitro fertilization procedures. J Ultrasound Med. 2001;20:125-34.

SECTION 4

Ovulation Induction Protocols: Oral Ovulogens

10. **Selective Estrogen Receptor Modulators**
    Gunjan Gupta Govil, Anshu Dhar

11. **Aromatase Inhibitors in Ovulation Induction**
    Lavanya Kiran, Sowparnika SN

12. **Insulin Sensitizers: Where We Stand?**
    Bushra Khan

CHAPTER 10

Selective Estrogen Receptor Modulators

Gunjan Gupta Govil, Anshu Dhar

■ INTRODUCTION

The development of selective estrogen receptor modulators (SERMs) has been a remarkable odyssey, with origins dating back to the 1950s. Initially, the primary quest was to discover a compound that could effectively inhibit estrogen's actions, particularly in the context of breast cancer therapy. However, this narrative took an unexpected turn when these compounds, initially explored for their potential as antifertility agents, serendipitously revealed their ability to induce ovulation in subfertile women.

SERMs, or selective estrogen receptor modulators, are a class of compounds designed to interact with intracellular estrogen receptors (ERs) within target organs. These compounds can act as either agonists or antagonists, depending on the specific context, and their selective action at the receptor level has yielded a wide array of therapeutic effects. These range from managing postmenopausal symptoms and cancer treatment to aiding in the induction of ovulation.

Among the many SERMs, clomiphene citrate (CC) stands as a pioneering figure. Synthesized for the first time in 1956, it took a significant leap forward in 1961 when Greenblatt and his colleagues made a groundbreaking discovery. They observed that clomiphene stimulated the ovaries of anovulatory women.[1] This discovery culminated in the Food and Drug Administration (FDA) approval of clomiphene for use in infertile patients in 1967.

■ CHEMICAL COMPOSITION (FIG. 1)

Clomiphene citrate is a nonsteroidal derivative of triphenyl chloroethylene. It is characterized by the replacement of four hydrogen atoms in the ethylene core with three phenyl rings and a chloride anion. Additionally, one of the three phenyl rings features an aminoalkoxy [OCH_2-CH_2-$N(C_2K_2)_2$] side chain. This configuration results in a white or pale-yellow, odorless powder. CC exhibits instability in air and light, and its melting point is within the range of 116–118°C.

Despite not being a steroid, CC shares a steric configuration remarkably similar to estradiol. This similarity enables CC to effectively bind to ERs. The compound's structural resemblance to estradiol likely contributes to its ability to interact with ERs,

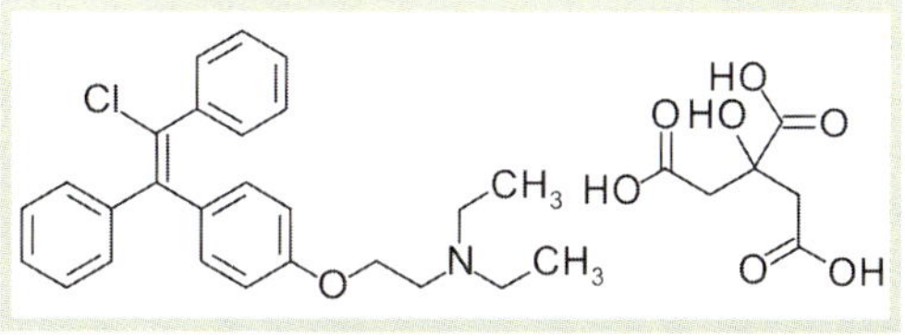

Fig. 1: Structure of clomiphene.

highlighting its significance in biological systems and potential applications in research or therapeutic contexts.

Commercially available CC exists as a racemic mixture comprising two stereochemical isomers: 38% Zu-clomiphene and 62% En-clomiphene. Notably, En-clomiphene exhibits greater potency, making it a significant contributor to the overall clinical efficacy of the drug.[2,3]

Each isomer displays distinct pharmacokinetic profiles. En-clomiphene is characterized by faster absorption and more complete elimination compared to Zu-clomiphene. The primary route of excretion for both isomers is through the feces, although minor amounts are also excreted in the urine.

Understanding the differential pharmacokinetics of Zu-clomiphene and En-clomiphene is crucial for optimizing the therapeutic effects and ensuring appropriate dosing regimens in clinical settings.

Zu-clomiphene is excreted more slowly and can be detected in the circulation for more than a month and has a tendency to accumulate over successive cycles of administration. This, however, has not been shown to have any significant clinical effects.[4] This explains the fact that even though its biological half-life is 5–6 days, the metabolites of clomiphene have been detected in stools up to 5–6 weeks.[5]

■ MECHANISM OF ACTION (FIG. 2)

Due to structural similarity to estrogen, it binds to nuclear ERs with agonistic and antagonistic actions at different sites. The agonistic actions are manifested only at low-endogenous estrogen concentration. Clomiphene has antagonistic effects at hypothalamus, pituitary, uterine endometrium, and cervix. Clomiphene citrate binds to the ERs at the level of hypothalamus and depletes them by interfering with receptor recycling hence preventing the negative feedback action of estrogen at the level of hypothalamus. This leads to an increase in the levels of circulating follicle-stimulating hormone (FSH) and luteinizing hormone (LH) which start falling as the 5-day course of treatment ends[6,7] with development of one or more dominant follicles. This stimulation to the ovary takes

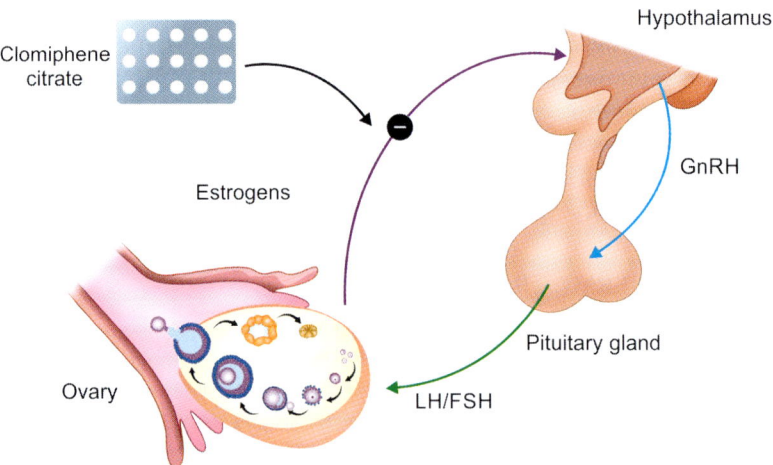

Fig. 2: Action of clomiphene at HPO axis. (FSH: follicle-stimulating hormone; GnRH: gonadotropin-releasing hormone; HPO: hypothalamic-pituitary-ovarian; LH: luteinizing hormone)

care of the subtle ovulatory disturbances which might be contributing to infertility. It has been seen that in cases of polycystic ovary syndrome (PCOS) with anovulation where the gonadotropin-releasing hormone (GnRH) pulse frequency is already abnormally raised, clomiphene causes an increase in pulse amplitude without affecting the frequency.[8,9] However, the rise of LH with FSH under the influence of clomiphene may lead to a delay in ovulation.

The advantage of clomiphene citrate lies in the lack of progestational, corticotropic, androgenic, or antiandrogenic properties.

■ INDICATIONS OF TREATMENT

- Anovulatory infertility
- Empirical therapy of males with idiopathic infertility with limited results[10]
- Unexplained infertility for superovulation
- Mild stimulation regimen in in vitro fertilization (IVF)
- Stimulated frozen embryo cycles in IVF
- Prevention of premature LH surge.

■ CONTRAINDICATIONS

- Ovarian cysts
- Malignancy
- Hypogonadotropic hypogonadism
- Hypothalamic amenorrhea
- Liver disease
- Visual disturbances
- Pregnancy
- Hypersensitivity.

■ TREATMENT REGIMEN

Standard Therapy

Clomiphene can be administered from day 2 to day 5 of spontaneous or hormone-induced menstruation. No difference in the outcome was seen irrespective of the day of starting treatment, if it was done between and including day 2 to day 5 of menses.[11] The empirical starting dose of clomiphene is usually 50 mg/day which has been shown to induce ovulation in up to 52% of the cases.[12] In cases which fail to ovulate, clomiphene is given in incremental doses of 50 mg/cycle over subsequent cycles till ovulation is achieved up to a dose of 250 mg/day. However, doses higher than 100 mg/day are not approved by the FDA[13] and do little in terms of improving the outcome.

Among anovulatory women who achieve ovulation with CC, the cumulative pregnancy rates vary based on the dosage administered. For the 50 mg/day dosage, the 3-month cumulative pregnancy rate is reported at 50%, followed by a 62% conception rate at 6 months. The 100 mg/day dosage exhibits a 45% cumulative pregnancy rate at 3 months, increasing to a 66% conception rate at 6 months. Lastly, for the 150 mg/day dosage, the 3-month cumulative pregnancy rate is 33%, with a small increase to a 38% conception rate at 6 months.[14,15] Obesity has been shown to reduce the success rates in anovulatory women taking clomiphene with live birth rate of 16% in women with body mass index (BMI) >35 kg/m^2 compared to 28% for women with BMI <30%.[16]

Pregnancy with clomiphene usually occurs within 3–6 months of treatment. It is not recommended to continue therapy beyond 6 months.

Stair Step Protocol (Fig. 3)

The stair-step protocol (described in **Fig. 3**) was introduced as an alternative to the traditional protocol. Here, instead of canceling the cycle in case a patient does not respond to a particular dose of clomiphene, given for a duration of 5 days and starting afresh, an incremental dose of clomiphene

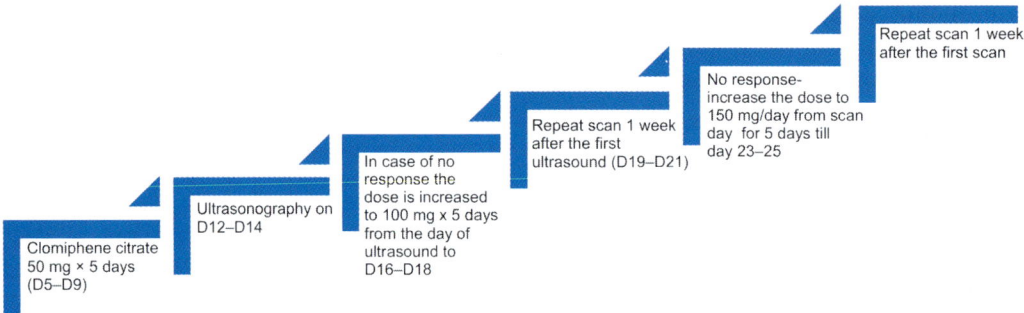

Fig. 3: Clomiphene citrate: stair-step protocol.

is administered in the same cycle. In a randomized-controlled trial (RCT) conducted by Deveci et al., 60 patients with PCOS who did not respond to the standard 50 mg/day for 5 days of CC treatment in one cycle were assigned randomly to either the traditional protocol or the stair-step protocol groups. Several endpoints were assessed, including ovulation and pregnancy rates, duration of treatment, and potential uterine and systemic side effects.

The results revealed that the rates of ovulation were similar between the stair-step and the control group (43.3 vs. 33.3%, respectively), as were the pregnancy rates (16.7 vs. 10%). Interestingly, the stair-step protocol demonstrated a shorter duration of treatment compared to the traditional protocol (20.5 ± 2.0 vs. 48.6 ± 2.4 days, respectively).

Moreover, the analysis of systemic side effects between the two groups did not show any significant differences. Additionally, there were no significant variations in uterine effects, as assessed by parameters such as endometrial thickness and uterine artery Doppler, between the two protocols.

These findings suggest that the stair-step protocol may offer comparable ovulation and pregnancy rates to the traditional protocol, with the added advantage of a shorter treatment duration. Furthermore, the absence of significant differences in systemic side effects and uterine effects indicates that the stair-step protocol may be a viable alternative with potential benefits for certain patients with PCOS who do not respond to the standard CC treatment.[17]

Efficacy of Treatment

The rates of ovulation with clomiphene range from 70 to 92% in anovulatory women. However, the pregnancy rates are lower. Several reasons have been proposed to explain the challenges and difficulties associated with CC treatment in achieving successful pregnancies. These reasons include:
1. Estrogen antagonist effects on the endometrium and cervical mucus
2. Decrease of uterine blood flow
3. Impaired placental protein 14 synthesis
4. Subclinical pregnancy loss
5. Effect on tubal transport
6. Detrimental effects on the oocytes.

These various factors highlight the complex interactions and potential challenges associated with CC treatment in fertility.

Clomiphene citrate resistance: Failure to ovulate even after administration of maximum 150 mg dose of clomiphene citrate for three cycles. The strategies to deal with clomiphene resistance will be discussed in subsequent pages.

Clomiphene failure: The patient ovulates with CC but fails to conceive even after three ovulatory cycles. In such patients, management consists of switching over to other ovulation inducing agents including aromatase inhibitors, gonadotropins or more aggressive forms of treatment.

ADJUNCTIVE THERAPIES IN CLOMIPHENE RESISTANCE

Various modalities of treatment have been used in cases of clomiphene resistance in conjunction with clomiphene to improve the response to clomiphene. However, it is not always necessary to follow a set sequence with a trial of adjunctive therapies before switching over to the most effective gonadotropins. However, these therapies may be tried especially where the resources do not permit the administration and monitoring of gonadotropin cycles.

Use of Metformin with Clomiphene

In cases which have failed to respond to clomiphene alone, addition of metformin has been suggested as a means to induce ovulation.[18,19]

In the RCT, the live birth rates observed in women treated with CC alone were comparable to those treated with a combination of CC and metformin, indicating no significant difference in live births between the two groups.[16] However, several randomized-controlled studies have demonstrated that administering metformin as a pretreatment at doses ranging from 1,500 to 1,700 mg daily resulted in significantly improved ovulation rates[19-23] and pregnancy rates[24-29] in women who previously showed no response to clomiphene treatment. It is important to note that these studies often had limitations due to small sample sizes.

Moreover, when metformin is given to obese women in combination with dietary adjustments and exercise, it may contribute to weight loss and potentially enhance the response to clomiphene.

Despite its potential benefits, metformin is associated with gastrointestinal side effects and, in some cases, may lead to hepatotoxicity or induce lactic acidosis. Thus, it is advisable to monitor liver and renal functions both before initiating metformin treatment and regularly once treatment begins. This monitoring helps in early detection of any adverse effects and ensures the safe administration of metformin in conjunction with CC for fertility treatment.

Use of Clomiphene with Glucocorticoids

Glucocorticoids are sometimes prescribed to induce ovulation in women who fail to ovulate with clomiphene alone. In a triple-blinded randomized control trial, 60 patients of PCOS were randomly allocated to dexamethasone + CC or CC + placebo. 21 out of 30 (70%) women ovulated in dexamethasone + CC group which was not significantly different from the rate of ovulation in the CC + placebo group (17 out of 30 women ovulated amounting to an ovulation rate of 56.7%. The pregnancy rate was 16.7% in the dexamethasone + CC group and 10% in the CC + placebo group which was not significantly different. However, the number of follicles ≥18 mm were significantly more in the dexamethasone + CC group (p <0.05). This study concluded that addition of dexamethasone to CC significantly increased the number of mature follicles, without any significant increase in ovulation and pregnancy rates.[30]

In another large RCT with 230 clomiphene-resistant women, a comparison was done between treatment with CC 200 mg daily over days 5–9 along with dexamethasone 2 mg daily over days 5-14 and CC 200 mg and placebo for the same amount of time. Ovulation rate in the combination group was 88% which was significantly more than the rate of 20% in the control group. The cumulative pregnancy rate in the combined treatment group was also significantly higher (40.5 vs. 4.2%) than the control group ($p < 0.0001$).[31]

The exact mechanism by which glucocorticoids act has been a matter of much contemplation with theories ranging from effect by lowering the levels of dehydroepiandrosterone sulfate (DHEAS) in the group of patients with elevated levels of the same. However, the effect has also been seen in cases where no such rise is present. Multiple theories have been proposed to elucidate this effect, encompassing the suppression of hyperandrogenism, synergistic actions with the direct effects of FSH on oocyte development, as well as indirect influences stemming from intrafollicular growth factors and cytokines.[32]

However, it is not advocated to coadminister steroids with clomiphene for extended periods of time to avoid the side effects associated with the same.

Clomiphene and Gonadotropins

Some CC-resistant women may benefit from sequential CC/gonadotropin therapy. However, since the use of gonadotropins is associated not only with additional costs but also entails closer monitoring, this treatment should be given only by clinicians who have requisite experience in the same. The treatment consists of standard CC regimen, followed by administration of low-dose human menopausal gonadotropin (hMG) or FSH (75–150 IU/day for 3 days). Following this, further treatment is decided based on serial transvaginal ultrasound examinations. Many[33-35] but not all[36] studies have reported the chances of conception with the combination to be similar to gonadotropins alone. The combination may offer benefit in terms of reducing the dose and hence the cost of gonadotropins. The aim of the therapy should be tailored to induce ovulation of a single mature follicle.

Alternative treatments for clomiphene citrate resistance: Other options that can be explored in the cases of clomiphene resistance are aromatase inhibitors, tamoxifen, insulin-sensitizing agents, laparoscopic ovarian drilling, gonadotropins, and lastly use of IVF.

Clomiphene Citrate Treatment Monitoring

Documentation of ovulation forms an important part of treatment especially when clomiphene is being used in combination with intrauterine insemination (IUI) as in cases of unexplained infertility.

Various modalities of monitoring may be used to achieve this end including the use of ovulation predictor kits, ultrasound, and serum measurements of estradiol, LH, and/or progesterone. Sometimes administration of human chorionic gonadotropin (hCG) can be used for synchronization of ovulation with IUI, eliminating the requirement for an endogenous LH surge. Urinary ovulation predictor kits pinpoint the midcycle LH surge, corresponding to the interval of peak fertility.[37,38] Ovulation can occur at any time within 2 days thereafter.[39,40]

The surge is mostly seen between 5 and 12 days after the last dose of clomiphene.[41] Serial folliculometry can tell us the size and number of follicles that are developing and can give us presumptive evidence of ovulation in the form of progressive follicular growth, followed by collapse of the preovulatory follicle, accompanied by an increase in cul-de-sac fluid volume with crenation of follicular margins and appearance of internal echoes. However, ultrasound being expensive is used for monitoring of clomiphene cycles when it is not possible to use less complicated methods for documentation of ovulation.

Human chorionic gonadotropin is sometimes used to trigger ovulation in clomiphene cycle. According to Cochrane meta-analysis, there is inadequate evidence to recommend or refute the use of urinary hCG as an ovulation trigger in anovulatory women treated with CC.[42] Hence, the use of hCG is reserved for cases where IUI is planned or where monitoring with LH is unreliable. Pregnancy rates are higher when the leading follicle sizes as measured by ultrasound are 23–28 mm in diameter.[43]

Side Effects

The side effects associated with the use of clomiphene include:
- Hot flushes (10%)
- Abdominal distention, bloating, or discomfort (5%)
- Breast discomfort (2%)
- Nausea and vomiting (2%)
- Visual symptoms and headache (1.5%)
- Rise in basal body temperature.

It is important to note that CC may rarely cause more serious visual symptoms, including floaters, flashes, or abnormal perception, as well as optic neuropathy. However, these effects are usually temporary and tend to disappear once the treatment is discontinued.

Association with Multiple Pregnancy

Due to growth of more than one follicle, multiple pregnancy may occur up to 8% overall for anovulatory women and 2.6–7.4% in women treated for unexplained infertility.[13] The overwhelming majority of multiple pregnancies that result from CC treatment are twin gestations; triplet and higher-order pregnancies are rare (0.08–1.1%) but may occur.[44]

Association with Ovarian Cancer

There have been controversial reports linking CC with the risk of ovarian cancer. There have been a few studies with limited number of cases without adequate information on the dose and type of infertility drugs to suggest that infertility drugs may increase the risk of ovarian cancer slightly in subfertile women as compared to the general population or to subfertile women who have not been treated with the risk being slightly higher for nulliparous than multiparous women, and that too for borderline ovarian tumors.[45]

Association with Congenital Malformations

Many old studies had pointed out the association of ovulation induction with neural tube defects especially with clomiphene citrate. However, a recent meta-analysis has failed to show any such increase.[46,47]

POLYCYSTIC OVARY SYNDROME: THE LATEST VERDICT FOR SELECTIVE ESTROGEN RECEPTOR MODULATORS

In present times, the first-line ovulation induction agent in PCOS is letrozole. Since the use of letrozole is still banned in some countries, the American Society for Reproductive Medicine (ASRM) recommends that in situations where letrozole cannot be used due to restrictions or nonavailability, other ovulation induction agents can be used. Though not the most effective agent, metformin could be used alone in the cases where there is PCOS with anovulatory infertility and other infertility factors have been ruled out with improved clinical pregnancy and live birth rate. In comparison to metformin in such scenarios, CC used alone could lead to improve ovulation, clinical pregnancy, and live birth rates with increased multiple pregnancy, hence, clomiphene cycles may need ultrasound monitoring. The use of CC along with metformin in comparison to CC alone in such women may lead to improved ovulation and clinical pregnancy rates.[48]

COMPARISON OF AROMATASE INHIBITORS AND SELECTIVE ESTROGEN RECEPTOR MODULATORS

Polycystic Ovary Syndrome

According to the Cochrane analysis by Franik et al., letrozole demonstrates a notable improvement in live birth and pregnancy rates for infertile women with anovulatory PCOS compared to SERMs when employed for ovulation induction followed by intercourse. The evidence suggests a high level of certainty that rates of ovarian hyperstimulation syndrome (OHSS) are similar with letrozole or SERMs. Furthermore, there is high-certainty evidence indicating no significant differences in miscarriage rate and multiple pregnancy rate between the two approaches. Based on the evidence, the recommendation is for the use of letrozole over clomiphene citrate in women with PCOS experiencing anovulatory infertility and no other infertility factors, aiming to enhance ovulation, clinical pregnancy, and live birth rates.[49] The latest evidence-based international guidelines on PCOS also recommend letrozole as first-line ovulation induction drug in PCOS.[48]

Unexplained Infertility

The conventional treatments for unexplained infertility have typically involved the administration of gonadotropins or CC. However, to address unexplained infertility while concurrently mitigating the risk of multiple births, the utilization of letrozole has been suggested. In a multicenter RCT, normally ovulating women, aged between 18 and 40 years, possessing at least one patent fallopian tube, were randomly allocated to receive ovarian stimulation, spanning up to four cycles, with gonadotropin (301 women), clomiphene (300 women), or letrozole (299 women). The primary endpoint assessed was the incidence of multiple gestations among women with clinical pregnancies. The study concluded that in women experiencing unexplained infertility, ovarian stimulation (OS) with letrozole led to a significantly reduced occurrence of multiple gestations, albeit with a lower frequency of live births when compared to gonadotropin, but not clomiphene.[50]

Tamoxifen

Another SERM which has been used for ovulation induction but not as widely is tamoxifen. The mechanism of action of tamoxifen is similar to that of clomiphene, i.e., it blocks the action of estrogen at the level of hypothalamus thus releasing the feedback inhibition, in turn increasing the levels of GnRH and consequently FSH and LH.

Dose

Tamoxifen is administered in a dosage of 40 mg daily for 5 days starting between day 2 and day 5 of natural or hormone-induced menses.

The advantage of tamoxifen lies in the fact that it does not have an adverse effect on cervical mucus and endometrium unlike clomiphene. Ovulation rates of 50–90% and pregnancy rates of 30–50% have been reported with tamoxifen.[51-53] Some studies have shown it to be effective in cases of clomiphene failure.[51]

Use of tamoxifen for shorter durations does not appear to increase the risk of endometrial or ovarian cancer.

In a prospective study involving 104 women diagnosed with PCOS and randomly assigned to receive either tamoxifen or clomiphene, comparable ovulation rates were observed in both groups (66.6 vs. 70%, $p = 0.715$). Despite a slightly elevated pregnancy rate per treatment cycle and per ovulatory cycle in the tamoxifen group (14.81 and 22.22%, respectively), in comparison to the clomiphene group (14 and 20%, respectively), these differences did not achieve statistical significance ($p > 0.05$). Notably, the tamoxifen group demonstrated a significantly higher endometrial thickness.[54] These findings align with a meta-analysis conducted by Steiner et al., which also reached similar conclusions.[55]

OTHER USES OF SELECTIVE ESTROGEN RECEPTOR MODULATORS IN INFERTILITY

Male Infertility

The role of clomiphene has been investigated in idiopathic male infertility.[56] Clomiphene therapy is cheap and requires an intact hypothalamic pituitary testicular axis. GnRH produced from the hypothalamus stimulates LH and FSH from the anterior pituitary gland promoting the production of testosterone and in turn spermatogenesis. This testosterone is then converted into estradiol by the action of aromatase enzyme. Similar to the action in females, testosterone in the normal physiological state exerts negative feedback mechanism on the male reproductive axis by binding to the hypothalamus, causing inhibition of GnRH. CC acts at hypothalamic ER level and blocks the negative feedback mechanism and results in increased GnRH. This action has been utilized for empirical treatment of male infertility. According to ASRM, it can be considered an alternative to other therapies in idiopathic hypogonadotropic hypogonadism.[10]

Endometrial Preparation using Stimulated Cycle

Mild OS with an oral agent (CC or letrozole) and/or exogenous gonadotropins may be used to prime the endometrium for frozen embryo transfer (FET). According to recent Cochrane by Ghobara et al., there is insufficient evidence to support the use of one cycle regimen in preference to another in preparation for FET in subfertile women with regular ovulatory cycles.[57] Hence, endometrial preparation using stimulated regimen is a viable option.

Mild Stimulation In Vitro Fertilization

It essentially denotes OS for IVF using a daily gonadotropin dose of ≤150 IU, with or without the addition of oral medication (CC or letrozole) in a GnRH antagonist cycle.[58] Addition of oral agents has not only been shown to have similar efficacy but also reduces the total dose of gonadotropins used in IVF cycle and hence the cost per

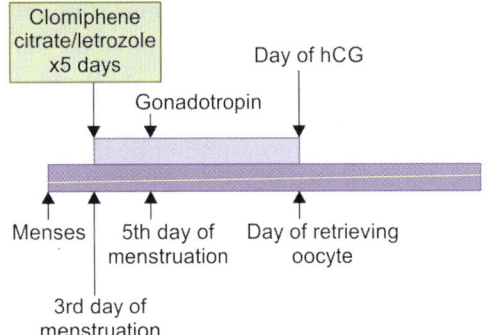

Fig. 4: Mild stimulation protocol for in vitro fertilization (IVF). (hCG: human chorionic gonadotropin)

cycle. This has been confirmed in multiple RCTs[59,60] **(Fig. 4)**.

In the RCT conducted by Ragni et al., comparing CC with high doses of gonadotropins for IVF in women with compromised ovarian reserve, it was observed that women assigned to high doses of gonadotropins yielded more oocytes and had a higher probability of undergoing embryo transfer. However, the likelihood of achieving a successful pregnancy was found to be similar. The delivery rate per started cycle for women receiving CC and high-dose gonadotropins was 3% ($n = 5$) and 5% ($n = 7$), respectively ($p = 0.77$). Notably, the clomiphene cycle was more cost-effective compared to the gonadotropin cycle. Consequently, this study concluded that in women with compromised ovarian reserve, OS with either CC or high-dose gonadotropins resulted in comparable chances of achieving pregnancy, with the added advantage of cost-effectiveness associated with the clomiphene cycle.[61]

Clomiphene for Prevention of Premature Luteinizing Hormone Surge in Intrauterine Insemination Cycles

With os for IUI cycles, especially for PCOS patients, there may be a premature rise in serum LH levels in response to rising estrogen levels. Some studies have shown the advantage of suppressing this premature LH surge using antagonist. However, this increases the cost of treatment. The same results have been obtained by administration of clomiphene and has been attributed to its antiestrogenic effect. In the RCT studying the effect of clomiphene administration on premature LH surge, the incidence of premature LH surge was significantly lower in those who received CC (3.0 vs. 14.9%; $p = 0.021$). Patients who received CC had higher number of mature follicles >18 mm when compared to controls (3.85 ± 1.3 vs. 2.94 ± 1.01; $p < 0.001$).[62]

Clomiphene Citrate for Prevention of Premature Luteinizing Hormone Surge in In Vitro Fertilization Cycles

Similar to the action described above for IUI cycles, it has been postulated that clomiphene continued till the day of ovulation trigger can be used in place of antagonist to prevent premature LH surge.[63-65] In a study comparing CC versus antagonist for the prevention of premature LH surge, it was found that the serum estradiol levels were significantly raised in the clomiphene group ($p < 0.001$) with similar pregnancy rates.[66] This area of clomiphene use requires further research.

Other Uses

Selective estrogen receptor modulators especially the newer molecules like ospemifene, lasofoxifene, bazedoxifene, and arzoxifene are being studied for amelioration of postmenopausal symptoms and osteoporosis. Bazedoxifene recently got FDA approval for the same.

In the year 2005, a mini review by Homberg[67] boldly proclaimed the potential end of an era for CC. Enumerating various candidates that might replace it, the review hinted at a transformative shift in the landscape of reproductive medicine. However, nearly 2 decades later, clomiphene's resilience persists, defying the prediction of its obsolescence.

Despite facing mounting competition from aromatase inhibitors and gonadotropins, SERMs, including clomiphene, continue to hold their ground in clinical practice, fuelled by factors such as cost-effectiveness, widespread availability, and the deep-seated familiarity that older clinicians have with the drug.

Far from fading into obscurity, the use of clomiphene is undergoing a metamorphosis. Once celebrated for its traditional role for ovulation induction, it now stands at the forefront of innovation, adapting to the evolving landscape of modern medicine. It gracefully bows out from its classic era, embracing the winds of change and finding renewed purpose, particularly in the realm of assisted reproductive technologies.

■ CONCLUSION

In 2005, in a mini review titled *Clomiphene citrate—end of an era?* Homberg[67] enumerating the various potential candidates which may replace clomiphene had declared that it might be the beginning of end of clomiphene. However, almost 2 decades down the lane, SERMs are still being used due to their cheaper cost, easy availability, and familiarity of the older clinicians with the drug, though they are facing increasing competition from aromatase inhibitors and gonadotropins. Clomiphene, a versatile medication once renowned for its traditional role, is now paving the way for newer horizons as its classic era gracefully bows out, embracing the winds of medical innovation carving a niche for itself in the modern medicine with newer uses especially in assisted reproductive technologies.

■ KEY LEARNING POINTS

- Selective estrogen receptor modulators (SERMs) constitute a class of compounds extensively employed for inducing ovulation.
- Despite the heightened ovulation rates associated with clomiphene, the corresponding pregnancy rates appear to be diminished, likely attributable to the antagonistic actions of clomiphene on the endometrium and cervix.
- Although there is a notable shift toward adopting aromatase inhibitors for ovulation induction, the decision to persist with SERMs over aromatase inhibitors often hinges on considerations of financial constraints, ease of availability, and the established comfort level of healthcare providers with these medications.

■ REFERENCES

1. Greenblatt RB, Barfield WE, Jungck EC, Ray AW. Induction of ovulation with MRL/41: Preliminary report. J Am Med Assoc. 1961; 178:101-4.
2. Charles D, Klein T, Lunn SF, Loraine JA. Clinical and endocrinological studies with the isomeric components of clomiphene citrate. J Obstet Gynaecol Br Commonw. 1969;76:1100-10.
3. Pandya G, Cohen MR. The effect of cis-isomer of clomiphene citrate (cis-clomiphene) on cervical mucus and vaginal cytology. J Reprod Med. 1972;8:133-8.
4. Young SL, Opsahl MS, Fritz MA. Serum concentrations of enclomiphene and zuclomiphene across consecutive cycles of clomiphene citrate therapy in anovulatory infertile women. Fertil Steril. 1999;71:639-44.

5. MacLeod SC, Mitton DM, Parker AS, Tupper WR. Experience with induction of ovulation. Am J Obstet Gynecol. 1970;108:814-24.
6. Legro RS, Brzyski RG, Diamond MP, Coutifaris C, Schlaff WD, Casson P, et al. Letrozole versus clomiphene for infertility in the polycystic ovary syndrome. N Engl J Med. 2014;371:119-29.
7. Athar R, Mehrnoosh M, Masoumeh H, Hooshmand F, Fatemeh A. A clomiphene citrate and letrozol varsus tamoxifen and letrozole as an infertility treatment in women with polycystic ovary syndrome. Pak J Biol Sci. 2015;18:300-3.
8. Kettel LM, Roseff SJ, Berga SL, Mortola JF, Yen SS. Hypothalamic-pituitary ovarian response to clomiphene citrate in women with polycystic ovary syndrome. Fertil Steril. 1993;59:532-8.
9. Rebar R, Judd HL, Yen SSC, Rakoff J, VandenBerg G, Naftolin F. Characterization of the inappropriate gonadotropin secretion in polycystic ovary syndrome. J Clin Invest. 1976;57:1320-9.
10. Practice Committee of the American Society for Reproductive Medicine. Management of nonobstructive azoospermia: a committee opinion. Fertil Steril. 2018;110(7):1239-45.
11. Wu CH, Winkel CA. The effect of initiation day on clomiphene citrate therapy. Fertil Steril. 1989;52:564-8.
12. Gysler M, March CM, Mishell DR Jr, Bailey EJ. A decade's experience with an individualized clomiphene treatment regime including its effect on the postcoital test. Fertil Steril. 1982;37:161-7.
13. Practice Committee of the American Society for Reproductive Medicine. Use of clomiphene citrate in infertile women: a committee opinion. Fertil Steril. 2013;100(2):341-8.
14. Imani B, Eijkemans MJ, te Velde ER, Habbema JD, Fauser BC. Predictors of chances to conceive in ovulatory patients during clomiphene citrate induction of ovulation in normogonadotropic oligoamenorrheic infertility. J Clin Endocrinol Metab. 1999; 84:1617-22.
15. The Thessaloniki ESHRE/ASRM-Sponsored PCOS Consensus Workshop Group. Consensus on infertility treatment related to polycystic ovary syndrome. Fertil Steril. 2008;89:505-22.
16. Legro RS, Barnhart HX, Schlaff WD, Carr BR, Diamond MP, Carson SA, et al. Clomiphene, metformin, or both for infertility in the polycystic ovary syndrome. N Engl J Med. 2007;356:551-66.
17. Deveci CD, Demir B, Sengul O, Dilbaz B, Goktolga U. Clomiphene citrate 'stair-step' protocol vs. traditional protocol in patients with polycystic ovary syndrome: a randomized controlled trial. Arch Gynecol Obstet. 2015;291(1):179-84.
18. Heard MJ, Pierce A, Carson SA, Buster JE. Pregnancies following use of metformin for ovulation induction in patients with polycystic ovary syndrome. Fertil Steril. 2002;77:669-73, 35.
19. Zain MM, Jamaluddin R, Ibrahim A, Norman RJ. Comparison of clomiphene citrate, metformin, or the combination of both for first-line ovulation induction, achievement of pregnancy, and live birth in Asian women with polycystic ovary syndrome: a randomized controlled trial. Fertil Steril. 2009;91:514-21.
20. Creanga A, Bradley H, McCormick C, Witkop CT. Use of metformin in polycystic ovary syndrome: a meta-analysis. Obstet Gynecol. 2008;111:959-68.
21. Nestler JD, Jacubowicz DJ, Evans WS, Pasquali R. Effects of metformin on spontaneous and clomiphene induced ovulation in the polycystic ovary syndrome. N Engl J Med. 1998;338:1876-80.
22. Kocak M, Caliskan E, Simsir C, Haberal A. Metformin therapy improves ovulatory rates, cervical scores, and pregnancy rates in clomiphene citrate-resistant women with polycystic ovary syndrome. Fertil Steril. 2002;77:101-6.
23. Chaudhury K, Chaudhury S, Chowdhury S. Does metformin augment the ovulation inducing effects of clomiphene in non-obese

women with polycystic ovary syndrome? J Indian Med Assoc. 2008;106:643-8.
24. Ben Ayed B, Dammak dit Mlik S, Ben Arab H, Trabelssi H, Chahtour H, Mathlouthi N, et al. Metformin effects on clomifene-induced ovulation in the polycystic ovary syndrome. Tunis Med. 2009;87:43-9.
25. Vandermolen DT, Ratts VS, Evans WS, Stovall DW, Kauma SW, Nestler JE. Metformin increases the ovulatory rate and pregnancy rate from clomiphene citrate in patients with polycystic ovary syndrome who are resistant to clomiphene citrate alone. Fertil Steril. 2001;75:310-5.
26. Sahin Y, Yirmibes U, Kelestimur F, Aygen E. The effects of metformin on insulin resistance, clomiphene-induced ovulation and pregnancy rates in women with polycystic ovary syndrome. Eur J Obstet Gynecol Reprod Biol. 2004;113:214-20.
27. Hwu YM, Lin SY, Huang WY, Lin MH, Lee RK. Ultra-short metformin pretreatment for clomiphene citrate-resistant polycystic ovary syndrome. Int J Gynaecol Obstet. 2005; 90:39-43.
28. Khorram O, Helliwell JP, Katz S, Bonpane CM, Jaramillo L. Two weeks of metformin improves clomiphene citrate-induced ovulation and metabolic profiles in women with polycystic ovary syndrome. Fertil Steril. 2006;85:1448-51.
29. Kazerooni T, Ghaffarpasand F, Kazerooni Y, Kazerooni M, Setoodeh S. Short-term metformin treatment for clomiphene-resistant women with polycystic ovary syndrome. Int J Gynaecol Obstet. 2009; 107:50-3.
30. Esmaeilzadeh S, Amiri MG, Basirat Z, Shirazi M. Does adding dexamethasone to clomiphene citrate improve ovulation in PCOS patients? A triple—blind randomized clinical trial study. Int J Fertil Steril. 2011;5(1):9-12.
31. Parsanezhad ME, Alborzi S, Motazedian S, Omrani G. Use of dexamethasone and clomiphene citrate in the treatment of clomiphene citrate-resistant patients with polycystic ovary syndrome and normal dehydroepiandrosterone sulfate levels: a prospective, double-blind, placebo-controlled trial. Fertil Steril. 2002;78:1001-4.
32. Keay SD, Jenkins JM. Adjunctive use of dexamethasone in Clomid resistant patients. Fertil Steril. 2003;80:230-1.
33. March CM, Tredway DR, Mishell DR Jr. Effect of clomiphene citrate upon the amount and duration of human menopausal gonadotropin therapy. Am J Obstet Gynecol. 1976;125:699-704, 54.
34. Ron-el R, Soffer Y, Langer R, Herman A, Weintraub Z, Caspi E. Low multiple pregnancy rate in combined clomiphene citrate—human menopausal gonadotrophin treatment for ovulation induction or enhancement. Hum Reprod. 1989;4:495-500.
35. Lu PY, Chen AL, Atkinson EJ, Lee SH, Erickson LD, Ory SJ. Minimal stimulation achieves pregnancy rates comparable to human menopausal gonadotropins in the treatment of infertility. Fertil Steril. 1996;65:583-7.
36. Ransom MX, Doughman NC, Garcia AJ. Menotropins alone are superior to a clomiphene citrate and menotropin combination for superovulation induction among clomiphene citrate failures. Fertil Steril. 1996;65(6):1169-74.
37. Miller PB, Soules MR. The usefulness of a urinary LH kit for ovulation prediction during menstrual cycles of normal women. Obstet Gynecol. 1996;87:13-7.
38. Nielsen MS, Barton SD, Hatasaka HH, Stanford JB. Comparison of several one-step home urinary luteinizing hormone detection test kits to OvuQuick. Fertil Steril. 2001;76:384-7.
39. Pearlstone AC, Surrey ES. The temporal relation between the urine LH surge and sonographic evidence of ovulation: determinants and clinical significance. Obstet Gynecol. 1994;83:184-8.
40. McGovern PG, Myers ER, Silva S, Coutifaris C, Carson SA, Legro RS, et al. Absence of secretory endometrium after false-positive home urine luteinizing hormone testing. Fertil Steril. 2004;82:1273-7.
41. Opsahl MS, Robins ED, O'Connor DM, Scott RT, Fritz MA. Characteristics of gonadotropin response, follicular development, and

42. George K, Kamath MS, Nair R, Tharyan P. Ovulation triggers in anovulatory women undergoing ovulation induction. Cochrane Database Syst Rev. 2014;1:CD006900.
43. Palatnik A, Strawn E, Szabo A, Robb P. What is the optimal follicular size before triggering ovulation in intrauterine insemination cycles with clomiphene citrate or letrozole? An analysis of 988 cycles. Fertil Steril. 2012;97:1089-94.
44. Tallon N, Case A. Quintuplets: a rare event following clomiphene citrate therapy. J Obstet Gynaecol Can. 2012;34(3):217.
45. Rizzuto I, Behrens RF, Smith LA. Risk of ovarian cancer in women treated with ovarian stimulating drugs for infertility. Cochrane Database Syst Rev. 2019;6:CD008215.
46. Auffret M, Cottin J, Vial T, Cucherat M. Clomiphene citrate and neural tube defects: a meta-analysis of controlled observational studies. BJOG. 2019;126:1127-33.
47. Tulandi T, Martin J, Al-Fadhli R, Kabli N, Forman R, Hitkari J, et al. Congenital malformations among 911 newborns conceived after infertility treatment with letrozole or clomiphene citrate. Fertil Steril. 2006;85(6):1761-5.
48. Teede HJ, Tay CT, Laven JJE, Dokras A, Moran LJ, Piltonen TT, et al. Recommendations From the 2023 International Evidence-based Guideline for the Assessment and Management of Polycystic Ovary Syndrome. J Clin Endocrinol Metab. 2023;108(10):2447-69.
49. Franik S, Le QK, Kremer JAM, Kiesel L, Farquhar C. Aromatase inhibitors (letrozole) for ovulation induction in infertile women with polycystic ovary syndrome. Cochrane Database Syst Rev. 2022;9:CD010287.
50. Diamond MP, Legro RS, Coutifaris C, Alvero R, Robinson RD, Casson P, et al. NICHD Reproductive Medicine Network. Letrozole, Gonadotropin, or Clomiphene for Unexplained Infertility. N Engl J Med. 2015;373(13):1230-40.
51. Borenstein R, Shoham Z, Yemini M, Barash A, Fienstein M, Rozenman D. Tamoxifen treatment in women with failure of clomiphene citrate therapy. Austr NZ J Obstet Gynaecol. 1989;29:173-5.
52. Gulekli B, Ozaksit G, Turhan NO, Senoz S, Oral H, Gokman O. Tamoxifen: an alternative approach in clomiphene resistant polycystic ovarian syndrome patients. J Pak Med Assoc. 1993;43:89-91.
53. Williamson JG, Ellis JD. The induction of ovulation by tamoxifen. J Obstet Gynecol Brit Commonw. 1973;80:844-7.
54. Sharma S, Choudhary M, Swarankar V, Vaishnav V. Comparison of tamoxifen and clomiphene citrate for ovulation induction in women with polycystic ovarian syndrome: a prospective study. J Reprod Infertil. 2021;22(4):274-81.
55. Steiner AZ, Terplan M, Paulson RJ. Comparison of tamoxifen and clomiphene citrate for ovulation induction: a meta-analysis. Hum Reprod. 2005;20(6):1511-5.
56. Whitten SJ, Nangia AK, Kolettis PN. Select patients with hypogonadotropic hypogonadism may respond to treatment with clomiphene citrate. Fertil Steril. 2006;86:1664-8.
57. Ghobara T, Gelbaya TA, Ayeleke RO. Cycle regimens for frozen-thawed embryo transfer. Cochrane Database Syst Rev. 2017;7(7):CD003414.
58. Nargund G, Datta AK, Campbell S, Patrizio P, Chian RC, Ombelet W, et al. The case for mild stimulation for IVF: recommendations from The International Society for Mild Approaches in Assisted Reproduction. Reprod biomed online. 2022;45(6):1133-44.
59. Datta AK, Maheshwari A, Felix N, Campbell S, Nargund G. Mild versus conventional ovarian stimulation for IVF in poor responders: a systematic review and meta-analysis. Reprod Biomed Online. 2020;41:225-38.
60. Kamath MS, Maheshwari A, Bhattacharya S, Lor KY, Gibreel A. Oral medications including clomiphene citrate or aromatase inhibitors with gonadotropins for controlled ovarian stimulation in women undergoing in vitro

fertilisation. Cochrane Database Syst Rev. 2017;11:CD008528.
61. Ragni G, Levi-Setti PE, Fadini R, Brigante C, Scarduelli C, Alagna F, et al. Clomiphene citrate versus high doses of gonadotropins for in vitro fertilisation in women with compromised ovarian reserve: a randomised controlled non-inferiority trial. Reprod Biol Endocrinol. 2012;10:1-8.
62. Zarei A, Alborzi S, Askary E, Alborzi M, Shahbazi F. Effects of clomiphene citrate for prevention of premature luteinizing hormone surge in those undergoing intrauterine insemination outcome: a randomized, double-blind, placebo-controlled trial. J Adv Pharm Technol Res. 2018;9(3):87-93.
63. Zhang J, Chang L, Sone Y, Silber S. Minimal ovarian stimulation (mini-IVF) for IVF utilizing vitrification and cryopreserved embryo transfer. Reprod Biomed Online. 2010;21:485-95.
64. Kato K, Takehara Y, Segawa T, Kawachiya S, Okuno T, Kobayashi T, et al. Minimal ovarian stimulation combined with elective single embryo transfer policy: age specific results of a large, single centre, Japanese cohort. Reprod Biol Endocrinol. 2012; 10:35.
65. Bodri D, Kawachiya S, De Brucker M, Tournaye H, Kondo M, Kato R, et al. Cumulative success rates following mild IVF in unselected infertile patients: a 3-year, single-centre cohort study. Reprod Biomed Online. 2014;28:572-81.
66. Singh A, Bhandari S, Agrawal P, Gupta N, Munaganuru N. Use of clomiphene-based stimulation protocol in oocyte donors: a comparative study. J Hum Reprod Sci. 2016;9(3):159-63.
67. Homburg R. Clomiphene citrate—end of an era: a mini-review. Hum Reprod. 2005;20(8):2043-51.

CHAPTER 11

Aromatase Inhibitors in Ovulation Induction

Lavanya Kiran, Sowparnika SN

■ OVERVIEW

Ovulation induction remains a milestone in the treatment of women with anovulatory infertility. Clomiphene citrate (CC) is considered the first-line treatment for induction of ovulation in women with polycystic ovary syndrome (PCOS), while it may be used for ovulation induction in unexplained infertility. Aromatase inhibitors (AIs) have been introduced as a new treatment option that could challenge CC for ovulation induction. A systematic review of the literature was conducted in order to highlight the efficacy and safety of AI in female infertility. Current data from randomized and nonrandomized trials suggest that AI may have a role in ovulation induction regimens in PCOS patients, as well as for ovarian stimulation, since they achieve comparable clinical pregnancy rates to CC. Furthermore, when combined with gonadotropins, AI improves the ovarian response of poor responders and reduces the gonadotropin dose required. However, the current review is based on small trials with a limited number of patients.

If solid data from future large adequately powered randomized trials support current evidence regarding efficacy and safety, AI might offer a new treatment choice for infertile women.

■ INTRODUCTION

A small story from mythology, Brihadratha, A powerful king of Magadha was suffering from primary infertility. He had two wives who were having irregular cycles. He worshipped Moolapurush, and got a fruit, which he divided into two parts and gave to his wives. This led to the birth of Jarasandha. Ages passed, drugs we used have changed, but the concept remains the same—ovulation induction.

Ovulation induction is the prime modality of treatment for anovulation, which constitutes almost 25% of infertility.[1] Many drugs have been used for ovulation induction. About 20% of the female fertility seeking patients are anovulatory. Though CC as always been the first line of therapy for ovulation induction due to its antiestrogenic effects, alternative agents have been used for ovulation induction like aromatase inhibitors (AIs) instead of gonadotropins like human menopausal gonadotropin (hMG) or pure follicle-stimulating hormone (FSH), have been used due to the higher risk of ovarian hyperstimulation and in turn multiple pregnancy.

Aromatase Inhibitors were initially used in the treatment for the postmenopausal women diagnosed with breast cancer and endometrial cancer, as a maintenance therapy postoperatively. As they suppress the estrogen in the plasma, they have been widely used in the field of reproductive medicine for ovulation induction, among them, AIs have gained lots of importance off late. There were many ups and downs, and finally they have reached the stable first line of management among the oral ovulogens used for ovulation induction.

MECHANISM OF ACTION

Aromatase inhibitor acts at the peripheral level. In a normal ovarian physiology, the androgens synthesized by theca cells are converted to estradiol and estrone with the help of aromatase enzyme. Aromatase is a microsomal cytochrome P450 (CYP P450) enzyme. This estradiol (converted androgen) causes negative inhibition on hypothalamus causing decreased secretion of gonadotropin-releasing hormone (GnRH), thus allowing the FSH window to close **(Fig. 1)**.

These AIs inhibit the aromatase enzyme, thus preventing the conversion of androgen to estrogen, and the inhibition to the hypothalamus is lost. Hence, there is increased GnRH pulsatility which indirectly causes the recruitment of the follicles, making the FSH window open for a longer duration. Once the dominant follicle starts growing, causes the inhibition by secretion of ample amount of estrogen **(Fig. 2)**. Thus, AIs usually lead to limited rather a single mature follicle.

CLASSIFICATION OF AROMATASE INHIBITORS

Aromatase inhibitors are classified based on what it is made of (steroidal or nonsteroidal) and drug-to-drug interactions. Third-generation AIs, which are nonsteroidal with least drug interactions; Letrozole and anastrozole are the most used ones. The classification of AIs goes as in **Table 1**.

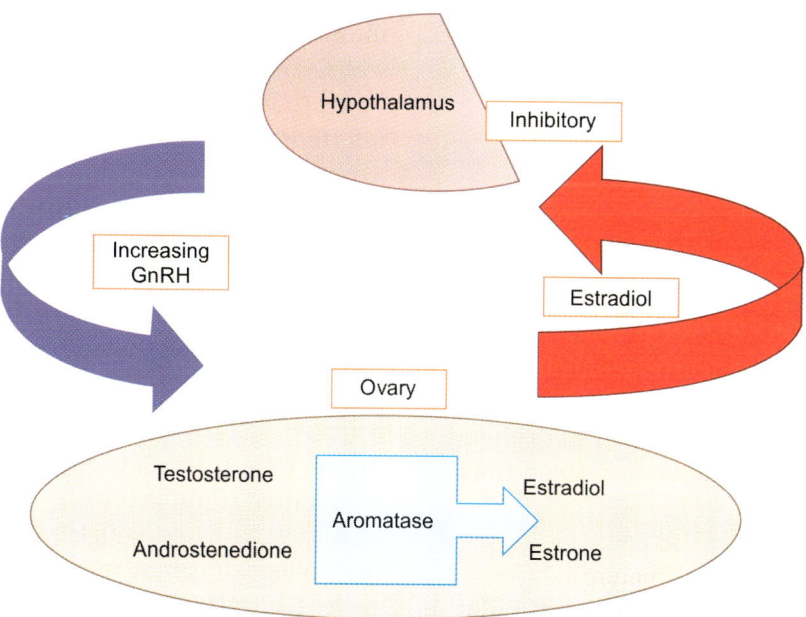

Fig 1: Function of aromatase enzyme. (GnRH: gonadotropin-releasing hormone)

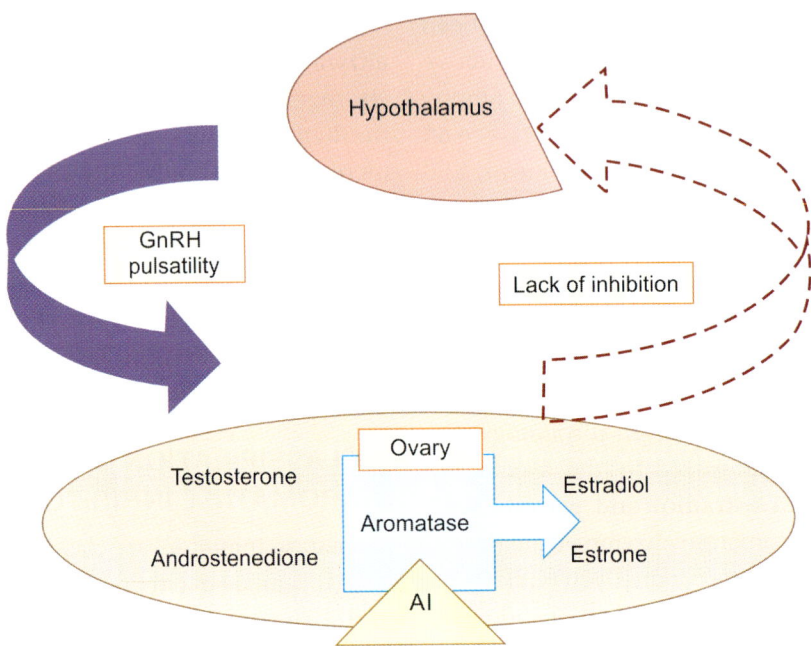

Fig. 2: Aromatase inhibitors. (AI: aromatase inhibitor; GnRH: gonadotropin-releasing hormone)

TABLE 1: Classification of aromatase inhibitors (AIs).

Generation	Type 1/ steroidal	Type 2/ nonsteroidal
First	None	Aminoglutethimide
Second	Formestane	• Fadrozole • Rogletimide
Third	Exemestane	• Anastrozole • Letrozole • Vorozole

Advantages of Aromatase Inhibitor

- No adverse antiestrogenic effect on the endometrium or cervical mucus.
- Absence of estrogen receptor depletion
- Rapid elimination from the body (half-life of 45 hours)
- Better uterine blood flow
- Limited number of mature follicles
- Decrease ovarian hyperstimulation syndrome (OHSS) and multiple pregnancies.

Letrozole when used in PCO patients, there has been better endometrial thickness with increased ovulation rate leading into better live birth rate when compared with CC.

In contrary when used in unexplained infertility (UI), the results were same for letrozole and CC, none were superior.

When compared to laparoscopic ovarian drilling (LOD), both proved to be effective enough in terms of ovulation, ovarian hyperstimulation, miscarriage, the live birth rates, and multiple pregnancy rates.

Clinical Indications

There have been publication of large randomized controlled trials demonstrating higher live birth rates with letrozole than with clomiphene, it is now regarded the drug of choice for ovulation induction in anovulatory infertile women with PCOS. The drug has also been tested in ovulatory women with unexplained infertility [in combination with intrauterine insemination (IUI)].

Similar to clomiphene, letrozole is ineffective in women with hypogonadotropic hypogonadism [World Health Organization (WHO) Group 1], who already have low serum estrogen concentrations and a dysfunctional hypothalamic-pituitary-ovarian axis.

In patients with endometriosis (minimal to mild) who could not achieve pregnancy despite 6–12 months of LOD treatment, the superovulation and pregnancy rates were comparable with letrozole and CC.

As per literature in poor responders letrozole has improved ovulation when combined with gonadotropins and also requiring lesser doses of gonadotropins with decreased cancellation rates and at a lesser treatment cost per cycle.

PROTOCOLS USED FOR OVARIAN STIMULATION (FLOWCHART 1)

Letrozole is administered in a dose of 5 mg starting from the day 2 or 3 of menstrual cycle. Letrozole when used in a dose of 2.5 mg twice daily causes monofollicular development. Recent Cochrane 2022 readings, letrozole appears to improve the live birth rate and pregnancy rates in infertile women, when used for ovulation induction compared to selective estrogen receptor modulators (SERMs) (CC). There was no difference in miscarriage rates and multiple pregnancy rates. There is uncertainty that whether letrozole improves the live birth rate when compared to LOD.[2] Many studies convey that letrozole has an equal efficacy[3,4] as of CC in inducing ovulation and pregnancy rate, with similar side effect profile, fewer studies show better pregnancy rate with letrozole when compared to CC,[5,6] hence, the American Society for Reproductive Medicine (ASRM) recommends to use letrozole as the first line of drug while inducing a patient with PCOS. Because, few studies have reported higher multiple pregnancy rates with CC than letrozole, though statistically nonsignificant.[6] The ovulation induction protocol is as given in **Figure 3**.

In cases of unexplained infertility, the CC is known to have same efficacy[7] or reduce efficacy with respect to conception rates,[8] and might be because of the antiestrogenic effect which the SERM is having on the endometrium and also on the cervical mucus. The multiple pregnancy rates are lower with letrozole without compromising the pregnancy rates.[8] The extended letrozole regime is superior to CC in inducing superovulation in unexplained infertility.[9]

Ovarian stimulation is of three types, In anovulatory cycles like PCOS, letrozole

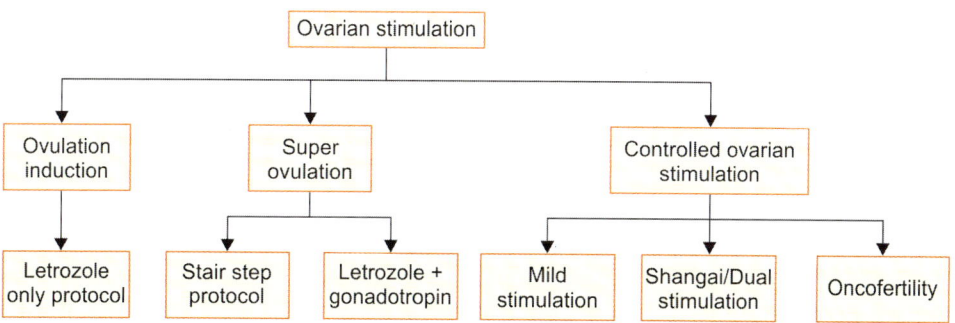

Flowchart 1: Ovarian stimulation protocols.

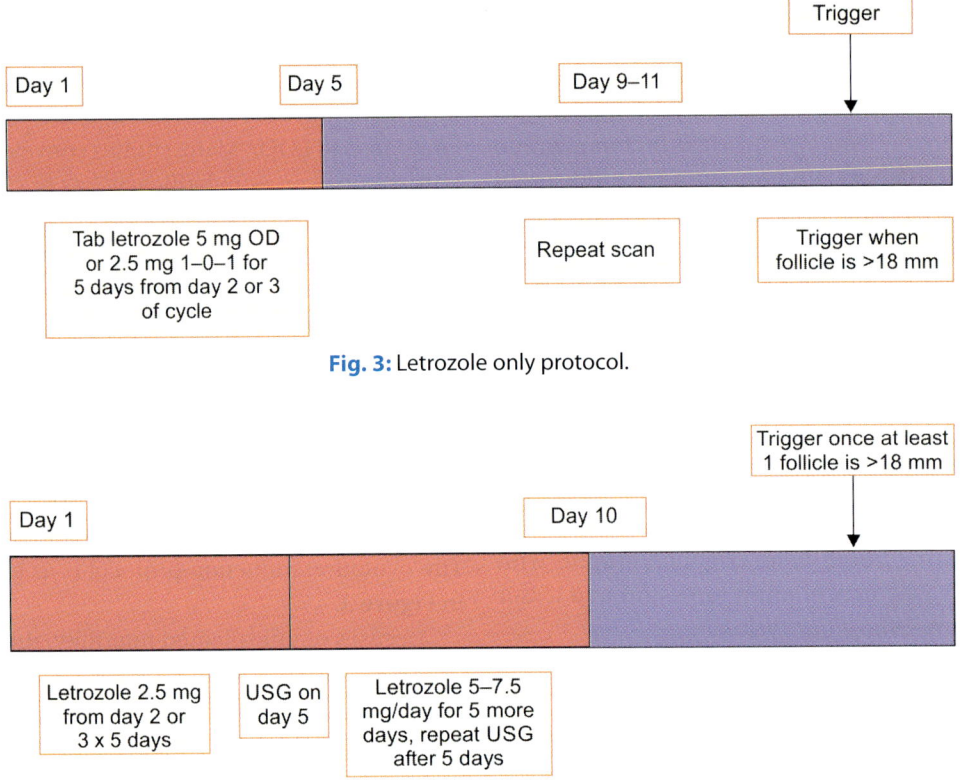

Fig. 3: Letrozole only protocol.

Fig. 4: Stair step protocol of letrozole.

is used as the first line of drug for ovulation induction. The extended letrozole or the stair step protocol induces superovulation and increases the probability of pregnancy in unexplained infertility or in mild-to-moderate degree of endometriosis. The regimen of stair step protocol includes 2.5 mg of letrozole per day for 5 days from day 2/3 of the cycle and later increased to 5 mg and if needed increased to 7.5 mg/day for another 5 days (**Fig. 4**) and the extended protocol includes administering the letrozole 2.5 mg for almost 10 days of cycle/till the dominant follicle is witnessed.[10]

Yet another protocol for superovulation is usage of letrozole with gonadotropin. This will increase the FSH window and allows the recruitment of multiple follicles. This not only increases the number of preovulatory follicle but also improves the pregnancy rate in case of unexplained infertility with IUI. The chances of OHSS with gonadotropin and letrozole are little higher than just letrozole alone. The regimen goes as in **Figure 5**.

The gonadotropin can also be used on alternative days. The dose of the gonadotropin needs to be titrated as per the patient's characteristics, and incrementally increasing the dose as and when required with ultrasound follow up. Always be watchable about OHSS, if three or more follicle is measuring 14 mm, then the cycle needs to be converted to in vitro fertilization (IVF) cycle or cancel the cycle. This method is to prevent the OHSS. The oocyte and endometrial synchrony is the most important thing which

CHAPTER 11: Aromatase Inhibitors in Ovulation Induction

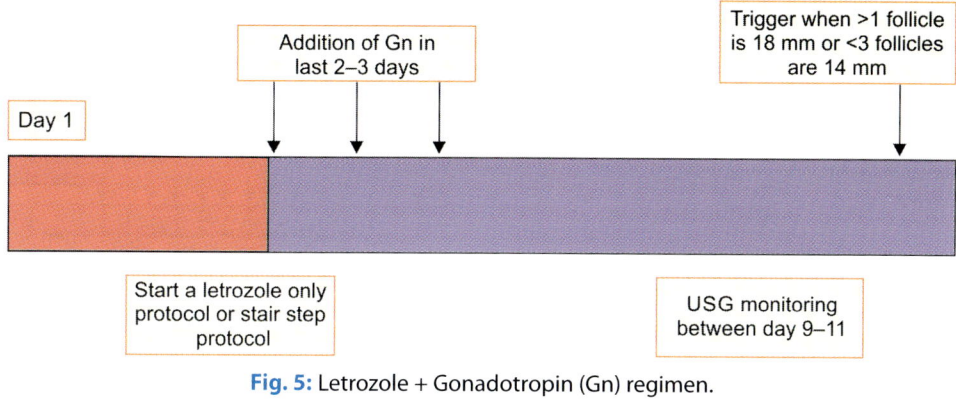

Fig. 5: Letrozole + Gonadotropin (Gn) regimen.

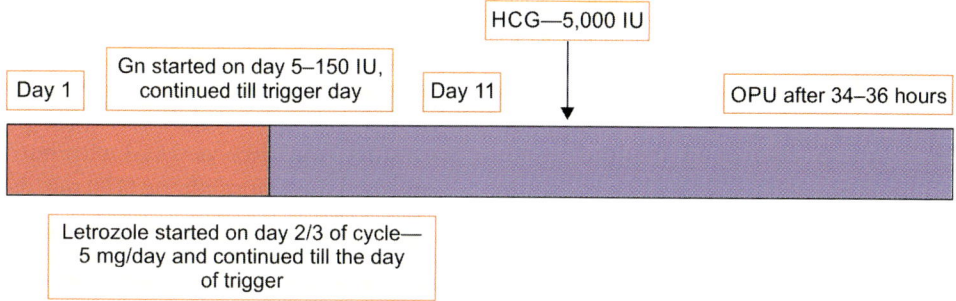

Fig. 6: Minimal or mild stimulation protocol. (HCG: human chorionic gonadotropin; OPU: oocyte pickup)

fetches us a clinical pregnancy which needs to be visualized.

Letrozole is also used in mild stimulation and costless protocols to keep the luteinizing hormone (LH) surge in check. They are as follows:

Using of letrozole in mild stimulation has many advantages. It decreases the estrogen levels and keeps the LH surge in check, and only if necessary through the monitoring of LH, antagonist injection to be added if necessary. This cuts down the cost of the cycle. Mild stimulation also gives a good quality oocyte.

The decrease in the estrogen levels makes it wonder drugs for its usage in oncofertility, after all that was the main reason why it was prepared in the first go. The protocol can be followed as per **Figure 6**, antagonist needs to be added if there is increase of LH. It is advisable to continue the letrozole post pickup also for 10 days or till the women menstruates, whichever earlier. This decreases the estrogen levels even after ovum pickup, which will not trigger the underlining carcinoma, which might be estrogen-dependent like breast cancer, ovarian cancer, or endometrial cancer. Hence, AIs are most important drugs used for fertility preservation.

Another indication is in case of thromboembolism in the prior history. A woman will surpass supraphysiologic level of estrogen during controlled ovarian stimulation. Estrogen being a potential trigger for this thromboembolic episode. Keeping the estrogen levels low will reduce the risk of thromboembolism where the same protocol as shown in **Figure 6**.

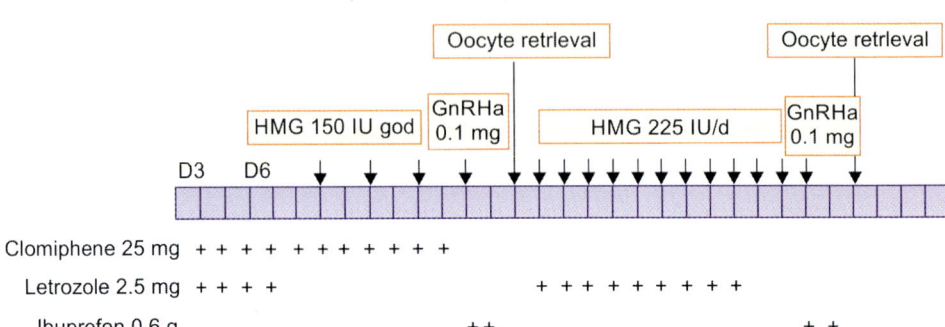

Fig. 7: Double stimulation protocol. (GnRHa: gonadotropin-releasing hormone agonist; HMG: human menopausal gonadotropin; MPA: medroxyprogesterone acetate)

Letrozole is also used in dual stimulation or Shangai protocol as in the following figure.

Letrozole is also used in double stimulation or Shanghai protocol as shown in **Figure 7**.

Results with Aromatase Inhibitors

The largest trial involved 750 patients who were randomized to receive letrozole (2.5 mg daily increased up to a maximum of 7.5 mg/day in case of anovulation) or clomiphene (50 mg daily increased up to a maximum of 150 mg/day), without ovulation trigger, up to five treatment cycles.

In the letrozole group, a significantly higher proportion of women achieved ovulation [88.5% vs. 76.6%, relative risk (RR): 1.16; 1.08–1.24] and the proportion of ovulations over total treatment cycles was significantly higher (61.7% vs. 48.3%, RR: 1.28; 1.19–1.37).

Cumulative pregnancy (27.3% vs. 21.5%) and live birth (27.5% vs. 19.1%, RR: 1.44; 1.10–1.87) rates were also significantly higher with letrozole treatment.

One randomized trial, which recruited 100 anovulatory women with PCOS who had never received ovulation induction, also reported significantly higher ovulation (60% vs. 32%) and a nonsignificant increase in pregnancy rate (26% vs. 14%) with letrozole (5 mg/day) than clomiphene (100 mg/day).

A 2018 systematic review reported significantly higher live birth rates with letrozole than clomiphene [odds ratio (OR): 1.79; 1.42–2.25].

The beneficial effect of letrozole seems independent of body mass index (BMI), that is, despite decreasing overall live birth rates with increasing BMI, letrozole outperforms clomiphene across categories of BMI.

Miscarriage per pregnancy (OR: 0.96; 0.65–1.42) and multiple pregnancy rates (OR: 0.61; 0.41–1.16) are also similar between letrozole- and clomiphene-induced cycles.

Available evidence suggests that letrozole should be considered the first-line agent for ovulation induction in anovulatory women with PCOS.

In anovulatory clomiphene-resistant women, 9/12 of patients (75%) ovulated after treatment with letrozole (2.5 mg daily) and hCG (lead follicle >20 mm), three conceived (resulting in two singleton births), and normal endometrial proliferation was observed in all. AIs can also be effective in anovulatory women who fail to ovulate in response to clomiphene treatment.

Letrozole is associated with a significantly thicker endometrium, and can also be considered in women who respond to clomiphene but exhibit poor endometrial growth.[11]

ADVERSE EFFECTS

The risk of multiple pregnancies is about 3–7%, with the vast majority of multiples limited to twins. There is no evidence suggesting letrozole is any more teratogenic than clomiphene. One case series comparing the incidence of congenital malformations in 911 newborns of women who conceived after treatment with letrozole (14/514, 2.4%) or clomiphene (19/397, 3.0%) found no difference. Previously, it was reported in that the drug letrozole causes teratogenic cardiovascular abnormalities in the children. Later an extended study was done for 11 months; which did not show any cardiovascular risk in additional. Hence, it can be used safely in planning for pregnancy.

The risk of clinically significant OHSS is very low when letrozole is used cautiously in an incremental manner.

Common side effects associated with letrozole are hot flushes, difficult sleeping, mood swings, night sweats, nausea, bone pain, tiredness, and hair fall.

Anastrozole is known to increase the incidence of ischemic cardiovascular disease.

Aromatase inhibitors approved by the Food and Drug Administration (FDA) as ovulation-inducing agent: Anastrozole, letrozole, and exemestane.

LETROZOLE VERSUS ANASTROZOLE

Many studies show equal efficacy with regards to ovulation rate and clinical pregnancy rate with both letrozole and anastrozole.[12]

CONCLUSION

The available data suggest that letrozole is more effective than clomiphene as a first-line treatment for ovulation induction in anovulatory women with PCOS, without a significant increase in complications or side effects. In summary, the letrozole the AI is an effective and inexpensive oral ovulogen for induction which has a potentially replaced the first line of treatment of the CC. Letrozole gives good clinical pregnancy rate when compared with CC, hence used as a first-line drug in PCOS and unexplained infertility. It can be used in all types of ovarian stimulation.

KEY LEARNING POINTS

- Aromatase inhibitors are the peripheral estrogen blockers which revolutionised the ovarian stimulation.
- Letrazole is the first drug of choice in PCOS as it results in mono follicular development.
- Letrozole is used in all types of ovulation induction with the help of different protocols.
- Drug was primarily discovered for the treatment of Breast cancer and takes its prime position in onco fertility.
- The efficacy is comparable with other oral ovulogens with a benefit of decreased risk of Multiple pregnancy and considerable reduction of OHSS.

REFERENCES

1. Franik S, Le QK, Kremer JA, Kiesel L, Farquhar C. Aromatase inhibitors (letrozole) for ovulation induction in infertile women with polycystic ovary syndrome. Cochrane Database Syst Rev. 2022;9(9):CD010287.

2. Bayar U, Basaran M, Kiran S, Coskun A, Gezer S. Use of an aromatase inhibitor in patients with polycystic ovary syndrome: a prospective randomized trial. Fertil Steril. 2006;86(5):1447-51.
3. Practice Committee of the American Society for Reproductive Medicine; Practice Committee of the American Society for Reproductive Medicine. Interpretation of clinical trial results: a committee opinion. Fertil Steril. 2020;113(2):295-304.
4. Kar S. Clomiphene citrate or letrozole as first-line ovulation induction drug in infertile PCOS women: a prospective randomized trial. J Hum Reprod Sci. 2012; 5(3):262-5.
5. Legro RS, Brzyski RG, Diamond MP, Coutifaris C, Schlaff WD, Casson P, et al. Letrozole versus clomiphene for infertility in the polycystic ovary syndrome. N Engl J Med. 2014;371(2):119-29. Erratum in: N Engl J Med. 2014;317(15):1465.
6. Diamond MP, Legro RS, Coutifaris C, Alvero R, Robinson RD, Casson P, et al. Letrozole, Gonadotropin, or Clomiphene for Unexplained Infertility. N Engl J Med. 2015;373(13):1230-40.
7. Eskew AM, Bedrick BS, Hardi A, Stoll CRT, Colditz GA, Tuuli MG, et al. Letrozole compared with clomiphene citrate for unexplained infertility: a systematic review and meta-analysis. Obstet Gynecol. 2019; 133(3):437-44.
8. Fouda UM, Sayed AM. Extended letrozole regimen versus clomiphene citrate for superovulation in patients with unexplained infertility undergoing intrauterine insemination: a randomized controlled trial. Reprod Biol Endocrinol. 2011;9:84.
9. Pavone ME, Bulun SE. The use of aromatase inhibitors for ovulation induction and superovulation. J Clin Endocrinol Metab. 2013;98(5):1838-44.
10. Badawy A, Mosbah A, Tharwat A, Eid M. Extended letrozole therapy for ovulation induction in clomiphene-resistant women with polycystic ovary syndrome: a novel protocol. Fertil Steril. 2009;92(1):236-9.
11. Badawy A, Mosbah A, Shady M. RETRACTED: Anastrozole or letrozole for ovulation induction in clomiphene-resistant women with polycystic ovarian syndrome: a prospective randomized trial. Fertil Steril. 2008;89(5):1209-12.
12. Lee VC, Ledger W. Aromatase inhibitors for ovulation induction and ovarian stimulation. Clin Endocrinol (Oxf). 2011; 74(5):537-46.

CHAPTER 12

Insulin Sensitizers: Where We Stand?

Bushra Khan

INTRODUCTION

Polycystic ovary syndrome (PCOS) is the most common endocrine disorder, affecting approximately 5–10% of the female population, especially in reproductive age group.[1] Causes of PCOS are still unknown but genetics and poor lifestyle seems to be the two main culprits. PCOS is commonly associated with hormonal and metabolic imbalances resulting in hyperandrogenism, insulin resistance, hyperinsulinemia, obesity, dyslipidemia, and type 2 diabetes. These patients may also suffer from sleep disorders, sleep apnea, or depression.[2-4] On the whole, there is increased risk of long-term effects, such as diabetes, cardiovascular diseases, and other illnesses. All of them raise the risk of diabetes, cardiovascular disease, and other illnesses.

From a historical perspective, PCOS was one of the earliest diagnosed conditions causing female infertility, being described in 1935 by Irving Freiler Stein and Michael Leventhal as amenorrhea associated with polycystic ovaries.

Among the various treatment modalities, insulin sensitizers are the most popular ones.

Various insulin sensitizers for infertile PCOS women are:
- Biguanides such as metformin
- Thiazolidinediones such as rosiglitazone and pioglitazone
- Inositols such as D-chiro-inositol (DCI) and myoinositol (MI)
- Chromium picolinate (CrP)
- α-glucosidase inhibitors such as acarbose.

PATHOPHYSIOLOGY OF POLYCYSTIC OVARY SYNDROME AND INSULIN RESISTANCE

Infertility is very common among obese PCOS, especially when time to pregnancy is more. Insulin can increase the frequency and amplitude of gonadotropin hormone-releasing hormone (GnRH) and luteinizing hormone (LH) pulse secretion. Insulin directly triggers androgen production in ovarian theca cells, in turn, ovarian steroidogenesis is stimulated **(Box 1)**.[5-7]

> **BOX 1:** Pathogenesis of polycystic ovary syndrome.
>
> - Hypothalamic-pituitary axis abnormalities cause abnormal secretion of gonadotropin-releasing hormone and luteinizing hormone, resulting in increased ovarian androgen production
> - An enzymatic defect of ovarian (adrenal) steroidogenesis favors excess androgen production
> - Insulin resistance drives the metabolic and reproductive abnormalities in polycystic ovary syndrome

Ovarian Physiology

Ovary as an organ remains immune to insulin resistance, hence, effects of insulin are evident in ovary. Hyperinsulinemia alters the follicle-stimulating hormone (FSH) to LH shift, preventing the selection of a dominant follicle. Insulin increases granulosa cell sensitivity to LH, thus increasing ovarian androgen production as well. This is mediated by a stimulation of cytochrome P450c17α. Ovarian theca cells produce abundant testosterone.

Hyperinsulinemia inhibits ovulation too. Insulin activates pathways in ovary, which increases production of androgens. Hyperandrogenemia worsens insulin resistance, accentuating a vicious cycle, by interfering with insulin signaling directly as well as indirectly.

Androgens also reduce the proportion of highly oxidative, insulin-sensitive type I muscle fibers, in comparison with glycolytic, insulin-resistant type II muscle fibers. This vicious cycle is promoted by obesity, which enhances androgen synthesis in both ovaries and adrenals, and promotes leptin-mediated inflammation.[8]

■ METFORMIN

Metformin is an oral biguanide insulin-sensitizing agent also known as oral hypoglycemic drug, specifically used in type 2 diabetes mellitus. It belongs to Food and Drug Administration (FDA) category B.

Mechanism of Action

- Glucose production in the liver is inhibited without hypoglycemia.
- It does not increase insulin secretion.[9,10]
- The effects of insulin on glucose uptake in skeletal muscles and adipocytes are enhanced, which increase peripheral utilization of glucose (Hundal et al., 1992; Klip et al., 1992; Wiernsperger and Bailey, 1999).
- It decreases intestinal absorption of glucose (Wilcock and Bailey, 1991; Ikeda et al., 2000).
- Potentiation of insulin actions.
- Lowering of circulating total and free androgen levels with improvement of the clinical sequelae of hyperandrogenism.
- Facilitating weight loss.

Dose

It is given 500 mg once a day initially, then step up weekly to twice and then thrice a day after food. Maximum dose: 2–3 g/day as an antidiabetic drug and 1.5–2 g/day in PCOS.

Side Effects

- The most common side effect of metformin is gastrointestinal upset, which can be reduced by taking metformin with meals and increasing the dose slowly to the effective dose of 1.5–2 g/day.
- Lactic acidosis, a serious side effect, is extremely rare and has only been seen in women with renal insufficiency, which causes lactate to accumulate to high concentrations, or serious medical problems.

Contraindication

- Hypersensitivity
- Severe renal/hepatic impairment
- Cardiac failure
- Recent myocardial infarction
- Congestive cardiac failure
- Severe infection
- Acute/chronic metabolic acidosis
- Severe thyroid dysfunction
- Dehydration
- Acute or chronic alcoholism.

Adverse Reactions

- Anorexia
- Weight loss
- Nausea
- Flatulence
- Vomiting
- Occasional metallic taste
- Diarrhea
- Weakness
- Hypoglycemia
- Rash
- Malabsorption of vitamin B_{12}.

Uses in Gynecology

- In infertile women with PCOS either alone or in combination with ovulation induction.
- Regularization of menstrual cycle
- Metformin is effective for anovulatory infertility and is associated with restoration of monofollicular ovulation, but there is no consensus on dose and duration.[11-14]
- To reduce hyperinsulinemia and hyperandrogenism[9,10,15-17]
- Metformin improves ovulation in women with PCOS by reducing gluconeogenesis, improving insulin sensitivity, and reducing ovarian androgen production.[18]

Use of Metformin in Infertility Treatment

- *Metformin versus placebo:* The evidence suggests that metformin may improve live birth rates compared with placebo in PCOS women but some gastrointestinal discomfort is experienced.[19]
- *Metformin along with clomiphene versus only clomiphene:* There was no conclusive evidence of a difference in live births when metformin in combination with clomiphene citrate was compared with clomiphene citrate alone. In subgroup analysis, there was no difference between obese group and nonobese group. There was evidence of more frequent gastrointestinal side effects in the metformin group including nausea and vomiting. Although evidence showed a beneficial effect in ovulation rates in metformin group. However, there was no significant evidence in miscarriage rate or multiple pregnancy rates.[19]
- *Only metformin versus only clomiphene:* Overall, there was no significant difference in live birth rates in both the groups but, in subgroup analysis, clomiphene alone group showed benefit among obese patients.[19]
- *Metformin as a first line treatment in infertile PCOS women:* There have been number of advocates for the use of insulin sensitizing agents, not only to restore ovulation but to facilitate weight loss, counteract androgenic symptoms, prevent long-term complications, decrease the risk of early pregnancy loss, decrease the risk of ovarian hyperstimulation syndrome (OHSS), and even improve the outcome of in vitro fertilization therapy.

  There is a significant improvement in insulin concentrations, insulin sensitivity, and serum androgen concentrations accompanied by decreased LH and increased sex hormone-binding globulin (SHBG) concentration.[20]

- *Rationale for metformin treatment:* Metformin is used widely for all the women with PCOS wishing to conceive because:
  • Difficulty to accurately measure serum insulin levels
  • Lack of set criteria to define hyperinsulinism
  • Direct androgen-lowering action of metformin on the ovary

- *Metformin as an adjuvant to clomiphene in clomiphene-resistant PCOS:* In a randomized controlled trial performed on clomiphene resistant infertile patients with PCOS, compared with placebo, metformin markedly improved ovulation and pregnancy rates with clomiphene treatment.[21]

  Other studies[10,22] evaluating the combined effect of metformin and clomiphene have shown that:
  - Ovulation rate significantly improved in metformin and clomiphene group (group B) compared to clomiphene alone (group A) (83.3–90% vs. 8–11.8%)
  - Pregnancy rate was also higher in metformin and clomiphene group (group B) compared to clomiphene alone (group A) (26.8–58.3 vs. 5.9–22.5%).
  - Addition of metformin helps in reducing abortion rate
  - Addition of metformin helps in reducing multiple pregnancy rate (6% vs. 3.1%).

Metformin as an Adjuvant to Gonadotropins in Clomiphene-resistant PCOS

When women with clomiphene-resistant PCOS were administered gonadotropins with or without pretreatment with metformin for 1 month, in randomized controlled trial, those receiving metformin developed significantly smaller follicles, produced less estradiol and had fewer cycles canceled due to excessive follicular development. The reduction of insulin concentrations induced by metformin seemed to favor a more orderly follicular growth in response to exogenous gonadotropins for ovulation induction.

These studies confirm that insulin-resistant women with PCOS have a much greater tendency to a multifollicular response and thus a relatively high cycle cancellation rate on low-dose FSH stimulation. This can be avoided or reduced by metformin.[19]

However, Cochrane review suggests that metformin alone may be beneficial over placebo for live birth, although the evidence quality was low. When metformin was compared with clomiphene citrate, data for live birth were inconclusive, and these findings were limited by lack of evidence. Results were different by body mass index (BMI), emphasizing the importance of stratifying results by BMI. An improvement in clinical pregnancy and ovulation suggests that clomiphene citrate remains preferable to metformin for ovulation induction in obese women with PCOS. An improved clinical pregnancy and ovulation rate with metformin and clomiphene citrate versus clomiphene citrate alone suggests that combined therapy may be useful although Cochrane do not mention whether this translates into increased live births. Women taking metformin alone or with combined therapy should be advised that there is no evidence of increased miscarriages, but gastrointestinal side effects are more likely.

Metformin as an Alternative to Laparoscopic Ovarian Drilling in Clomiphene Citrate-resistant PCOS

Surgical ovarian wedge resection was the first established treatment for women with anovulatory PCOS but was largely abandoned due to the risk of postsurgical adhesions and the introduction of medical ovulation induction with clomiphene and gonadotropins. There is no randomized study comparing metforimin with laparoscopic ovarian drilling.[23]

Combined therapy with insulin sensitizers (metformin) and ovulation induction agents (clomiphene) gives effective, cheaper, noninvasive, and safer alternative to ovarian drilling with no risk of premature ovarian failure.

■ THIAZOLIDINEDIONES

Thiazolidinedione is a selective ligand of the nuclear transcription factor perioxisome proliferator activated receptor T. These are widely available, standard medications for the treatment of noninsulin-dependent diabetes mellitus (NIDDM). While they lower elevated sugar levels in people with diabetes, when given to nondiabetic people, insulin levels are lowered but blood glucose levels remain unchanged.

Troglitazone had been used as a therapy for people with diabetes and in some trials involving women with PCOS. However, rare cases of liver damage were reported during its marketed use. The liver damage was usually reversible but very rare cases of hepatic failure, leading to death or liver transplant, were reported (Graham 2003). Injury occurred after short- and long-term troglitazone treatment, leading to its withdrawal from the market in March 2000 (FDA 2002).

Rosiglitazone and pioglitazone are considered relatively safer as compared to other thiazolidinediones. However, they are classified as pregnancy category C drugs according to the FDA due to the potential risk of causing fetal growth restriction in animal experiments (Yki-Jarvinen 2004). A high incidence of weight gain among the users further hampers their use in obese women with PCOS (Baillargeon 2004). Rosiglitazone is currently available in the USA but has been suspended from use in the European Union by the European Medicines Agency (EMA) and has also been withdrawn from India, New Zealand, and South Africa.

Pioglitazone has been withdrawn from some countries due to an association with bladder cancer reported with long-term use (EMA 2011).

In a large randomized controlled trial, troglitazone improved glycemic measures, ovulation, hirsutism, and free testosterone levels in women with PCOS.[24] More recently, smaller trials of rosiglitazone and pioglitazone have had promising results. However, these benefits need to be confirmed in larger trials.

■ ROSIGLITAZONE

Rosiglitazone is only active in the presence of insulin. It should not be used in type 1 diabetes mellitus or for the treatment of *diabetic ketoacidosis (DKA)*.

Combination therapy of rosiglitazone with insulin or other oral hypoglycemic agents may increase the risk for hypoglycemia.

Dose

It is given 4 mg PO once daily or 2 mg PO twice daily, initially. It may increase dose to 8 mg/day after 12 weeks, if needed.

Contraindication

- Diabetic ketoacidosis
- Cardiac disease, especially *New York Heart Association (NYHA) Class III or IV heart failure.*

Precautions

- Acute heart failure
- Anemia
- Angina
- Bone fractures
- Breastfeeding
- Cardiac disease
- Children
- Contraception requirements
- Edema

- Geriatric
- Hepatic disease
- Hypoglycemia.

Rosiglitazone versus Placebo or No Treatment

Due to withdrawal of troglitazone, studies have included only rosiglitazone and pioglitazone. Not enough data is available for live birth rates, but a slight improvement is noted in menstrual cycle.

■ INOSITOLS

The inositol stereoisomers, MI and DCI, are hexahydroxy cyclohexane, with the same molecular formula as glucose. They are the two most abundant members of a family of nine steroisomeric inositols, and are found widely in nature. Myoinositol (myo-ins) acts as second messengers, which accumulate rapidly and transiently in response to external or endocrine signals.[25,26]

Noticeably, inositol is involved in the transduction of several endocrine signals, such as insulin thyroid hormones, gonadotropins, lipids, and many other endocrine systems. There is a growing body of evidence that states that inositols may be effective in reversing some clinical, metabolic, or biochemical features of PCOS. Myoinositol, alone or in combination with DCI, showed to exert a variable—albeit significant—effect in improving both symptoms and outcome in PCOS patients (**Fig. 1**).[27]

Types of Inositol

- Myoinositol
- D-chiro-inosotol

Mechanism of Action

Evidence suggests that DCI can directly regulate steroidogenic enzyme genes in human granulosa cells, reducing the mRNA expression of both aromatase and cytochrome P450.[29] Furthermore, DCI increases testosterone levels in theca cells from PCOS women.[30]

▌NOVEL MOLECULES FOR INSULIN SENSITIZERS

Glucagon-like Peptide-1 Analogs

Glucagon-like peptide-1 (GLP-1) analogs such as semaglutide are more expensive than metformin. The available data suggests that GLP-1 analogs might be more effective at improving insulin sensitivity and reducing weight as compared with metformin but it shows more side effects such as nausea and vomiting.[31]

α-Glucosidase Inhibitors Like Acarbose

Some of the initial studies were in early 2000s as this molecule showed promising results in hyperandrogenic PCOS patients. At a dose of 300 mg/day for 3 months, there was significant difference noted in acne and few patients even resumed normal menstrual rhythm. Most common side effects remained to be abdominal discomfort and diarrhea. Biochemically changes were noted in levels of LH, testosterone, and androstenedione as they reduced and SHBG levels increased. But, mostly of these studies were of low power, hence more robust clinical evidence is needed still. However, use of acarbose is justifiable as an adjuvant.

■ CHROMIUM PICOLINATE

Trivalent chromium (Cr^{3+}) is found naturally in foods and is associated with nutritional supplements in various forms, the most popular of which is CrP. It improves insulin sensitivity at the insulin receptor level,[32]

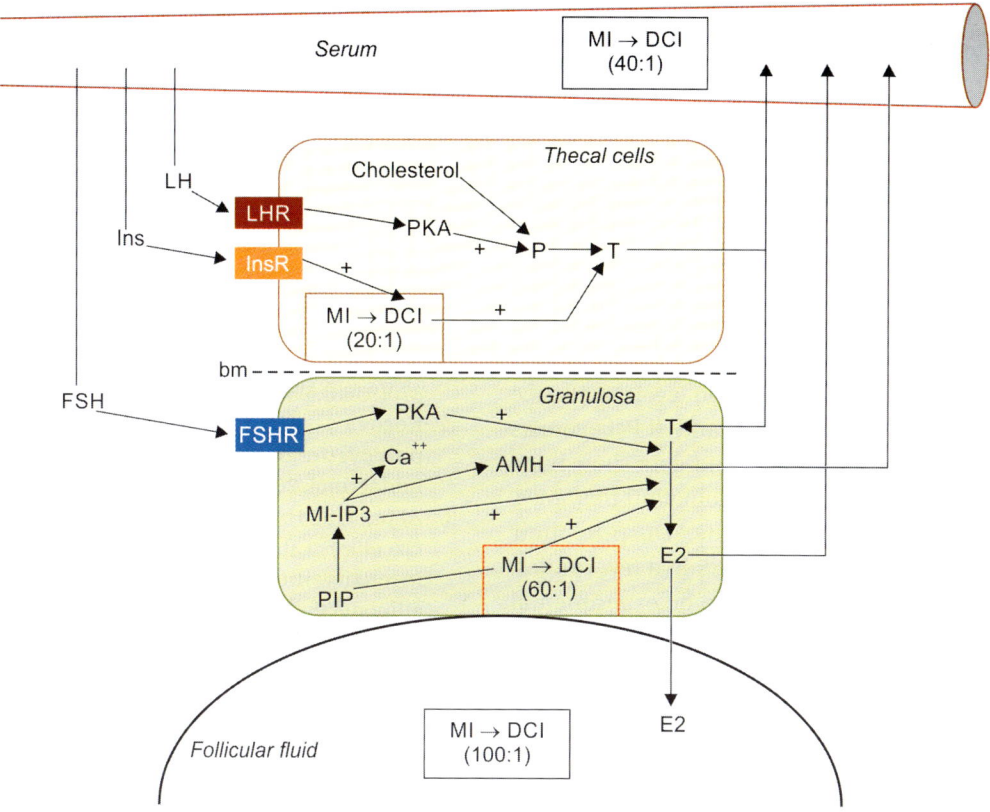

Fig. 1: Roles of myoinositol (MI) in the ovary.[28] [AMH: anti-Müllerian hormone; bm: basalis membrane; DCI: D-chiro-inositol; E2: estradiol; INs: insulins; InsR: insulin receptor; IP3: inositide triphosphate; LHR: LH receptor; MI: myoinositol; P: progesterone; PIP: phospho-inositide phosphate; PKA: protein kinase A; T: testosterone; +: stimulating effect; (40:1): MI/DCI ratio]

which should theoretically help with the IR and the obesity seen in PCOS. Few studies have been found comparing effects of CrP with metformin in PCOS women, CrP decreased fasting blood sugar (FBS) and insulin levels and, thus, increased insulin sensitivity in clomiphene citrate-resistance PCOS women. Overall, CrP was better tolerated compared to metformin. But due to limited research, results are in conclusive.

■ CONCLUSION

Hyperinsulinemia and insulin resistance play a pivotal role in the pathophysiology of PCOS. In addition to lifestyle changes, insulin sensitizers have been used as a therapeutic option for the past few decades. Insulin sensitizers are extensively being used these days not only for regularization of menses and hyperandrogenism but also in infertile women. Only metformin has shown promising results in patients with PCOS in terms of its combined metabolic and endocrine effects; however, its use in PCOS is off label. After lifestyle changes, it is the first-line insulin sensitizer in PCOS patients who have glucose intolerance or type 2 diabetes mellitus or who develop gestational diabetes. Metformin may improve fertility outcomes in patients with PCOS; however, it has not shown to be superior to clomiphene or letrozole in terms of ovulation induction and fertility outcomes. The other insulin sensitizer, thiazolidinedione, may improve endocrine and metabolic outcomes but can cause weight gain and should be avoided in those who wish to conceive. Inositol and alpha-lipoic acids (ALAs) may improve insulin sensitivity, menstruation, and ovulation rate. GLP-1 agonists are incretins that result in weight loss, thus helping to improve insulin sensitivity, menstruation, and androgen levels. Evidence suggests that inositol, ALA, and GLP-1 agonists are mostly experimental and data show huge variations in terms of combination therapies, dose, and target subjects. Despite their promising clinical outcomes in a few studies, these agents are deemed to be experimental in patients with PCOS.

■ KEY LEARNING POINTS

- There is an established role of insulin resistance in pathogenesis of PCOS.
- There are no clear guidelines regarding role of insulin-sensitizing drugs in PCOS.
- In lean PCOS, there is moderate-quality evidence which indicates a beneficial role of metformin, whereas in obese PCOS, metformin and clomiphene cotherapy has shown better reproductive outcomes.
- Metformin/clomiphene combination therapy has been found useful in CC-resistant women.
- In assisted reproductive technology like in vitro fertilization (IVF) metformin, adjuvant therapy has shown to reduce OHSS; however, no improvement in clinical pregnancy rate, miscarriages, or live birth rate.
- Some poor-quality evidence is available implying role of inositols in ameliorating symptoms of androgen excess, namely, hirsutism and acne.
- Very limited data is available supporting role for metformin therapy in reducing the incidence of type 2 diabetes mellitus, coronary artery disease, or endometrial cancer in women with PCOS.
- Low-quality evidence for other insulin sensitizing agents and their uses in PCOS.

■ REFERENCES

1. Norman RJ, Dewailly D, Legro RS, Hickey TE. Polycystic ovary syndrome. Lancet. 2007; 370(9588):685-97.
2. Kosova G, Urbanek M. Genetics of the polycystic ovary syndrome. Mol Cell Endocrinol. 2013;373(1-2):29-38.
3. Aktaş HŞ, Uzun YE, Kutlu O, Pençe HH, Özçelik F, Çil EÖ, et al. The effects of high intensity-interval training on vaspin, adiponectin and leptin levels in women with polycystic ovary syndrome. Arch Physiol Biochem. 2022;128(1):37-42.
4. Medeiros LR, Colonetti T, Nagib EC, Rodrigues Uggioni ML, Denoni Junior JC, Ceretta L, et al. Anti-Müllerian Hormone levels after metformin treatment in polycystic ovary syndrome: a systematic review and meta-analysis. Obes Res Clin Pract. 2023;17(4):288-97.
5. Bannigida DM, Nayak BS, Vijayaraghavan R. Insulin resistance and oxidative marker in women with PCOS. Arch Physiol Biochem. 2020;126(2):183-6.
6. Wang YW, He SJ, Feng X, Cheng J, Luo YT, Tian L, et al. Metformin: a review of its potential indications. Drug Des Dev Ther. 2017;11:2421-9.
7. Zhang C, Hu J, Wang W, Sun Y, Sun K. HMGB1-induced aberrant autophagy contributes to insulin resistance in granulosa cells in PCOS. FASEB J. 2020;34(7):9563-74.
8. Kalra B, Kalra S, Sharma JB. The inositols and polycystic ovary syndrome. Indian J Endocr Metab. 2016;20:720-4.
9. Vel'azquez E, Acosta A, Mendoza SG. Menstrual cyclicity after metformin therapy in polycystic ovary syndrome. Obstet Gynecol. 1997;90(3):392-5.

10. Nestler JE, Jakubowicz DJ, Evans WS, Pasquali R. Effects of metformin on spontaneous and clomiphene-induced ovulation in the polycystic ovary syndrome. N Engl J Med. 1998;338(26):1876-80.
11. Legro RS, Arslanian SA, Ehrmann DA, Hoeger KM, Murad MH, Pasquali R, et al. Diagnosis and treatment of polycystic ovary syndrome: an Endocrine Society clinical practice guideline. J Clin Endocrinol Metab. 2013;98(12):4565-92.
12. American College of Obstetricians and Gynecologists' Committee on Practice Bulletins—Gynecology. ACOG Practice Bulletin No. 194: Polycystic Ovary Syndrome. Obstet Gynecol. 2018;131(6):e157-e171.
13. Ding H, Zhang J, Zhang F, Zhang S, Chen X, Liang W, et al. Resistance to the insulin and elevated level of androgen: a major cause of polycystic ovary syndrome. Front Endocrinol (Lausanne). 2021;12:741764.
14. Jahromi BN, Dabbaghmanesh MH, Bakhshaie P, Parsanezhad ME, Anvar Z, Alborzi M, et al. Assessment of oxytocin level, glucose metabolism components and cutoff values for oxytocin and anti-mullerian hormone in infertile PCOS women. Taiwan J Obstet Gynecol. 2018;57(4):555-9.
15. Morin-Papunen LC, Koivunen RM, Ruokonen A, Martikainen HK. Metformin therapy improves the menstrual pattern with minimal endocrine and metabolic effects in women with polycystic ovary syndrome. Fertil Steril. 1998;69(4):691-6.
16. Glueck CJ, Wang P, Fontaine R, Tracy T, Sieve-Smith L. Metformin-induced resumption of normal menses in 39 of 43 (91%) previously amenorrheic women with the polycystic ovary syndrome. Metabolism. 1999;48(4):511-9.
17. Moghetti P, Castello R, Negri C, Tosi F, Perrone F, Caputo M, et al. Metformin effects on clinical features, endocrine and metabolic profiles, and insulin sensitivity in polycystic ovary syndrome: a randomized, double-blind, placebo-controlled 6-month trial, followed by open, long-term clinical evaluation. J Clin Endocrinol Metab. 2000; 85(1):139-46.
18. Shaw RJ, Lamia KA, Vasquez D, Koo SH, Bardeesy N, Depinho RA, et al. The kinase LKB1 mediates glucose homeostasis in liver and therapeutic effects of metformin. Science. 2005;310(5754):1642-6.
19. Morley LC, Tang T, Yasmin E, Norman RJ, Balen AH. Insulin-sensitising drugs (metformin, rosiglitazone, pioglitazone, D-chiro-inositol) for women with polycystic ovary syndrome, oligo amenorrhoea and subfertility. Cochrane Database Syst Rev. 2017;11(11):CD003053.
20. Nestler JE, Stovall D, Akhter N, Luorno MJ, Jacubwicz DJ. Strategies for the use of insulin sensitising drugs to treat infertility in women with polycystic ovary syndrome. Fertil Steril. 2002;77:209-15.
21. Vandermolen DT, Ratts VS, Evans WS, Stovall DW, Kauma SW, Nestler JE. Metformin increases the ovulatory rate and pregnancy rate from clomiphene citrate in patients with polycystic ovary syndrome who are resistant to clomiphene citrate alone. Fertil Steril. 2001;75(2):310-5.
22. Legro RS, Barnhart HX, Schlaff WD, Carr BR, Diamond MP, Carson SA, et al. Clomiphene, metformin, or both for infertility in the polycystic ovary syndrome. N Engl J Med. 2007;356(6):551-66.
23. Donesky BW, Adashi EY. Surgical Ovulation Induction: the role of ovarian diathermy in polycystic ovary syndrome. Bailliers Clin Endocrinol Metab. 1996;10:293-310.
24. Azziz R, Ehrmann D, Legro RS, Whitcomb RW, Hanley R, Fereshetian AG, et al. 2001 PCOS/Troglitazone Study Group. Troglitazone improves ovulation and hirsutism in the polycystic ovary syndrome: a multi-center, double-blind, placebo-controlled trial. J Clin Endocrinol Metab. 2001;86:1626-32.
25. Hughes AR, Horstman DA, Takemura H, Putney JW Jr. Inositol phosphate metabolism and signal transduction. Am Rev Respir Dis. 1990;141(3 Pt 2): S115-8.
26. Chakraborty A, Kim S, Snyder SH. Inositol pyrophosphates as mammalian cell signals. Sci Signal. 2011;4(188):re1.
27. Lagana AS, Garzon S, Casarin J, Franchi M, Ghezzi F. Inositol in polycystic ovary

28. Merviel P, James P, Bouée S, Le Guillou M, Rince C, Nachtergaele C, et al. Impact of myo-inositol treatment in women with polycystic ovary syndrome in assisted reproductive technologies. Reprod Health. 2021;18(1):13.
29. Sacchi S, Marinaro F, Tondelli D, Lui J, Xella S, Marsella T, et al. Modulation of gonadotrophin induced steroidogenic enzymes in granulosa cells by d-chiroinositol. Reprod Biol Endocrinol. 2016;14(1):52.
30. Monastra G, Vucenik I, Harrath AH, Alwasel SH, Kamenov ZA, Laganà AS, et al. PCOS and inositols: controversial results and necessary clarifications. Basic differences between D-Chiro and Myo-Inositol. Front. Endocrinol. 2021;12:660381.
31. Han Y, Li Y, He B. GLP-1 receptor agonists versus metformin in PCOS: a systematic review and meta-analysis. Reprod Biomed Online. 2019;39(2):332-42.
32. Suksomboon N, Poolsup N, Yuwanakorn A. Systematic review and meta-analysis of the efficacy and safety of chromium supplementation in diabetes. J Clin Pharm Ther. 2014;39:292-306.

(Note: reference 27 continues from previous page) syndrome: restoring fertility through a pathophysiology-based approach. Trends Endocrinol Metab. 2018;29(11):768-80.

SECTION 5
Ovulation Induction Protocols: Gonadotropins

13. **Gonadotropins in Intrauterine Insemination**
    Ameet Patki, Mrinmayi Dharmadhikari

14. **Use of Gonadotropin-releasing Hormone: Analogs in Intrauterine Insemination**
    Seema Pandey, Aanchal Garg

CHAPTER 13

Gonadotropins in Intrauterine Insemination

Ameet Patki, Mrinmayi Dharmadhikari

INTRODUCTION

Gonadotropin therapy plays an integral role in ovarian stimulation (OS) for infertility treatment. Even though it was introduced a century ago, it is the last few years which have seen a revolution in the use of gonadotropins in infertility treatment. The use of gonadotropins to stimulate follicular growth in anovulatory women began as early as the 1960s. We have come a long way since then with numerous formulations now available for fertility treatment, especially use of gonadotropins in in vitro fertilization cycles for ovarian stimulation. In this chapter, we will be discussing the use of gonadotropin stimulation in intrauterine insemination (IUI) cycles.

OVARIAN STIMULATION AND INTRAUTERINE INSEMINATION

Intrauterine insemination itself has seen a long path of development in semen processing methods as well as in stimulation methods. The rationale behind IUI is to reduce the distance traveled by the sperms to reach the oocyte thereby increasing their concentration at the site of fertilization despite the sperm or cervical mucous abnormalities. This bypasses a number of barriers thereby improving pregnancy rate. IUI is now increasingly being used for unexplained infertility as well as male factor infertility consequent to refinement of techniques for sperm processing.

Natural cycle IUI was a practice followed for purely male factor infertility; however with the introduction of ovarian stimulation in IUI cycles, natural cycle IUI has shown to have lower pregnancy rates. There are numerous studies supporting this. IUI with ovarian stimulation improves the rate of pregnancy in couples with infertility as compared to IUI in a natural cycle.[1] According to the Practice Committee of the American Society for Reproductive Medicine, 2020, for unexplained infertility in subfertile couples, IUI with ovarian stimulation is now considered a first-line management option. The committee has given a strong recommendation to not perform IUI in natural cycles for the treatment of unexplained infertility as it appears to be less effective than ovarian stimulation with IUI and likely no more effective than expectant management.

Ovarian stimulation increases the conception rates by increasing the number of dominant follicles stimulated per cycle, which, in turn, is achieved by increasing the serum levels of follicle-stimulating hormone (FSH).

This brings into picture—gonadotropins, letrozole, clomiphene citrate (CC), and a combination of them as well for ovarian stimulation.

Several ovarian stimulation protocols have been used for ovarian stimulation in IUI cycles, but it is still not clear which stimulation protocol and dose is the most cost-effective with highest pregnancy rates.

Ovarian stimulation with CC has traditionally remained the mainstay treatment, especially in women with polycystic ovarian syndrome (PCOS). With the introduction of letrozole, numerous studies have been undertaken to compare the two. A recent meta-analysis[2] showed improved ovulation, pregnancy, and live-birth rates with letrozole as compared with CC. Letrozole, however, is still an off-label agent for ovarian stimulation in infertility treatment in many countries, resulting in its unavailability, although it has been widely used today with no evidence of an increased risk of congenital fetal malformation for which it had gone into disrepute.[3] These ovarian stimulation agents have been compared with each other in numerous studies in women with unexplained infertility undergoing IUI.

In the current era, various drugs available for ovarian stimulation are used in combination with gonadotropins to give better results.

This concept of minimal stimulation in infertility cycles for ovarian stimulation, was first proposed by Kistner in 1972. He used CC followed by administration of human menopausal gonadotropin (hMG). The idea was to increase the pregnancy rate by increasing the number of dominant follicles compared to the use of CC alone and to reduce the amount of hMG required for stimulation thereby making it apparently safer and cost-effective.

Research has continued in this, wherein, variable agents are combined with various doses and types of gonadotropin to improve conception rates and reduce cost. There is still lack of evidence regarding the ideal regimen to be selected. A study by Yun BH et al.[4] found that a dose of 100 mg/day CC or 5 mg/day letrozole was administered on days 3–5 of the menstrual cycle for 5 days. Along with this fixed schedule of CC or letrozole, patients also received two different regimens of hMG namely, a 2-day regimen or a 3-day regimen. In the former 150 IU hMG was administered on day 6 and 8 of the menstrual cycle on alternate days or 150 IU was administered on days 5, 7, and 9 of the menstrual cycle on alternate days. There is no recommendation to the ideal regimen as yet and more studies are needed in this aspect.

The use of minimal stimulation in IUI cycles was aimed to get better results with cost-effectiveness. This reduces the cost of the cycle overall as compared to stimulation with gonadotropins only, however, is it as beneficial?

Ransom et al. compared and found that menotropin used alone in ovarian stimulation is superior to the use of a combination of clomiphene and menotropin for ovulation induction among patients with previous CC failures.[5]

In women with normogonadotropic anovulation and CC failure, starting treatment with gonadotropins alone increased the chance of live birth as compared to continuing treatment with CC.[6]

GONADOTROPIN STIMULATION IN INTRAUTERINE INSEMINATION

An important question was addressed by Peeraer K et al.[7] wherein the ovarian stimulation was compared in IUI cycles. Controlled ovarian stimulation with low-dose hMG was compared with ovarian stimulation with CC in IUI program for infertile couples. Their results were as follows:

As compared to ovarian stimulation with CC, hMG stimulation was found to result in:
- Higher clinical pregnancy rate [hMG 48/334 (14.4%) vs. CC 29/323 (9.0%)]

- Higher live birth rate [hMG 46/334 (13.8%) vs. CC 28/323 (8.7%)]
- Low and comparable multiple live birth rate [hMG 3/46 (6.5%) vs. CC 1/28 (3.6%), $p > 0.99$]
- Increased endometrial thickness [hMG 8.5 mm vs. CC 7.5 mm, $p < 0.001$]
- Lower cancellation rate per started cycle [hMG 15/322 (4.7%) vs. CC 46/298 (15.4%), $p < 0.001$].

In a Cochrane Database Systematic Review,[8] in which 43 trials involving 3,957 women were included, the author concluded that gonadotropins might be the most effective drugs when ovarian hyperstimulation is used in IUI cycles. Some of the other conclusions highlighted in this review were that the use of gonadotropins might be done on a daily basis. When gonadotropins are used, low doses are advisable for ovarian stimulation as the outcome in terms of pregnancy rates do not differ from those which result from higher doses. In addition, the chance of ovarian hyperstimulation syndrome and multiple pregnancies is also reduced when low doses are used.

Of these trials, in seven trials involving 556 couples with unexplained infertility, mild male factor, and mild endometriosis, pregnancy rates were again shown to be higher with gonadotropins alone than with antiestrogens. Moreover, no significant difference in conception rates were seen when different types of gonadotropins were used for ovarian stimulation. Taking into consideration, the available results of the studies mentioned, gonadotropins might be the most effective drugs for ovarian stimulation in IUI cycles when the dose and regimen is tailored as per patient characteristics and individual response.

In a similar comparative study[9] in patients with unexplained infertility, gonadotropins increased the chance of a live birth compared to both CC and letrozole. It also suggested that gonadotropins may increase the chance of a multiple pregnancy, especially for triplet pregnancy. However, the quality of evidence for this was low. Gonadotropins, it was observed, reduced the time to pregnancy leading to live birth as compared to both CC and letrozole. Gonadotropin stimulation resulted in a significantly higher number of dominant follicles though also a significantly higher risk of cycle cancellation.

Drawbacks of Gonadotropin Stimulation

Intrauterine insemination with gonadotropins increases live birth and/or ongoing pregnancy rates as shown in several studies but there were concerns about multiple pregnancy rates rising as compared to other oral ovarian stimulation agents. An inherent disadvantage of ovarian stimulation is an increased risk of multiple pregnancies with its consequent maternal and neonatal complication risks. IUI with gonadotropin stimulation when done within a protocol which strictly adheres to a cancellation criteria, like not inseminating if more than three dominant follicles have developed, led to an acceptable multiple pregnancy rate without having an impact on the overall effectiveness of the treatment strategy.[10] The solution seems to be IUI with ovarian stimulation using gonadotropins within a protocol that includes strict cancellation criteria which would decrease risk of multiple gestations without really compromising the effectiveness.

Another drawback of gonadotropin stimulation is the need for daily injections and regular monitoring in patients. This can be cumbersome for patients and may add to the physical and emotional stress which infertility patients are already under. The need for regulating temperatures of the injections to optimal levels, especially when patients carry them for administration at hospitals in their vicinity is also a parameter which may affect the injection efficacy, ultimately hampering outcome.

In the end, the cost of these injections also makes the cycle more expensive and cost-effectiveness is another concern in these gonadotropin-stimulated IUI cycles.

Even though success of these cycles is seen to be higher than with other ovarian stimulation drugs, an unsuccessful cycle may dissuade patients from trying again given the physical, emotional, and financial burden.

Luteinizing Hormone Surge

The midcycle luteinizing hormone (LH) surge is a phenomenon which can affect the success of a stimulated cycle. Though LH surge at follicular maturation is a necessary endocrinological phenomenon for final oocyte maturation, luteinization, and follicle rupture, a premature LH surge can have a negative effect on the oocyte quality. The rising estradiol levels secreted from the growing follicles send out a positive feedback and via the hypothalamo-pituitary-gonadal axis the LH surge occurs from the pituitary which acts on the ovaries. Most data concur to this fact that it is the ovaries which indicate that the timing of the LH surge.[11] The positive feedback of estradiol in a progressive and time-dependent manner along with pituitary sensitization to gonadotropin-releasing hormone (GnRH) results in the LH surge.

A premature LH surge can be defined as rise in LH (>10 IU/L) prematurely during the cycle along with a simultaneous rise in progesterone (>1 μg/L–3.2 nM/L).[12] Premature LH surge in the natural cycles is uncommon and may be seen in older women where the follicle size is smaller at the time of ovulation. Premature LH surges, however, do occur in 25–30% of stimulated IUI cycles.[12] In stimulated cycles with gonadotropins, especially with multifollicular growth, there are high circulating levels of estradiol which can result in a premature LH surge before adequate maturation of the growing oocytes leading to premature luteinization and ultimately affecting oocyte quality and cycle outcome.

It may also interfere with timing of the IUI, result in cancellation of the cycle as well as unsuccessful outcome.

Administration of a GnRH antagonist almost completely abolishes premature luteinization and like in IVF cycles is now being used in IUI cycles with varying success reports. Some studies argue that premature luteinization may not be the cause of poor oocyte quality but in fact a consequence of the same.[12] There is conflicting evidence with respect to the addition of GnRH antagonist stimulated IUI cycles. A recent prospective randomized controlled trial (RCT) conducted in India center with 730 women concluded that the addition of GnRH antagonists to controlled ovarian stimulation cycles followed by IUI, significantly decreased the incidence of premature LH surge and also increased the clinical pregnancy as well as live birth rates.[13]

Hormones

A number of gonadotropins are available to the clinician today for use. These include recombinant human follicle-stimulating hormone (r-hFSH) and urinary hMG including urinary highly purified hMG (hMG HP). r-hFSH is produced by recombinant DNA technology containing purified FSH activity. Follitropin-α (r-hFSH-α) is a more purified form with a purity of >99%.[14] On the other hand, hMG HP is extracted from the urine of postmenopausal women and it contains both FSH and LH activity. In addition, it also contains traces of other proteins.[15,16]

Reflecting differences in manufacturing methods, the FSH content of r-hFSH differs from that of hMG HP as is seen in the difference in their manufacturing. This further is reflected in differences in glycosylation pattern (including sialylation) and isoelectric coefficient.[15,16] The glycosylation pattern of r-hFSH is very similar to that seen at the middle of the menstrual cycle. The glycosylation pattern of hMG HP is that seen in menopausal women.[15,16]

These differences could translate to differences in efficacy of these formulations and therefore many RCTs comparing these treatments have been undertaken. These have reported conflicting results. A few RCTs and meta-analyses have found no difference between r-hFSH and urinary gonadotropins [hMG, purified FSH (P-FSH) and highly purified FSH (HP-FSH)].[17-19] Certain others, however, have reported a difference in live birth and clinical pregnancy rates between r-hFSH and urinary hMG.[20-23] The most recent meta-analysis[24] included 28 RCTs and compared r-hFSH with urinary-gonadotropins in 7,553 women. In this meta-analysis, there was no significant difference between the groups in cumulative live birth rate.

In conclusion, the European Society of Human Reproduction and Embryology (ESHRE) 2019 guidelines equally recommend the use of r-hFSH or hMG for ovarian stimulation.[25]

TRIGGER

The trigger to induce final oocyte maturation and rupture can be an hCG trigger, GnRH agonist trigger especially to prevent ovarian hyperstimulation syndrome or a dual trigger depending on the cycle characteristics and number of growing follicles. However, strict cancellation criteria should be kept in mind to prevent multiple pregnancies.

COUNSELING

Counseling couples for gonadotropin-stimulated IUI cycles forms an important aspect of management. This includes counseling with respect to higher pregnancy rates seen with this treatment strategy, need for daily injections, monitoring the cycle closely needing regular and more frequent follow-ups, cost of the cycle as well as risk of multiple pregnancy, cycle cancellation, and ovarian hyperstimulation syndrome. This counseling is an absolute must so that couples are more in control of their own treatment and they are well informed and prepared with respect to what to expect from the treatment cycle. Treatment cycles where the couple is as involved in their own treatment, helps to reduce the emotional stress which the couple may undergo at times and helps to build trust between the couple and clinician as well.

CONCLUSION

- In cases of anovulatory infertility resistant to clomiphene, unexplained infertility, and previous cycle failures with clomiphene, gonadotropins can be tried for stimulation in IUI cycles.
- Gonadotropin stimulated IUI cycles have been found to give better pregnancy rates as well as cumulative live birth rates in numerous studies as mentioned previously.
- Strict monitoring is important to prevent ovarian hyperstimulation syndrome.
- Low-dose regimens give equal pregnancy rates without added risks of ovarian hyperstimulation syndrome and multiple births.

- Adherence to strict cancellation criteria is important to prevent these risks without compromising on effectiveness.
- There are various gonadotropin preparations available and all have been found to be equally effective in numerous studies. ESHRE 2019 guidelines recommend rFSH or urinary hMG equally for ovarian stimulation.[25]
- The ultimate success rates with gonadotropin-stimulated IUI cycles do depend on appropriate patient selection as well as patient characteristics, namely, age of the female partner, duration of subfertility, sperm quality, and tubal patency.
- Couple counseling forms an important aspect of all infertility treatments, especially in terms of need for daily injections, risk of ovarian hyperstimulation syndrome, multiple pregnancies, cycle cancellation, cost involved, and individual success rate.

KEY LEARNING POINTS

- In cases of anovulatory infertility resistant to clomiphene, unexplained infertility, and previous cycle failures with clomiphene, gonadotropins can be tried for stimulation in IUI cycles.
- Gonadotropin-stimulated IUI cycles have been found to give better pregnancy rates as compared to stimulation with other oral agents.
- Strict monitoring is important to prevent ovarian hyperstimulation syndrome.
- Low-dose regimens give equal pregnancy rates without added risks of ovarian hyperstimulation syndrome and multiple births
- Adherence to strict cancellation criteria is important to prevent these risks without compromising effectiveness.
- The ultimate success rates with gonadotropin-stimulated IUI cycles do depend on appropriate patient selection.
- Couple counseling forms an important aspect of all infertility treatments.

REFERENCES

1. Streda R, Stepán J, Zadrobílková I, Cermáková E. Indukce ovulace zvysuje tehotenský index u intrauterinní inseminace [Ovulation induction increases pregnancy rate during intrauterine insemination compared with natural cycles]. Ceska Gynekol. 2007;72(6):397-402.
2. Liu Z, Geng Y, Huang Y, Hu R, Li F, Song Y, et al. Letrozole compared with clomiphene citrate for polycystic ovarian syndrome: a systematic review and meta-analysis. Obstet Gynecol. 2023;141(3):523-34.
3. Pundir J, Achilli C, Bhide P, Sabatini L, Legro RS, Rombauts L, et al. Risk of foetal harm with letrozole use in fertility treatment: a systematic review and meta-analysis. Hum Reprod Update. 2021;27:474-85.
4. Yun BH, Chon SJ, Park JH, Seo SK, Cho S, Choi YS, et al. Minimal stimulation using gonadotropin combined with clomiphene citrate or letrozole for intrauterine insemination. Yonsei Med J. 2015;56(2):490-6.
5. Ransom MX, Doughman NC, Garcia AJ. Menotropins alone are superior to a clomiphene citrate and menotropin combination for superovulation induction among clomiphene citrate failures. Fertil Steril. 1996;65(6):1169-74.
6. Weiss NS, Nahuis MJ, Bordewijk E, Oosterhuis JE, Smeenk JM, Hoek A, et al. Gonadotrophins versus clomifene citrate with or without intrauterine insemination in women with normogonadotropic anovulation and clomifene failure (M-OVIN): a randomised, two-by-two factorial trial. Lancet. 2018;391(10122):758-65.
7. Peeraer K, Debrock S, De Loecker P, Tomassetti C, Laenen A, Welkenhuysen M, et al. Low-dose human menopausal gonadotrophin versus clomiphene citrate in subfertile couples treated with intrauterine insemination: a randomized controlled trial. Hum Reprod. 2015;30(5):1079-88.
8. Cantineau AEP, Cohlen BJ. Ovarian stimulation protocols (anti-oestrogens,

gonadotrophins with and without GnRH agonists/antagonists) for intrauterine insemination (IUI) in women with subfertility. Cochrane Database Syst Rev. 2007;(2):CD005356.
9. Wessel JA, Danhof NA, van Eekelen R, Diamond MP, Legro RS, Peeraer K, et al. Ovarian stimulation strategies for intrauterine insemination in couples with unexplained infertility: a systematic review and individual participant data meta-analysis. Hum Reprod Update. 2022;28(5):733-46.
10. Danhof NA, Wang R, van Wely M, van der Veen F, Mol BWJ, Mochtar MH. IUI for unexplained infertility—a network meta-analysis. Hum Reprod Update. 2020b;26:1-15.
11. Knobil E. Discovery of the hypothalamic gonadotropin-releasing hormone pulse generator and of its physiologic significance. Endocrinology. 1992;131(3):1005-6.
12. Lambalk CB, Leader A, Olivennes F, Fluker MR, Andersen AN, Ingerslev J, et al. Treatment with the GnRH antagonist ganirelix prevents premature LH rises and luteinization in stimulated intrauterine insemination: results of a double-blind, placebo-controlled, multicentre trial. Hum Reprod. 2006;21:632-9.
13. Gopal L, Sudhakar P, Kandaswami D, Manivannan S. Addition of gonadotropin releasing hormone antagonist for women undergoing intrauterine insemination: a randomized controlled trial. Int J Reprod Contracept Obstet Gynecol. 2023;12:1101-5.
14. Leao Rde B, Esteves SC. Gonadotropin therapy in assisted reproduction: an evolutionary perspective from biologics to biotech. Clinics. 2014;69(4):279-93.
15. Lunenfeld B, Bilger W, Longobardi S, Alam V, D'Hooghe T, Sunkara SK. The development of gonadotropins for clinical use in the treatment of infertility. Front Endocrinol. 2019;10:429.
16. Niederberger C, Pellicer A, Cohen J, Gardner DK, Palermo GD, O'Neill CL, et al. Forty years of IVF. Fertil Steril. 2018;110(2):185-324.e5.
17. NCC-WCH. Fertility: assessment and treatment for people with fertility problems. Clinical guideline. London: RCOG Press; 2004.
18. Al-Inany H, Aboulghar M, Mansour R, Serour G. Meta-analysis of recombinant versus urinary-derived FSH: an update. Hum Reprod. 2003;18(2):305-13.
19. Larizgoitia I, Estrada MD, Garcia-Altes A. Recombinant FSH as adjuvant in assisted reproduction: some data on the efficacy and efficiency of recombinant FSH urinary FSH. Barcelona: Catalan Agency for Health Technology Assessment and Research (CAHTA); 2000. pp. 1-16.
20. van Wely M, Kwan I, Burt AL, Thomas J, Vail A, Van der Veen F, et al. Recombinant versus urinary gonadotrophin for ovarian stimulation in assisted reproductive technology cycles. Cochrane Database Syst Rev. 2011;2:Cd005354.
21. Al-Inany HG, Abou-Setta AM, Aboulghar MA, Mansour RT, Serour GI. Efficacy and safety of human menopausal gonadotropins versus recombinant FSH: a meta-analysis. Reprod BioMed Online. 2008;16(1):81-8.
22. Coomarasamy A, Afnan M, Cheema D, van der Veen F, Bossuyt PM, van Wely M. Urinary hMG versus recombinant FSH for controlled ovarian hyperstimulation following an agonist long down-regulation protocol in IVF or ICSI treatment: a systematic review and meta-analysis. Hum Reprod. 2008;23(2):310-5.
23. Van Wely M, Westergaard LG, Bossuyt PM, Van der Veen F. Human menopausal gonadotropin versus recombinant follicle stimulation hormone for ovarian stimulation in assisted reproductive cycles. Cochrane Database Syst Rev. 2003;1:CD003973.
24. Bordewijk EM, Mol F, van der Veen F, Van Wely M. Required amount of rFSH, HP-hMG and HP-FSH to reach a live birth: a systematic review and meta-analysis. Hum Reprod Open. 2019;2019(3):hoz008.
25. ESHRE. (2019). Guideline on Ovarian Stimulation in IVF/ICSI. [online] Available from: https://www.eshre.eu/Guidelines-and-Legal/Guidelines/Ovarian-Stimulation-in-IVF-ICSI [Last accessed January, 2024].

CHAPTER 14

Use of Gonadotropin-releasing Hormone: Analogs in Intrauterine Insemination

Seema Pandey, Aanchal Garg

INTRODUCTION

Intrauterine insemination (IUI) cycles since its inception have not been given similar kind of sincerity as in vitro fertilization-embryo transfer (IVF-ET) has received. Though it is very much clear that at any given point of time IUI is less invasive, more patient friendly and if done properly can decrease the burden of more invasive, expensive, and emotionally draining IVF treatment. The proponents of this thought compare the results and find it useless but looking at the increasing burden of infertility worldwide the need of hour is reappraisal of IUI cycles and a serious drive toward optimizing its results.

The success rate of IUI with ovulation induction varies widely, with pregnancy rates ranging between 8 and 18% per cycle.[1] These discrepancies in pregnancy rates are due to the selection of patients, duration of infertility, etiology of infertility, sperm preparation, total number of motile sperm inseminated, number of inseminations, monitoring of the cycle, timing of IUI, and protocols of ovarian stimulation. The best results of IUI we get when it is combined with controlled ovarian stimulation (COS) with gonadotropins as compared with natural cycle or oral ovulogens (**Fig. 1**).[2] COH with IUI ensures maximum number of available ova at the site of fertilization by ensuring 2–3 dominant follicles.[2] However, the recruitment of multiple follicles following COS also increases the serum estradiol (E2) levels, and brings the risk of a premature surge of luteinizing hormone (LH) and leads to premature luteinization (PL) in some cycles. PL has been reported to be detrimental to oocyte quality, fertilization, and embryo implantation. Approximately 20% of COS/IUI cycles have been shown to undergo PL.[1,3]

The exact time at which ovulation occurs post-LH surge cannot be recognized earlier. It varies from 24 to 56 hours. Oocyte-fertilization capacity and sperm lifetime are <1 day and 1.4 days, respectively. To get the best results, insemination needs to be performed close to ovulation time, and accurate synchronization is mandatory. The LH surge can occur at different follicular sizes in different age groups and diseases, various tests available to diagnose it are not up to the mark and it leads to treatment failure.[4]

Why do intrauterine insemination (IUI) cycles fail?

Figure 2 describes few key reasons of IUI failure.

PREMATURE LUTEINIZING HORMONE SURGE

- When there is rise in LH >10 IU/l accompanied by a concomitant rise in progesterone (>1 μg/l–3.2 nM/L) it is called premature LH-surge.[5]

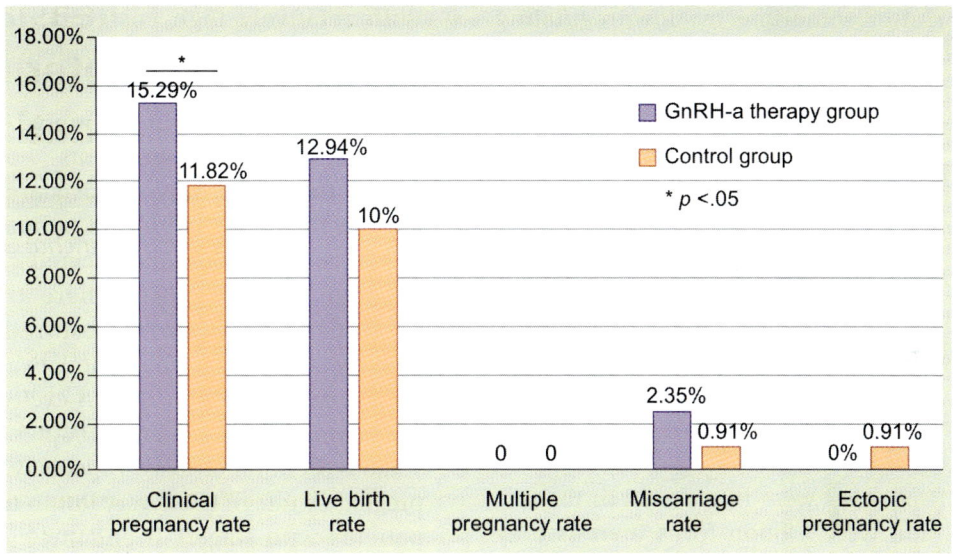

Fig. 1: Comparison of clinical pregnancy outcome per IUI cycle in endometriosis patients. (IUI: intrauterine insemination)

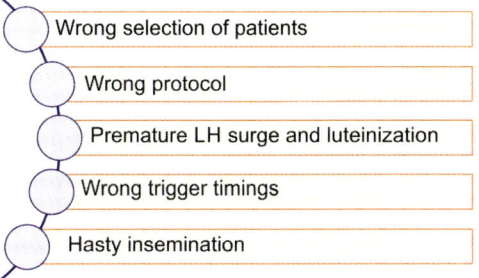

Fig. 2: Causes of IUI cycle. (LH: luteinizing hormone; IUI: intrauterine insemination)

- Premature LH surge in the natural cycle seems very rare but may be more frequent in older women since their maximum follicle diameter at the time of ovulation is substantially smaller.
- One of the challenges to optimizing the COS/IUI outcomes is to prevent the occurrence of the premature LH rise and consequent luteinization which, as is well known, is a possible complication of stimulated cycles. Like IVF cycles we can downregulate our IUI cycles with gonadotropin-releasing hormone (GnRH)-analogs though it takes away the very essence of it by being more invasive and more expensive.

GONADOTROPIN-RELEASING HORMONE ANALOGS

GnRH-analogs are substances which block or downregulate the GnRH receptors on pituitary to prevent further GN release.[5]

Why do we want GnRH-analogs in IUI cycles?

- Very low success rate of the IUI cycle is the main reason of lack of enthusiasm in its reappraisal.
- Premature LH surges also occur in 25–30% of stimulated IUI cycles and theoretically may interfere with timing of the IUI or result in cancellation and more treatment failures.
- Their suppressive effect on the secretion of gonadotropins from the pituitary is mediated either immediately after administration as in GnRH-antagonist

or after sometime by downregulating the receptors as in GnRH-agonists and rescues the cycle from cancellation.

These are mainly of two types:
1. GnRH-agonists
2. GnRH-antagonists.

Since our aim in IUI cycle is to keep the COH shorter, less expensive and patient friendly we use antagonist more in our IUI cycles than GnRH-agonists.

Gonadotropin-releasing Hormone-agonists

GnRH-agonists were introduced in the late 1980 and were a boon forus then as they had the ability to downregulate endogenous pituitary gonadotropin secretion and thereby prevent premature LH surge.

When administered they first produce a flare effect which leads to a rise in follicle-stimulating hormone (FSH) and LH. On continuous administration there is suppression of hypothalamic-pituitary-ovarian (HPO) axis because of receptor downregulation and desensitization thus reducing the circulating levels of gonadotropins and sex steroids.

Available as daily injections, depot preparations, and nasal sprays.

They can be given intramuscular, subcutaneous or intranasal. Daily injections are used in IVF but depot preparation (leuprolide 3.75 mg, goserelin 3.6 mg or 11.8 mg) is used in endometriosis patients before IVF for downregulation.

Leuprorelin, buserelin, nafarelin, and decapeptyl are few molecules of agonists which are being used in our reproductive medicine for various indications.

Disadvantages of Agonists

- For the use of GnRH agonists, it requires 2–3 weeks for desensitization
- With relatively high costs due to an increased requirement for gonadotrophin injections, and
- The need for frequent hormonal and ultrasonographic measurements
- This is the reason why agonists are not used in IUI cycles to prevent premature LH-surge except certain selected cases of stage endometriosis where tubo-ovarian relationship is restored by surgery and patient has good ovarian reserve and wishes for the IUI cycle. IUI is recommended for infertile couples with stage I–II endometriosis. Especially, the pregnancy rate of IUI is very low in those patients with stage I–II endometriosis. It is therefore necessary to find chances to improve the clinical outcomes of IUI in infertile women with endometriosis. GnRH agonist (GnRH-a) could be applied to lower the level of gonadotropins which could inhibit the progression of endometriosis and prevent the formation of new lesions. In a recent meta-analysis, it has been concluded that both laparoscopy and GnRH-a alone could improve the clinical pregnancy outcomes of infertile women with endometriosis .

In a recent study patients treated with GnRH-a had a higher clinical pregnancy rate than those without [adjusted odds ratio (AOR) 23.190, 95% confidence interval (CI) 1.238–434.312]. The live birth rate per IUI cycle in the GnRH-a group was also higher than in the controls. They concluded that the administration of GnRH-a in patients with stage I–II endometriosis could be beneficial to the outcomes of IUI.[6]

Gonadotropin-releasing Hormone-antagonist

GnRH-antagonists are competitive pituitary GnRH-receptor blockers which cause and direct immediate and reversible block and no flare effect with a rapid decrease in LH and FSH, preventing LH surge. Therefore, treatment can be restricted to those days when a premature LH surge is likely to be expected.

This property allows their use at any time during the follicular phase. Two main molecules namely cetrorelix and ganirelix are the most widely used third generation GnRH antagonists devoid of histamine release activity and associated systemic edema. After it is stopped there is a short recovery phase of 2–4 days after stoppage. There are other antagonists molecules like degarelix and relugolix, but these are not used in IUI or assisted reproductive technology (ART) cycles as of now.[7,8]

The oral preparation of GnRH antagonist, relugolix 20 mg, has gained the attention of clinicians and has been used in ART cycles to check its effectivity and it was found that relugolix is effective in preventing premature ovulation when used as an ovarian stimulation method in ART. In addition, the clinical usefulness of relugolix was shown to be comparable with an injectable GnRH antagonist, cetrorelix, in terms of the number of oocytes retrieved, oocyte maturation rate, fertilization rate, blastocyst formation rate, and clinical pregnancy rate. Thus, relugolix, like injectable GnRH antagonists, could be utilized in an ovarian stimulation protocol.[9]

Gonadotropin-releasing Hormone-antagonist Protocol in Intrauterine Insemination Cycles (Fig. 3)

Single Dose
Flexible Continuous Dose

- Patient is called on day 2 of menses, transvaginal sonography (TVS) is done to rule out any residual follicle, cyst, or corpus luteum.
- Gonadotropin is started in minimal required dose from the same day.
- Patient is called again on day 6–8 of stimulation, scanning is done, if two or more lead follicles are seen and are above 12–14 mm, antagonist can be administered according to the daily-dose scheme.
- The optimal dose for daily dose is 0.25 mg for both cetrorelix and ganirelix and 3 mg for the single dose scheme (cetrorelix). Studies have proven that these are the minimal effective doses required for prevention of LH surge.

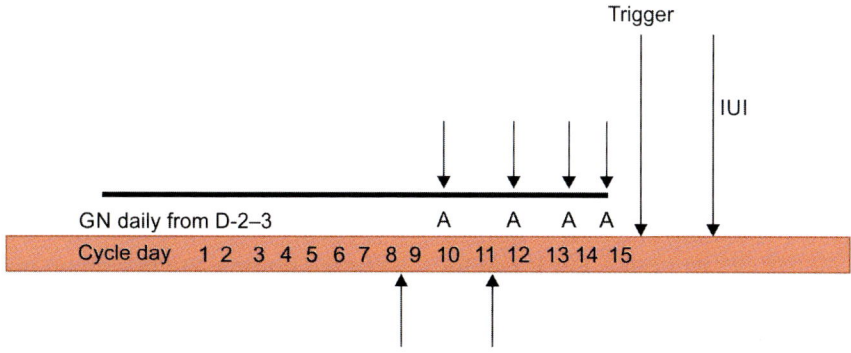

Fig. 3: Flexible continuous dose protocol in GN + antagonists. (GN: gonadotropin; IUI: intrauterine insemination)

- Once started ideally the antagonist should be used continuously till the day of trigger.
- A single-dose scheme where only one bolus dose of antagonist is given which inhibits the premature LH surge rise for 4 days is also used by certain people. But, many centers use a single-dose antagonist (0.25 mg) when they find two or more follicles beyond 16 mm, and they proceed to trigger when needed. The single-dose scheme can be combined with the daily-dose scheme if required.[10]

Advantages of Antagonists

- Antagonists are associated with lower risk of cycle cancellation due to spontaneous ovulation.
- GnRH antagonists make ovarian stimulation more patient friendly, requiring fewer days of treatment compared to GnRH agonists. They also constitute a more rational way to inhibit the premature LH surge compared to the agonists.
- It involves considerable cost as the therapy is expensive and it takes away the advantage of IUI being a simple and cost-effective treatment with minimal discomfort to the patient.

Though a Cochrane review done in 2014[11] concluded that GnRH-antagonists can effectively lower the incidence of PL and improve the clinical pregnancy rate (CPR) in patients without polycystic ovary syndrome (PCOS). A recent meta-analysis concluded that Gnrh antagonist use per se did not improve ongoing pregnancy rate/live birth rate (OPR/LBR) and CPR in women undergoing IUI + COH cycles, but it can be of use in decreasing the risk of premature luteinization and spontaneous ovulation.[12]

In subgroup analysis as per the mature follicle number on the human chorionic gonadotropin (hCG) day, the result for cycles with two or more mature follicles on the hCG day suggested that GnRH-antagonist tends to improve the clinical pregnancy outcome, although this was not statistically significant. But, there was no improvement in CPR if there was mono-follicular growth. Therefore, well-designed randomized-controlled trials (RCTs) with the same intervention protocol and evaluation criteria are required to draw a robust conclusion.

As per an Indian study, antagonists do not improve the IUI outcome in oral ovulogen cycles and combined gonadotropins with oral ovulogens while in another RCT again from India reported better pregnancy outcome in patients undergoing gonadotropin IUI.[10,13]

Indications of Antagonists in Intrauterine Insemination Cycles

Looking at the controversies in the usage of antagonist in the IUI cycles we should choose our patients carefully for this protocol which only optimizes our results without being a burden to the patient. **Figure 4** describes the population of patients who could get benefitted by using antagonist in their stimulation cycles.

Polycystic Ovary Syndrome

- Approximately 21–26% of women with PCOS undergoing COS with gonadotropin are at risk for premature luteinization.
- Due to the abnormal follicular environment, the physiology and the response to r-FSH treatment are generally different for patients with PCOS such that the findings based on non-PCOS women may not be reproducible in women with PCOS.
- Thus, PCOS especially CC-nonresponders where there is more frequent mono-follicular growth along with an

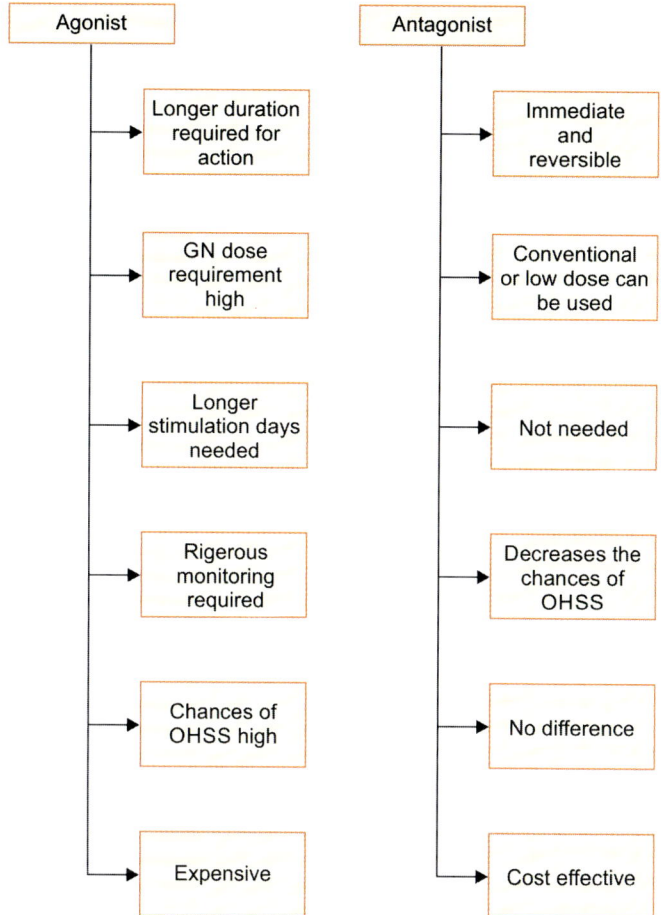

Fig. 4: Difference between agonist and antagonist. (OHSS: ovarian hyperstimulation syndrome)

improvement of hormonal levels, low premature LH-surge and slightly better pregnancy rate with antagonist addition is one subgroup where antagonist can be added safely in an IUI cycle.[13]

Where does antagonist work best?
- When a premature LH rise is expected, e.g., previous cycle of LH rises.
- Avoidance of weekend IUI.
- Where premature rupture at smaller size has been documented previously.
- PCOS population—especially CC nonresponders
- Older women with short follicular phase
- Reduced ovarian reserve
- Pure gonadotropin cycles with multi-follicular development.

Caution while prescribing GnRH-analogs:
- Patient has to be counseled properly.
- Counseling should be regarding increased cost, increased number of injections, and increased emotional stress.
- Realistic expectations in terms of success should be given. **Table 1** gives an expected highest pregnancy rate in different types of IUI cycles using different regimen.

TABLE 1: Pregnancy rates as per protocol.

Natural cycle	8%
Clomiphene citrate	8.9%
Letrozole	11.5%
Letrozole + gonadotropin	21%
Gonadotropin	25%
Gonadotropin + antagonist	38%

- Proper cost-benefit ratio has to be kept in mind.
- Antagonist timing of injection should be within 24 hours every day.

What does future hold?

IUI cycles would be utilized more as they become extremely effective and patient friendly where we could use long-acting preparation of gonadotropin given once a week along with oral antagonists like relugolix.[9]

CONCLUSION

Intrauterine insemination with controlled ovarian stimulation is the treatment of choice for subfertile couples as it is inexpensive, minimally invasive, requires minimal monitoring, it is safe, simple, and patient-friendly. If done properly, we can avoid IVF cycles. Using GnRH-analogs especially antagonist can optimize the success of IUI in certain selected group of population like PCOS mainly CC-non-responders and elderly couples but at the same time we have to look at cost-effectiveness, convenience, and its success rates in terms of livebirth rate and for that we need further future well-designed studies. The future seems brighter with advent of more friendly oral antagonistic preparations that could make IUI more sought after treatment.[14]

KEY LEARNING POINTS

- Use of GnRH-analogs in an IUI cycle prevents premature LH-surge.
- GnRH antagonist is preferred analogue and should be used in gonadotropin IUI cycles with multifollicular development where we find:
  - Previous premature LH-surge
  - Aged female partner
  - With history of short follicular phase
  - Selected PCOS population
- Once we start antagonist it has to be continued till the day of trigger.
- Theres no role of long GnRH-agonist suppression in IUI cycles except for rare endometriosis cases.
- Routine usage of antagonist in IUI cycles especially with oral ovulogens and gonadotropin is not recommended.

REFERENCES

1. Ragni G, Somigliana E, Vegetti W. Timing of intrauterine insemination: where are we? Fertil Steril. 2004;19:25-6.
2. Houmard BS, Juang MP, Soules MR, Fujinoto VY. Factors influencing pregnancy rates with a combined clomiphene citrate-gonadotropin protocol for non-assisted reproductive technology fertility treatment. Fertil Steril. 2002;77:384-6.
3. Verhulst SM, Cohlen BJ, Hughes E, Heineman MJ, Te Velde E. Intra-uterine insemination for unexplained subfertility. Cochrane Database Syst Rev. 2006;CD001838.
4. Guzick DS, Carson SA, Coutifaris C, Overstreet JW, Factor-Litvak P, Steinkampf MP, et al. Efficacy of superovulation and intrauterine insemination in the treatment of infertility. N Engl J Med. 1999;340:177-83.
5. Fleming R, Coutts JR. Induction of multiple follicular growth in normally menstruating women with endogenous gonadotropin suppression. Fertil Steril. 1986;45:226-30.

6. Zhang K, Huang S, Xu H, Zhang J, Wang E, Li Y, et al. Effectiveness of gonadotrophin-releasing hormone agonist therapy to improve the outcomes of intrauterine insemination in patients suffering from stage I-II endometriosis. Ann Med. 2022; 54(1):1330-8.
7. Lambalk CB, Leader A, Olivennes F, Fluker MR, Andersen AN, Ingerslev J, et al. Treatment with the GnRH antagonist ganirelix prevents premature LH rises and luteinization in stimulated intrauterine insemination: results of a double-blind, placebo-controlled, multicentre trial. Hum Reprod. 2006;21:632-9.
8. Coccia ME, Comparetto C, Bracco GL, Scarselli G. GnRH antagonists. Eur j obstet gynecol reprod biol. 2004;115(Suppl 1): S44-56.
9. Hamada M, Horikawa M, Franska C, Enomoto M, Ishi R, Toriumi R, et al. A novel orally active gonadotropin-releasing hormone antagonist, relugolix, is a potential substitute for injectable GnRH antagonists in controlled ovarian stimulation in assisted reproductive technology. Reprod Med Biol. 2021;21(1):e12424.
10. Wadhwa L, Khanna R, Gupta T, Gupta S, Arora S, Nandwani S. Evaluation of role of GnRH antagonist in intrauterine insemination (IUI) cycles with mild ovarian hyperstimulation (MOH): a prospective randomised study. J Obstet Gynaecol India. 2016;66(Suppl 1):459-65.
11. Luo S, Li S, Jin S, Li Y, Zhang Y. Effectiveness of GnRH antagonist in the management of subfertile couples undergoing controlled ovarian stimulation and intrauterine insemination: a meta-analysis. PLoS One. 2014;9(10):e109133.
12. Vitagliano A, Saccone G, Noventa M, Borini A, Coccia ME, Nardelli GB, et al. Pituitary block with gonadotrophin-releasing hormone antagonist during intrauterine insemination cycles: a systematic review and meta-analysis of randomised controlled trials. BJOG. 2019;126(2):167-75.
13. Ozelci R, Dilbaz S, Dilbaz B, Cırık DA, Yılmaz S, Tekin OM. Gonadotropin releasing hormone antagonist use in controlled ovarian stimulation and intrauterine insemination cycles in women with polycystic ovary syndrome. Taiwan J Obstet Gynecol. 2019;58(2):234-8.
14. Gopal L, Sudhakar P, Kandaswami D, Manivannan S. Addition of gonadotropin releasing hormone antagonist for women undergoing intrauterine insemination: a randomized controlled trial. Int J Reprod Contracept Obstet Gynecol. 2023;12(4): 1101-5.

SECTION 6

Ovulation Trigger

15. **Ovulation Trigger: Dose and Timing**
    Rajendra Shitole

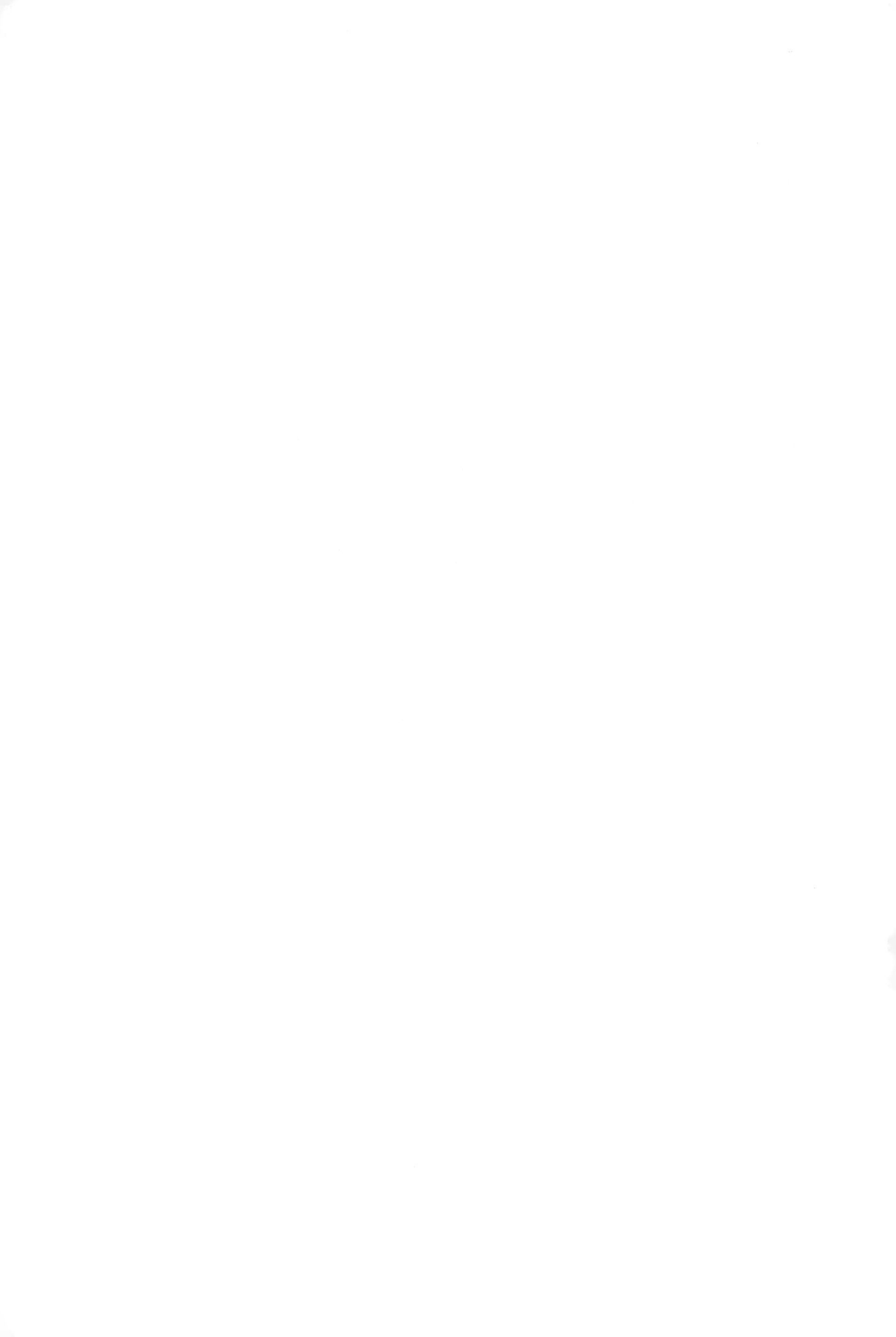

CHAPTER 15

Ovulation Trigger: Dose and Timing

Rajendra Shitole

■ INTRODUCTION

Intrauterine insemination (IUI) is the first treatment option for unexplained infertility, male factor, and a few other indications after the failure of expectant treatment and before in vitro fertilization (IVF) or ICSI. It is a more economical method than other assisted reproductive techniques. IUI is indicated for the treatment of unexplained infertility, mild male factor, minimal to mild endometriosis, cervical factor, and anovulation. The success rate of IUI is between 10% and 20% per treatment. Various steps are involved to increase the success rates of IUI, including ovarian stimulation, monitoring of follicles, sperm preparation, endometrial preparation, ovulation trigger, and luteal phase support. However, the dose and timing of ovulation triggers influence the success rate of IUI.

■ PHYSIOLOGY OF NORMAL MENSTRUAL CYCLE AND LUTEINIZING HORMONE SURGE[1]

Intrauterine insemination (IUI) is a method of assisted reproductive techniques (ARTs) that can be used for treatment of infertility in few infertile couples.

Normal menstrual cycle is an orchestra of events involving the hypothalamus, pituitary, ovary, and uterus. During the follicular phase, there is a rise in the level of follicle-stimulating hormone (FSH) which causes increase in estradiol (E2) and luteinizing hormone (LH) levels. Increase in LH causes androgen production in theca cells, which by the help of aromatase enzyme gets converted to E2. As the follicle grows and E2 levels rise, it causes negative feedback on FSH so that the growth of smaller follicles stops and dominant follicle emerges, having maximum E2 levels and highest number of FSH and LH receptors. E2 level rises causing FSH surge, which is followed by LH surge which leads of ovulation.[2]

For LH surge to cause ovulation, there should be sustained E2 levels of 200 pg/mL for 48–50 hours. The follicle must be at a stage of maturity to respond to the ovulatory stimulus. In a normal menstrual cycle, gonadotropin release and final maturity of the follicle coincides with the timing of FSH and LH surge. This is controlled by increasing E2 levels which in turn is the function of follicle growth and maturity.

Normal LH surge lasts for 36 hours. It has got three phases: the initial phase of acceleration lasting for 12 hours, plateau phase for 12 hours, and phase of deceleration lasting for 10–12 hours **(Fig. 1)**.

The starting of the LH surge occurs approximately 34–36 hours prior to ovulation and is a relatively good predictor for timing ovulation. The LH surge stimulates luteinization of the granulosa cells and stimulates the synthesis of progesterone

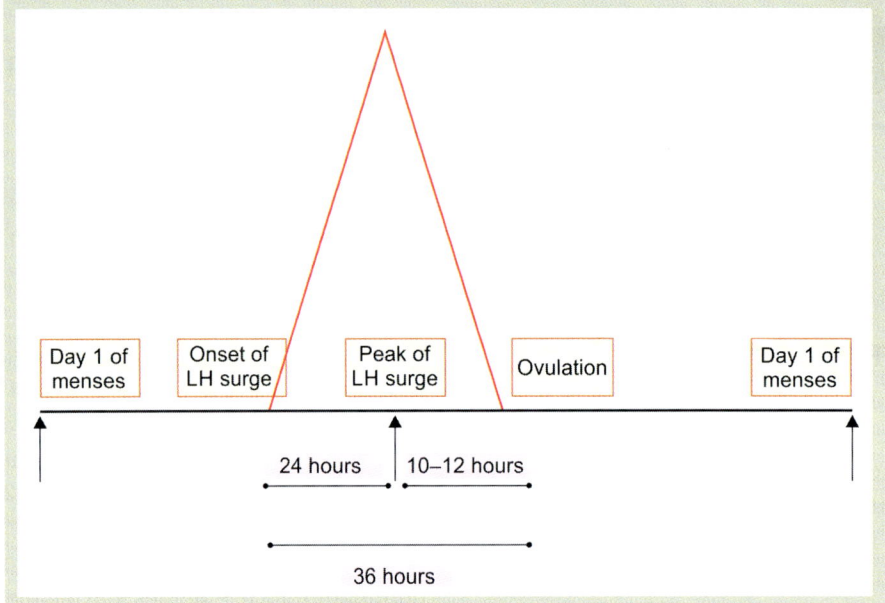

Fig. 1: The onset of luteinizing hormone (LH) surge usually occurs 36 hours before ovulation. The ovulation on the other hand occurs 10–12 hours after peak of LH surge.

responsible for the midcycle FSH surge. Also, the LH surge stimulates resumption of meiosis and the completion of reduction division in the oocyte with the release of the first polar body. The LH surge increases intrafollicular proteolytic enzymes, weakening the wall of the ovary, and allowing for the mature oocyte to pass through causing ovulation.

Why trigger is necessary?

The trigger injection is necessary as the LH secreted by the body is usually not high enough as would occur during a natural cycle. Furthermore, the body LH may not be adequate enough, to induce the necessary maturational changes in all oocytes, if there are many follicles in the ovary during superovulation done for IUI.[3]

When to give trigger for maturation?

Intrauterine insemination cycles are usually monitored by ultrasonography and if required with serum E2 values. Oral ovulogens or gonadotropins are usually used for ovulation induction in anovulatory cycles with aim of monofollicular growth or for superovulation in normo-ovulatory cycles with aim of multifollicular[2-3] growth.[4] Serial ultrasonography is performed from day 7 to decide the trigger timing. Sometimes cycles may get canceled due to multifollicular growth to avoid OHSS.

Usually trigger is given when:
- Dominant-rounded follicle with thin walls and no internal echogenicity is seen.
- Dominant follicle is 20–22 mm in cycles induced by oral ovulogens **(Fig. 2)**
- Dominant follicle is 18–20 mm in cycles induced by gonadotropins.
- Vascularity indices of follicle are favorable—three-fourths vascularity surrounding the follicle, peak systolic velocity (PSV) of follicle is >10 cm/s, resistivity index (RI) is 0.40–0.48.

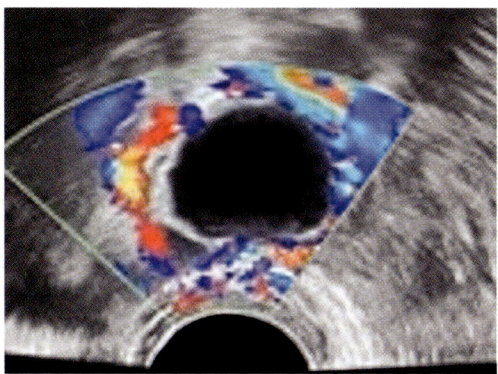

Fig. 2: Dominant follicle 20 mm with good vascularity.

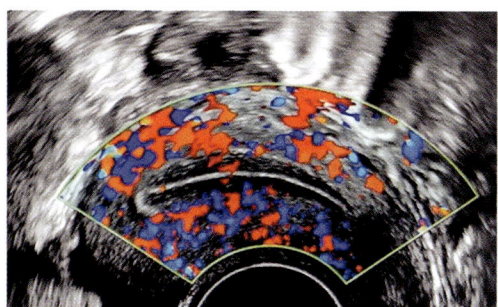

Fig. 4: Good endometrium with excellent zone 3–4 vascularity.

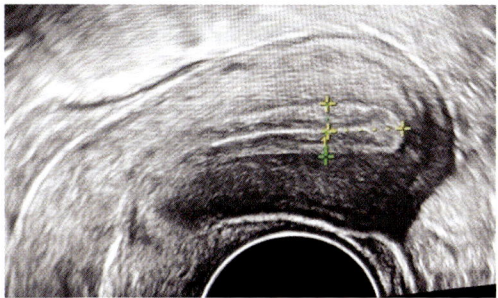

Fig. 3: Triple layer endometrium with good morphology.

- Endometrium is 7–14 mm triple line with good morphology and zone 3–4 vascularity **(Figs. 3 and 4)**.

Intrauterine insemination is usually carried out 36–40 hours after trigger.
- If the follicular vascular indices are not in the defined range, it means that the follicle is not yet physiologically mature and, therefore, stimulation still needs to be continued.
- The follicle is said to be functionally mature when PSV is 10 cm/s that is the time when the LH surge starts and under the effect of that LH, the perifollicular PSV keeps on rising constantly. Follicular blood flow velocity starts increasing approximately 26–29 hours before rupture and continues to 72 hours after rupture.

Rising PSV with steady low RI suggests that the follicle is close to rupture. Steady or decreasing PSV with rising RI suggests that the follicle is proceeding toward luteinized unruptured follicle (LUF).
- In patients with higher perifollicular pretrigger PSV, IUI done at 12–14 hours has been successful.
- Fertilization of a follicle with a PSV of <10 cm/s has a high chance of fertilizing into an embryo with a chromosomal abnormality.

VARIOUS PHARMACOLOGICAL OPTIONS FOR OVULATION TRIGGER

- *Human chorionic gonadotropin (hCG):* Urinary/recombinant
- Recombinant LH
- *Gonadotropin-releasing hormone (GnRH) agonist:* Triptorelin acetate or leuprolide acetate
- *Dual trigger:* GnRH agonist with hCG
- Kisspeptins.

Human Chorionic Gonadotropin

Human chorionic gonadotropin is a glycoprotein like LH with extended plasma half-life. It has two subunits α and β. The α subunit is similar to LH and it is the β subunit which is different in both of these molecules.

Unlike physiologic LH surge which lasts for 48–50 hours, the surge caused by hCG spans several days which leads to increased levels of E2 and progesterone along with vasoactive amines. This excessive amount of vasoactive amines and steroids leads to an increased OHSS incidence with hCG.[5]

- It is available as urinary or recombinant preparation.
- Recombinant preparations are associated with higher serum progesterone and serum hCG postadministration.
- Urinary hCG (u-hCG) still remains the first choice as it is cheap and easily available.
- No difference in terms of follicular maturation, risk of OHSS, and pregnancy outcome between the two.
- *Dose:* 5,000–10,000 IU of u-hCG intramuscularly or 250-375 µg of r-hCG subcutaneously.
- Usually avoided or combined with agonist trigger when more than two follicles are developed or risk of OHSS is high.

Recombinant Luteinizing Hormone

- It has a shorter half-life and is very physiological.
- *Dose:* Single dose of 15,000–30,000 IU with safety superior to hCG with respect to incidence of OHSS
- Availability and high cost limit its use for IUI cycles.

Gonadotropin-releasing Hormone Agonist

- GnRH agonist acts at the level of pituitary gland and activates GnRH receptor which causes a surge of gonadotropins LH and FSH which leads to ovulation. It is as close to natural menstrual cycle as possible. There is first FSH surge as in a natural cycle followed by LH surge which leads to resumption of meiosis. Unlike natural cycle LH surge, GnRH agonist surge is a short surge lasting for 24–36 hours with only two phases unlike three phases of LH surge. So, less amount of gonadotropins is released which leads to early demise of corpus luteum. This is one of the major drawbacks of GnRH triggering, there is deficient corpus luteum leading to deficient luteal phase. This leads to significantly lesser pregnancy rates. So good luteal phase support should be given to IUI patients where agonist trigger is used.
- It is usually used in polycystic ovary syndrome (PCOS) patients with high risk for OHSS. Patients having previous history of OHSS and repeated LUF in previous cycles with hCG trigger.

Types of Gonadotropin-releasing Hormone Agonist Trigger

- *Triptorelin acetate:* It is used in the doses of 0.2 mg subcutaneously.
- *Leuprolide acetate:* It is used in the doses of 2–4 mg subcutaneously.

Dual Trigger

- GnRH analog with low dose hCG 1,000–2,500 IU
- Adding the FSH component causing FSH surge which helps overcome any impairment in granulosa cell function, oocyte meiotic maturation, or cumulus expansion.
- Mainly indicated in patients with risk of OHSS, LUF, and where chances of luteal phase defect are more with agonist trigger alone.[6]

Kisspeptins

- Still in research
- Not routinely available or used
- Physiological but short acting.[7]

CONCLUSION

Ovulation trigger with hCG is associated with significantly higher clinical pregnancy rates in patients undergoing ovulation induction with IUI in comparison to GnRH agonist trigger. The size of the dominant follicle, PSV, RI of the dominant follicle, and endometrial thickness are important factors to be considered at the time of giving a trigger for IUI to have good success.

KEY LEARNING POINTS

- Intrauterine insemination therapy utilizes various treatments to simulate many of the physiological processes occurring in the normal human menstrual cycle.
- Oocyte maturation is a critical process to the success of IUI treatment, during which the oocyte gains competence for fertilization.
- Oocyte maturation is initiated by LH-like exposure that can be provided by hCG, GnRH agonist, recombinant LH, or kisspeptin.
- The mode by which oocyte maturation is induced has significant impact on the efficacy of follicular rupture, the chance of pregnancy, and the safety of IUI treatment.
- The size of follicles at time of trigger administration and the dose of trigger agent can impact the efficacy of drugs used for oocyte maturation.
- The risk of ovarian hyperstimulation syndrome, a potentially life-threatening complication of ART treatment that can affect otherwise healthy women undergoing fertility treatment, is strongly related to the agent used to induce oocyte maturation.
- Different agents like hCG (urinary or recombinant), GnRH agonists, recombinant LH, and kisspeptin can be used for final oocyte maturation during IUI.

REFERENCES

1. Reed BG, Carr BR. The Normal Menstrual Cycle and the Control of Ovulation. In: Feingold KR, Anawalt B, Blackman MR, Boyce A, Chrousos G, Corpas E, (Eds). Endotext [Internet]. South Dartmouth (MA): MDText.com, Inc.; 2000.
2. Erden M, Mumusoglu S, Polat M, Yarali Ozbek I, Esteves SC, Humaidan P, et al. The LH surge and ovulation re-visited: a systematic review and meta-analysis and implications for true natural cycle frozen thawed embryo transfer. Hum Reprod Update. 2022;28(5):717-32.
3. Kauffman AS. Neuroendocrine mechanisms underlying estrogen positive feedback and the LH surge. Front Neurosci. 2022;16:953252.
4. Singh S, Singh S, Ashraf C. Oral Ovulogens in IUI and IVF. In: Ghumman, S. (Ed). Principles and Practice of Controlled Ovarian Stimulation in ART. New Delhi: Springer; 2015. pp. 45-59.
5. Arici A, Byrd W, Bradshaw K, Kutteh WH, Marshburn P, Carr BR. Evaluation of clomiphene citrate and human chorionic gonadotropin treatment: a prospective, randomized, crossover study during intrauterine insemination cycles. Fertil Steril. 1994;61(2):314-8.
6. Vyrides AA, Mahdi EE, Lamnisos D, Giannakou K. Dual Trigger with Gonadotropin releasing hormone agonist and human chorionic gonadotropin of fresh autologous cycles in high responders: a systematic review. J Reprod Infertil. 2022; 23(1):3-17.
7. Masumi S, Lee EB, Dilower I, Upadhyaya S, Chakravarthi VP, Fields PE, et al. The role of Kisspeptin signaling in Oocyte maturation. Front Endocrinol (Lausanne). 2022;13:917464.

SECTION 7

Andrology and Laboratory Aspect

16. **Semen Analysis**
    Sunita Tandulwadkar, Darshan SM

17. **Sperm Functional Assays**
    Spondita Banerjee, Neena Malhotra

18. **Optimizing Sperm Preparation for Intrauterine Insemination**
    Keshav Malhotra

19. **Setting Up an Intrauterine Insemination Laboratory**
    Sonal Vaidya

20. **Assisted Reproductive Technology Act 2022: Level I Clinic**
    Ashwini Yelikar Kale, Ashish Kale

CHAPTER 16

Semen Analysis

Sunita Tandulwadkar, Darshan SM

■ INTRODUCTION

Sperm, the male reproductive gamete in anisogamous forms of sexual reproduction, is a unicellular motile structure. It is produced in the seminiferous tubules of the testes under the influence of follicular-stimulating hormone (FSH). The word "spermatozoon" is derived from the ancient Greek words (spérma) "seed" and and (zôion) "animal". It is a motile sperm cell, or moving form of the haploid cell that is the male gamete. We are all aware that spermatozoon joins an ovum to form a zygote. Sperm contributes approximately half of the nuclear genetic information to the diploid offspring. In mammals including humans, the sex of the offspring is determined by the sperm: a spermatozoon bearing an X chromosome will lead to a female (XX) offspring, while one bearing a Y chromosome will lead to a male (XY) offspring. Sperm was first observed in 1677 at Antonie van Leeuwenhoek's laboratory.[1,2]

For many years now, the World Health Organization (WHO) manuals have served as a primary resource for seminal fluid analysis procedures. The WHO laboratory manual for the examination of human semen was first published in 1980, in response to a growing need for standardization of procedures for the examination of human semen. The manual was revised four times,[1-5] widely read and translated into a number of languages. Indeed, over the past 40 years, the manual became a recognized standard, used extensively by clinical and research laboratories throughout the world. It is a procedural guide not only for those new to semen analysis, but a reference text for all who process semen and need to analyze and define sperm parameters for clinical practice or clinical and epidemiological research studies. The clinical assessment of the male together with the semen analyses can guide the clinician to determine how to proceed with further investigation and management of the subfertile couple. For an individual patient, a semen analysis is never prognostic of fertility, as it is the fertility potential of the couple that defines them as fertile or subfertile **(Fig. 1)**.[6]

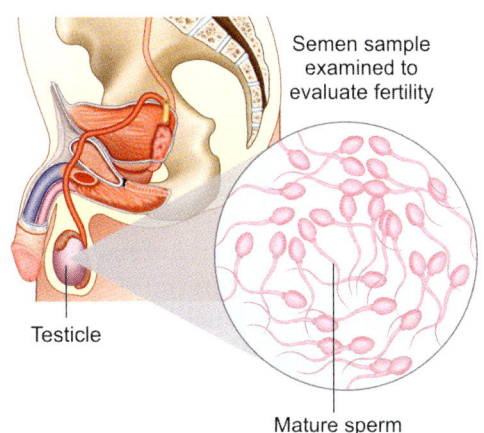

Fig. 1: Semen analysis.

Semen examination is important for different reasons:
- Assessment of male reproductive function and genital tract patency to enable appropriate treatment for male subfertility and to monitor treatment response.
- Appraisal of fertility potential and choice of suitable treatment modality for an infertile couple.
- Measure efficacy of male contraception (e.g., vas occlusion and interventions including hormonal male contraception and other potential methods).

Many known and unknown female factors hamper the value of using only semen examination parameters to predict the prognosis for the couple of spontaneous or assisted fertilization. A better prognostic value of semen examination can be obtained from using the combination of several parameters.[7-9]

WORLD HEALTH ORGANIZATION SIXTH EDITION

Comparison between 2010 and 2020 WHO manual semen analysis has been described in **Table 1**.

The first edition was published in 1980 and the latest, sixth edition in 2021. The sixth edition comprises three parts:
1. Semen examination
2. Sperm preparation and cryopreservation
3. Quality assessment and quality control.

Procedures for semen examination are divided into three chapters:
1. *Basic examination:* Robust routine procedures for determining semen variables that any laboratory performing a semen examination can follow.
2. *Extended analysis:* Used in certain situations by choice of the laboratory or by special request from the clinician.
3. *Advanced examination:* Currently not regarded as routine for use in the initial evaluation of a subfertile male.

TABLE 1: Comparison between 2010 and 2020 WHO manual semen analysis.

Semen parameters	WHO 2010	WHO 2020
Semen volume	1.5 mL	1.4 mL
Sperm concentration	15 million/mL	16 million/mL
Total motility	40%	42%
Progressive motility	32%	30%
Viability	58%	54%
Morphology (normal forms)	4%	4%

Notably, human cervical mucous tests were eliminated from this new edition as they are no longer used in the clinical practice. This new edition was written as an easy-to-follow procedural manual for those performing semen examination, with background information and rationale of the test separated from the description of the procedure.

- The re-introduction of the four-category distinction of sperm motility, which causes additional work for laboratories in changing reporting parameters but is clinically important.
- The widened focus from mainly a prognostic tool for medically assisted reproduction to additionally raising awareness of semen examination as a measure of male reproductive functions and general male health.
- The new edition of the manual includes step-by-step procedures and checklists to ensure it is user-friendly for laboratory technicians and scientists.
- 200 spermatozoa per replicate should be counted.
- Count is given more importance than the concentration.

- In addition, emerging new methods using sperm movement or changes in light may constitute the basis of measuring sperm motility without the need of a microscope.

SPERM EXAMINATION

Basic Examination

Basic examinations are those that any laboratory investigating human ejaculate is expected to perform. The ejaculate is produced from a concentrated suspension of spermatozoa, stored in the paired epididymis, mixed with, and diluted by, primarily the prostatic fluid in the urethra, followed by the emptying of the secretion of the seminal vesicles.[10] Approximately 90% of the volume is composed of secretions from the accessory organs,[11] mainly the prostate and seminal vesicles, with minor contributions from the bulbourethral (Cowper's) glands and epididymis.

Temporal Outline of Basic Semen Examination[6,12]

The preexamination procedures comprise:
- Patient information
- Sample collection
- Sample reception
- Initial sample handling.

In the first 5 minutes—Initial sample handling:
- Measuring semen volume by weight can preferably be done at the time the sample is received, and before liquefaction.
- Allow time for liquefaction to occur (usually no >30 minutes).

Between 30 and 60 minutes after ejaculate collection:
- Assess liquefaction and macroscopic appearance of the semen.
- Prepare a wet preparation for assessing microscopic appearance, sperm motility, and the dilution required for assessing sperm concentration.
- Measure semen pH (if indicated).
- Assess sperm vitality (if the percentage of motile cells is low).
- Make dilutions for assessing sperm concentration.
- Make smears for assessing sperm morphology, and fixing smears.
- Perform the mixed antiglobulin reaction (MAR) test for antisperm antibodies (if required).
- Assess the presence of leukocytes cells (if required).
- Centrifuge semen aliquots (if biochemical markers are to be assayed).

Within 3 hours of ejaculate collection:
- Determine sperm concentration (can be done later, preferably the same day).
- Send samples to the microbiology laboratory (if required).

Later, the same day or on a subsequent day:
- Stain and assess smears for sperm morphology.
- Biochemical analysis of accessory gland markers (optional).

Sample Collection
- Before ejaculate collection, the specimen container should be kept at ambient temperature, between 20 and 37°C, to avoid large changes in temperature that may affect the spermatozoa.
- The specimen container should be a clean, wide-mouthed container made of plastic, from a batch that has been confirmed to be nontoxic for spermatozoa.
- The specimen container, as well as corresponding manual worksheets, must be labeled with identifiers that in combination with the procedures for sample reception and further handling

eliminate the risk for mix-up of samples and worksheets. Legal requirements for container-identity markers may differ. It could be the man's name and identification number, the date and time of collection, or unique sample identifying numbers.
- The following information should be recorded at sample reception and presented in the final report.
- Identity of the man (e.g., name, date of birth, and personal code number) and ideally his confirmation that the sample is his own, the period of prior ejaculatory abstinence.
- The date and time of collection
- The completeness of the sample and any difficulties in producing the sample
- *Special conditions apply for some specific situations:* sterile collection for assisted reproduction or cryostorage, sterile collection for microbiological analysis.

MACROSCOPIC APPEARANCE OF THE EJACULATE[11-14]

- *Appearance:* Opalescent/turbid
- *Semen volume:* Weight in grams
- *Liquefaction:* ↑/↓
- *Consistency:* Viscous/watery
- Odor
- pH

Appearance

A normal liquefied ejaculate has a macroscopically homogeneous, cream/gray opalescent appearance. It may appear less opaque if the sperm concentration is very low; the color may also be different—i.e., slightly yellowish after longer abstinence times, red-brown when red blood cells are present (hemospermia), or clearer yellow in a patient with jaundice or taking certain vitamins or drugs. If the ejaculate appears viscous, totally clear and colorless, then it may be preejaculate from only the Cowper's glands, which men produce in varying quantity during arousal; in this scenario, this should be discussed with the patient to establish whether an orgasm-associated ejaculation occurred.

Volume

The volume is best measured by weighing the sample in the container in which it has been collected. This can preferably be done at reception of the ejaculation container before incubation for liquefaction. Other methods introduce greater inaccuracy (Cooper et al., 2007).

Liquefaction

Immediately after ejaculation into the collection vessel, the ejaculate is a semi-solid coagulated mass or a gel-like clump which begins to liquefy (become thinner) within minutes at room temperature, at which time a heterogeneous mixture of semi-solid lumps will be seen in the fluid. As liquefaction continues, it becomes more homogeneous and watery, but still with a higher viscosity than water. In the final stages, only small areas of coagulation remain. A temperature of 37°C facilitates liquefaction. A slow and swirling movement of the container will help liquefaction to complete. If a moving tray is not used during liquefaction, it is essential that the container is slowly swirled for 15–30 seconds before starting the macroscopic assessment.
- Complete liquefaction is normally achieved within 15–30 minutes at room temperature.
- If liquefaction is not complete within 30 minutes, this should be recorded, and noted in the final report. The ejaculate

could then be left in 37°C for another 30 minutes.
- If liquefaction is not complete after 60 minutes, this should also be included in the final report.
- Normal liquefied ejaculates may contain a few jelly-like granules (gelatinous bodies) which do not liquefy and do not appear to have any clinical significance. The presence of mucus strands though may interfere with ejaculate examination and should therefore be noted in the final report.

Viscosity

After liquefaction, the viscosity of the ejaculate can be estimated by gently aspirating it into a wide-bore (approximately 1.5 mm diameter) plastic disposable pipette (verified as nontoxic to sperm and, if needed, sterile), allowing the semen to drop by gravity and observing the length of any thread. A normal liquefied ejaculate falls as small discrete drops. If viscosity is abnormal, the drop will form a thread >2 cm long.

Ejaculate Odor

There is considerable variability in the ability of individuals to perceive the normal smell of a human ejaculate.[6] Information of a strong odor of urine or putrefaction is of clinical importance and therefore to note this in the report.

Ejaculate pH

The pH depends on the relative contribution of acidic prostatic secretion and alkaline seminal vesicular secretion. In the Ejaculate, there is no efficient control of the pH of the fluid. In vitro, there will be a continuous loss of CO_2 that causes a gradual increase in pH. The clinical interest of ejaculate pH is a low value. If pH is to be assessed, it should be done at a uniform time, preferably 30 minutes after collection, but in any case, within 1 hour of ejaculation.

For normal samples, pH test strips in the range 6.0–10.0 should be used.

A pH value <7.2 may be indicative of a lack of alkaline seminal vesicular fluid. It can also be due to urine contamination.

■ MICROSCOPIC EXAMINATION

- Motility
- Concentration and count
- Morphology.

For reliable results of microscopic investigation, it is essential that the aliquots examined are representative of the entire ejaculate. If the sample is not well mixed, analysis of two separate aliquots is unlikely to be representative of the entire ejaculate and can show marked differences in sperm concentration, motility, vitality, and morphology. Even if the liquefied ejaculate is macroscopically homogeneous, small aliquots can have very different composition.

Before removing an aliquot of semen for any assessment, the sample should be mixed well in the original container. Care should be taken so that no air bubbles are created.
- Use replicate aliquots of at least 50 μL for dilution for sperm concentration assessment.
- Use replicate aliquots of at least 10 μL for sperm motility assessment.

Motility

The extent of progressive sperm motility is related to pregnancy rates.[13,15,16] The total number of progressively motile spermatozoa in the ejaculate is of biological significance and is obtained by multiplying the total number of spermatozoa in the ejaculate by the percentage of progressively motile cells. The velocity of spermatozoa is temperature dependent. It is therefore essential to standardize the temperature during motility assessment. It is often easiest to control a temperature similar to body temperature, but that requires that the microscope is equipped with a temperature-controlled object stage, that microscope slides and coverslips are prewarmed, and that the sample is also warmed to 37°C before assessment.

Always start scanning several fields without counting to get an impression of how well spread spermatozoa are. This can be done at lower magnification (100–200 × total magnification).

- Avoid assessing areas close (<5 mm) to the edge of the coverslip to prevent drying artifacts affecting the assessment.
- Field choice should be random; avoid choosing fields based on the number of spermatozoa seen.
- Scan the slide systematically to avoid repeatedly viewing the same area. At least five different fields should be assessed, even if >200 spermatozoa have been counted in fewer than 5 fields.

Clinical data from both manual assessment of sperm motility as well as computer-aided sperm analysis demonstrate that the identification of rapidly progressive spermatozoa is important.[14,17-26] Therefore, the recommended categories are (with approximate velocity limits):

- *Rapidly progressive:* Spermatozoa moving actively, either linearly or in a large circle, covering a distance, from the starting point to the end point, of at least 25 μm (or half-tail length) in 1 second.
- *Slowly progressive:* Spermatozoa moving actively, either linearly or in a large circle, covering a distance, from the starting point to the endpoint, of 5 to <25 μm (or at least one head length to less than half-tail length) in 1 second.
- *Nonprogressive:* All other patterns of active tail movements with an absence of progression, i.e., swimming in small circles, the flagellar force displacing the head < 5 μm (one head length), from the starting point to the endpoint.
- *Immotile:* No active tail movements.

Sperm Vitality

Estimated by assessing the membrane integrity of the cells. In samples with poor motility (<40%), the vitality test is important to discriminate between immotile dead sperm and immotile live sperm. The presence of a large proportion of live but immotile cells may be indicative of structural defects in the flagellum,[27,28] a high percentage of immotile and dead cells may indicate epididymal pathology[29,30] or an immunological reaction due to an infection.

The percentage of live spermatozoa is assessed by identifying those with an intact cell membrane, by dye exclusion (dead cells have damaged plasma membranes that allow entry of membrane-impermeant stains) or by hypotonic swelling. The recommended test for diagnostic use is the eosin–nigrosin test.

It should be assessed as soon as possible after liquefaction of the semen sample, preferably at 30 minutes, but in any case, within 1 hour of ejaculation, to limit deleterious effects of dehydration or changes in temperature on vitality.

Count

There are various ways to measure the count:
- The hemocytometer with improved Neubauer ruling (Recommended)
- Mekler's chamber (Easy and faster)
- Cover slip (Easy)

The improved Neubauer hemocytometer has two separate counting chambers, each of which has a microscopic 3 mm × 3 mm pattern of grid lines etched on the glass surface. It is used with a special and thick cover slip (thickness #4, 0.44 mm), which lies over the grids and is supported by glass pillars 0.1 mm (100 µm) above the chamber floor. Each counting area is divided into nine 1 mm × 1 mm grids. Depending on the dilution and the number of spermatozoa counted, different areas of the chamber are used for determining sperm concentration. In general, the central grid is used for counting. The eight peripheral grids are used when fewer than 200 spermatozoa have been counted in the central grid.

Principles for counting in a hemocytometer grid:
- Count only whole spermatozoa (with a head and a tail).
- If there are many headless sperm tails (so-called "pinhead" spermatozoa) or heads without tails, their presence should be recorded in the report. The concentration can be estimated in relation to whole spermatozoa (for instance, "32 headless tails per 100 spermatozoa").
- The boundary of a large square is indicated by the middle line of the three.
- Whether or not a spermatozoon is counted is confirmed by the location of its head, the orientation of its tail is unimportant.
- All spermatozoa without contact with the boundaries (middle of triple line) of a large square are counted.
- Only those in contact with the lower or left boundaries are counted, not those in contact with the upper or right.
- Sperm number should be assessed in both chambers of the hemocytometer. If the two values agree sufficiently, the aliquots taken can be considered representative of the sample. It is important to remember that the absence of spermatozoa from the aliquot examined does not necessarily mean that they are absent from the rest of the ejaculate.

It is essential to calculate and report the total number of spermatozoa per ejaculate, as this parameter provides a much better measure of testicular sperm production and of the number of spermatozoa transferred to the female during coitus. This is obtained by multiplying the sperm concentration by the volume of the whole ejaculate.

- The total sperm number should be reported as an integer number (no decimal places) of millions of spermatozoa, with exception only for numbers below 10 million, where 1 decimal place may be acceptable for the sake of clarity in the lower range of results, although the analytical variability does justify the use of a decimal place.
- The sum of the two accepted replicate counts is divided by a factor that is determined by the dilution and number of large squares or grids assessed in both counting chambers (if three attempts have been done without reaching sufficient agreement between replicate counts, the average of the three sums is used).

Morphology

All human ejaculates contain spermatozoa with a wide range of different morphological appearances. Earlier definitions of sperm morphology were based primarily on experiences from veterinary medicine and microscope investigations.

Morphologically "Ideal" Spermatozoa

- Shorr-stained spermatozoa recovered from the zona pellucida in vitro.

- Papanicolaou-stained spermatozoa recovered from endocervical mucus after intercourse. Very few defects on the sperm head, midpiece, or principal piece are observed. Tails may be curved but not sharply angulated.

Categories of sperm abnormalities are:
- Head (%H)
- Neck and midpiece (%NM)
- Tail (%T)
- Excess residual cytoplasm (%C).

Report the presence and prevalence relative to spermatozoa of:
- Specific sperm defects, e.g., free sperm heads, pinheads (free tails), heads lacking acrosomes
- Immature germ cells
- Nonsperm cells.

ASSESSMENT OF SPERM CLUMPING

There are two different types of sperm clumping that is essential to assess separately.
1. *Sperm aggregates:* The adherence either of immotile spermatozoa to each other or of motile spermatozoa to mucous strands, nonsperm cells, or debris.
2. *Sperm agglutinates:* Agglutination specifically refers to motile spermatozoa sticking to each other, head-to-head, tail-to-tail, or in a mixed way. The motility is often vigorous, with a frantic shaking motion, but sometimes the spermatozoa are so agglutinated that their motion is limited. Any motile spermatozoa that stick to each other by their heads, tails or mid-pieces should be noted.

CONCLUSION

Semen Analysis should be the first investigation in the male sub-fertility work-up along with physical examination. A single normal report is enough to presume and rule out male factor as a cause while a single abnormal report cannot discern the male factor.

KEY LEARNING POINTS

- The clinical assessment of the male together with the semen analyses can guide the clinician to determine how to proceed with further investigation and management of the sub-fertile couple.
- For an individual patient, a semen analysis is never prognostic of fertility, as it is the fertility potential of the couple that defines them as fertile or sub-fertile.

REFERENCES

1. Collins English Dictionary. (2020). Spermatium definition and meaning. [online] Available from: www.collinsdictionary.com. [Last accessed January, 2024].
2. Belsey M, Eliasson R, Gallegos AJ, Moghissi KS, Paulsen CA, Prassad AMN. Laboratory Manual for the Examination of Human Semen and Semen-Cervical Mucus Interaction. Singapore: Press Concern; 1980.
3. World Health Organization. WHO laboratory manual for the examination of human semen and semen-cervical mucus interactions, 2nd edition. Cambridge, UK: Cambridge University Press; 1987. p. 67.
4. World Health Organization. WHO laboratory manual for the examination of human semen and sperm-cervical mucus interactions, 3rd edition. Cambridge, UK: Cambridge University Press; 1992. p. 107.
5. World Health Organization. WHO laboratory manual for the examination of human semen and sperm-cervical mucus interactions, 4th edition. Cambridge, UK: Cambridge University Press; 1999. p. 128.
6. Campbell MJ, Lotti F, Baldi E, Schlatt S, Festin MP, Bjorndahl L, et al. Distribution of Semen Examination Results 2020—a follow up of data collated for the WHO Semen Analysis Manual 2010. Andrology. 2021.

7. Björndahl L. What is normal semen quality? On the use and abuse of reference limits for the interpretation of semen analysis results. Hum Fertil (Camb). 2011;14(3):179-86.
8. Jedrzejczak P, Taszarek-Hauke G, Hauke J, Pawelczyk L, Duleba AJ. Prediction of spontaneous conception based on semen parameters. Int J Androl. 2008;31(5):499-507.
9. Guzick DS, Overstreet JW, Factor-Litvak P, Brazil CK, Nakajima ST, Coutifaris C, et al. Sperm morphology, motility, and concentration in fertile and infertile men. N Engl J Med. 2001;345(19):1388-93.
10. Mortimer D. Laboratory standards in routine clinical andrology. Reprod Med Rev. 1994;3:97-111.
11. Jouannet P, Ducot B, Feneux D, Spira A. Male factors and the likelihood of pregnancy in infertile couples. I. Study of sperm characteristics. Int J Androl. 1988;11(5):379-94.
12. Barratt CLR, Bjorndahl L, De Jonge CJ, Lamb DJ, Osorio Martini F, McLachlan R, et al. The diagnosis of male infertility: an analysis of the evidence to support the development of global WHO guidance-challenges and future research opportunities. Hum Reprod Update. 2017;23(6):660-80.
13. Barratt CL, Björndahl L, Menkveld R, Mortimer D. ESHRE special interest group for andrology basic semen analysis course: a continued focus on accuracy, quality, efficiency and clinical relevance. Hum Reprod. 2011;26(12):3207-12.
14. Mortimer D. Practical Laboratory Andrology. Oxford: Oxford University Press; 1994. p. 393.
15. Zinaman MJ, Brown CC, Selevan SG, Clegg ED. Semen quality and human fertility: a prospective study with healthy couples. J Androl. 2000;21(1):145-53.
16. Larsen L, Scheike T, Jensen TK, Bonde JP, Ernst E, Hjollund NH, et al. Computer-assisted semen analysis parameters as predictors for fertility of men from the general population. The Danish First Pregnancy Planner Study Team. Hum Reprod. 2000;15(7):1562-7.
17. Aitken RJ, Sutton M, Warner P, Richardson DW. Relationship between the movement characteristics of human spermatozoa and their ability to penetrate cervical mucus and zona-free hamster oocytes. J Reprod Fertil. 1985;73(2):441-9.
18. Mortimer D, Pandya IJ, Sawers RS. Relationship between human sperm motility characteristics and sperm penetration into human cervical mucus in vitro. J Reprod Fertil. 1986;78(1):93-102.
19. Comhaire FH, Vermeulen L, Hinting A, Schoonjans F. Accuracy of sperm characteristics in predicting the in vitro fertilizing capacity of semen. J In Vitro Fert Embryo Transf. 1988;5(6):326-31.
20. Barratt CL, McLeod ID, Dunphy BC, Cooke ID. Prognostic value of two putative sperm function tests: hypo-osmotic swelling and bovine sperm mucus penetration test (Penetrak). Hum Reprod. 1992;7(9):1240-4.
21. Irvine DS, Aitken RJ. Predictive value of in-vitro sperm function tests in the context of an AID service. Hum Reprod. 1986;1(8):539-45.
22. Bollendorf A, Check JH, Lurie D. Evaluation of the effect of the absence of sperm with rapid and linear progressive motility on subsequent pregnancy rates following intrauterine insemination or in vitro fertilization. J Androl. 1996;17(5):550-7.
23. Sifer C, Sasportes T, Barraud V, Poncelet C, Rudant J, Porcher R, et al. World Health Organization grade 'a' motility and zona-binding test accurately predict IVF outcome for mild male factor and unexplained infertilities. Hum Reprod. 2005;20(10):2769-75.
24. Van den Bergh M, Emiliani S, Biramane J, Vannin AS, Englert Y. A first prospective study of the individual straight-line velocity of the spermatozoon and its influences on the fertilization rate after intracytoplasmic sperm injection. Hum Reprod. 1998;13(11):3103-7.
25. Björndahl L. The usefulness and significance of assessing rapidly progressive spermatozoa. Asian J Androl. 2010;12(1):33-5.
26. Eliasson R. Semen analysis with regard to sperm number, sperm morphology and

functional aspects. Asian J Androl. 2010; 12(1):26-32.
27. Afzelius BA, Eliasson R, Johnsen O, Lindholmer C. Lack of dynein arms in immotile human spermatozoa. J Cell Biol. 1975;66(2):225-32.
28. Chemes EH, Rawe YV. Sperm pathology: a step beyond descriptive morphology. Origin, characterization and fertility potential of abnormal sperm phenotypes in infertile men. Hum Reprod Update. 2003; 9(5):405-28.
29. Wilton LJ, Temple-Smith PD, Baker HW, de Kretser DM. Human male infertility caused by degeneration and death of sperm in the epididymis. Fertil Steril. 1988;49(6): 1052-8.
30. Correa-Perez JR, Fernandez-Pelegrina R, Aslanis P, Zavos PM. Clinical management of men producing ejaculates characterized by high levels of dead sperm and altered seminal plasma factors consistent with epididymal necrospermia. Fertil Steril. 2004;81(4):1148-50.

CHAPTER 17: Sperm Functional Assay

Spondita Banerjee, Neena Malhotra

INTRODUCTION

Infertility is defined as the failure of couples to achieve pregnancy within 12 consecutive months of unprotected intercourse, affecting approximately 4–17% of couples of reproductive ages in India.[1] Fifty percent of these cases are solely due to male infertility. Factors affecting male infertility are varied including genetic and anatomical abnormalities, varicocele, endocrine disorders, systemic diseases, infections, immunological, environmental toxins, lifestyle, radiotherapy, chemotherapy, and medications.[2]

Semen analysis remains the gold standard for the evaluation of male factor infertility with the World Health Organization (WHO) guidelines providing the basis for procedural standardization and reference values worldwide.[3] Conventional semen analysis, based on sperm motility and macroscopic evaluation, may not accurately reflect the fertilization ability of the spermatozoa. Thus, it is essential to explore sperm function tests and overcome the limitations of conventional semen analysis.

IMPORTANCE OF SPERM FUNCTION TEST

Routine semen analysis is based on macroscopic evaluation, sperm count, motility, morphology, and vitality which does not accurately reflect the fertilization potential of the spermatozoa. Semen analysis may classify men as infertile according to the type and degree of spermatogenetic defect, but provides limited information about how well a sperm will function both in in vitro and in vivo. It has limited predictive value for pregnancy outcomes in couples trying to conceive with or without using assisted reproductive technology (ART). Therefore, sperm function tests that predict the fertilization potential of sperms are identified and focus on the steps spermatozoa must undergo before fertilization occurs **(Fig. 1)**. Therefore, sperm function tests directly or indirectly aim to evaluate the steps of fertilization including:[4]
- Process of capacitation of the spermatozoa
- Acquisition of sperm surface proteins required for zona binding and penetration
- Ability to fertilize the egg.

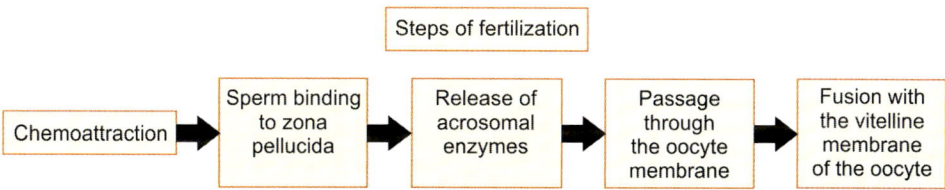

Fig. 1: Steps of fertilization.

The WHO Manual on Semen, 6th Edition, provides a detailed outline on the technical aspects of these tests and some guidance on the interpretation of the test results.[5]

Different Sperm Function Tests

These bioassays include the examination of sperm binding to the zona pellucida (ZP), acrosomal exocytosis, and fusion with the vitelline membrane of the oocyte. The binding of spermatozoa to the ZP initiates the acrosome reaction (AR), releases free, and exposes bound lytic acrosomal components, and allows the spermatozoa to penetrate through the zona matrix, driven by the increased flagellar thrusting of hyperactivated motility. The newly established manual also describes new sperm tests for the assessment of SDF and seminal ovarian stimulation (OS), while abandoning obsolete tests like human cervical mucus (**Flowchart 1**).[6]

Sperm Penetration Assay

Sperm penetration assay (SPA) is one of the first sperm function tests developed,[6] where human spermatozoa are subjected to the hamster oocytes which are devoid of ZP. SPA measures the capacitation ability of spermatozoa, AR, fusion, and penetration through the oolemma and de-condensation within the cytoplasm of hamster oocytes.[7] Vogiatzi et al. reported higher sensitivity (52–100%), specificity (0–100%), and positive predictive value (PPV: 18–100%) and negative predictive value (NPV: 0–100%) in terms of the diagnostic accuracy of SPA.[8]

The standardization and reproducibility of this assay is low. SPA differs from the physiological situation where ZP is absent during the procedure. This is expensive and time-consuming test should conceivably not be routinely used to determine fertility potential until the reproducibility and reliability of the test is improved. The SPA with zona-free hamster ova was widely used in the preintracytoplasmic sperm injection (ICSI) days.

Sperm-Zona Pellucida Binding Assays

The zona plays a major role in controlling fertilization and it is the most potent and only

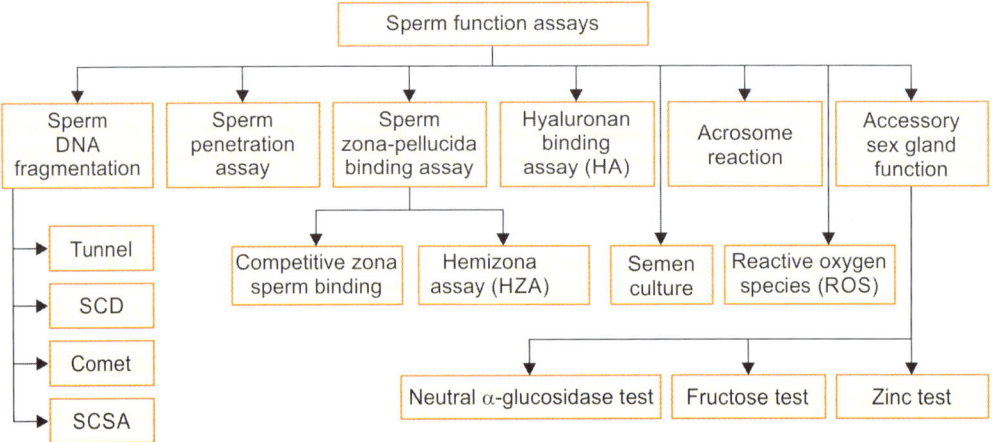

Flowchart 1: Flowchart of different sperm function tests.

(SCD: sperm chromatin dispersion; SCSA: sperm chromatin structure assay)

physiological inducer of the AR and reflects multiple sperm functions (i.e., completion of capacitation). To fertilize a human oocyte, sperm must recognize and tightly bind specific receptors on the zona, which are species specific. The two most commonly used sperm–ZP binding tests are:
1. Hemizona assay (HZA)
2. Competitive zona sperm binding.

Although both assays have different methodologies but they both use assessment of tight binding of sperm to the ZP as the primary endpoint. The HZA is indicated in cases where repeated poor or no fertilization is recorded during IVF therapy or in the presence of moderate-severe oligo-astheno-terato-zoospermia to determine clinical management.[9]

The HZA is an internally controlled bioassay that evaluates the ZP binding potential of the sperm population. The HZA provides a functional homologous test for sperm binding to the ZP during which populations of fertile and infertile spermatozoa are compared within the same assay. The assay uses matching halves of a human ZP from an oocyte with no developmental potential (salt-stored or cadaveric).

The HZA results are expressed as an index known as the hemizona index (HZI), calculated as follows:[10]

$$HZI = \frac{\text{Bound sperm from subfertile male}}{\text{Bound sperm from fertile male}} \times 100$$

In the HZA, sperms from fertile men are used as a control and typically exhibit significantly higher binding capacity to hemizona compared with sperm from infertile patients. Prospective clinical studies reported a cutoff HZI value of 35% as predictive of IVF outcome. Clinical results for IUI therapy showed that the HZI <30 was associated with a significantly lower pregnancy rate compared with patients with HZI >30. Consequently, results of this sperm function test are useful in counseling couples before allocating them into alternative therapeutic methods, that is, IUI versus ICSI.[11]

Patients with poor sperm-zona binding results should be referred to the ICSI. HZA has an excellent predictive power for the outcomes of IUI and IVF, and therefore the assay has a relevance in the clinical diagnostic setting in infertility.

■ ACROSOME REACTION

Sperm binding to the ZP triggers the release of hydrolyzing enzymes and is known as AR. The AR is an exocytotic process of spermatozoa and a prerequisite for fertilization. Only acrosome-reacted spermatozoa are able to pass through the ZP, bind the oocyte plasma membrane, and fuse with the oocyte. The physiological AR occurs at the ZP after sperm binding. The ZP-induced AR can be assessed on spermatozoa removed from the surface of the ZP or exposed to disaggregated human ZP proteins **(Fig. 2)**.[12]

These tests are limited by the restricted availability of human ZPs. Acrosomal status after induction of the AR can be assessed by microscopy, flow cytometry, or fluorescently labeled lectins. The zona-induced AR is calculated as the difference between the stimulated and the spontaneous (unstimulated) AR. Results of different meta-analysis also revealed a high-predictive power of the induced AR tests for the prediction of fertilization AR is currently used for research purposes rather than clinical purposes.[13]

■ HYALURONAN-BINDING ASSAY

Hyaluronic acid binding by human spermatozoa indicates cellular maturity,

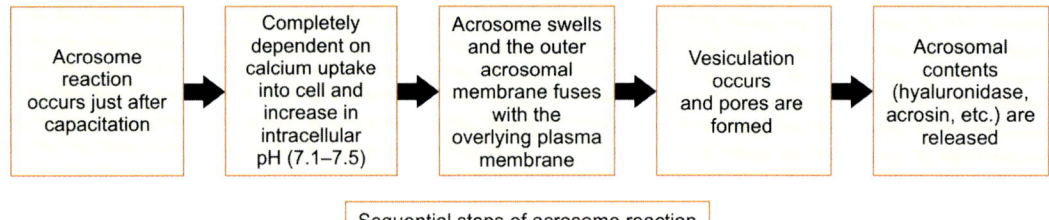

Fig. 2: Steps of acrosome reaction.

viability, and spermatozoa with intact acrosomes. Hyaluronic acid (HA) is a naturally occurring substance and is the major component of the cumulus oophorous matrix surrounds the human oocyte and acts as a natural spermatozoa selector. Human spermatozoa express HA receptors and only mature (completed spermatogenesis), motile spermatozoa bind to hyaluronan through specific receptors.[8]

The bound sperms are differentiated from unbound sperm by their beating tails with heads and make no progressive movement. Furthermore, hyaluronan-binding assay (HBA) represents a more convenient and reproducible laboratory test for identifying correct patient for ICSI or IVF.

Two methods have been examined for the selection of ideal sperm with high expression of HA activity: the HA culture dish [PICSI (physiological intracytoplasmic sperm injection) Sperm Selection Device] and viscous medium containing HA (sperm-slow). HA sperms are bound by the head to the bottom, however, in sperm-slow HA, spermatozoa have a very slow motility.

However, in clinical practice, the rates of achieving embryos of improved quality were similar between two groups.[14] Evidence is insufficient to show whether sperm selection by HA binding improves live birth or pregnancy rates in ART.

SEMEN CULTURE

Leukocytes, also known as polymorphonuclear leukocytes (neutrophils), are present in most human semen ejaculates. The size of the nucleus can further be used to help to distinguish between monocytes, lymphocytes (approximately 7 um), and macrophages (approximately 15 um), even if their functional changes cause an abnormal level of variability in this parameter.

The detection of leukocytes in human semen is performed by the use of cytochemistry to identify a peroxidase enzyme that is present in granulocytes. Leukocytospermia is a significant factor associated with high reactive oxygen species (ROS) levels, resulting in DNA damage and poor sperm quality. Quantification of leukocytes in the semen is important as they may indicate an underlying inflammation and infection of the male genitourinary tract.

A commercial kit LeukoChek*, CryoLab for this test is available. This technique has, however, two major disadvantages: (1) It does not detect activated granulocytes that have released their granules and (2) It does not detect other types of leukocytes that do not express peroxidase, such as lymphocytes, macrophages, and monocytes. The peroxidase staining by Endtz test, although is not the gold standard, is simple, practical, and provides reliable results and would certainly be helpful in the management of infertile men.[15]

BIOCHEMICAL ASSAYS FOR ACCESSORY SEX GLAND FUNCTION

Poor-quality semen may result from abnormal accessory gland secretions. Zinc has a probable role in protecting and stabilizing condensed sperm chromatin. Fructose is secreted by seminal vesicles and provides an energy source to spermatozoa for anaerobic metabolism. This is an important energy source for the sperm and exclusion of the seminal vesicular component from the ejaculate will result in almost completely immotile sperm.

Secretions from accessory glands can be measured to assess gland function, e.g., citric acid, zinc, glutamyl transpeptidase, and acid phosphatase for the prostate; fructose and prostaglandins for the seminal vesicles; and free L-carnitine, glycero-phosphocholine (GPC), and neutral α-glucosidase for the epididymis. An infection in any of the glands can sometimes cause a temporary decrease in the secretion of markers. An infection can also cause irreversible damage to the secretory epithelium, so that even after the acute infection the secretion may remain low.

- *Secretory markers of the prostate:* The amount of zinc, citric acid, or acid phosphatase in semen gives a reliable measure of prostate gland secretion, and there are good correlations between these markers. A spectrophotometric assay for zinc.
- *Secretory markers of the seminal vesicles:* Fructose in semen reflects the secretory function of the seminal vesicles. A spectrophotometric method for its estimation.
- *Secretory markers of the epididymis:* L-carnitine, GPC, and neutral α-glucosidase are epididymal markers used clinically. Neutral α-glucosidase has been shown to be more specific and sensitive for epididymal disorders than L-carnitine and GPC. There are two isoforms of α-glucosidase in the ejaculate: the major, neutral form originates solely from the epididymis, and the minor, acidic form mainly from the prostate.

A simple spectrophotometric estimation method is used for zinc, fructose, and neutral α-glucosidase. Fructose levels should be determined in any patient with azoospermia and especially in those whose ejaculate volume is <1 mL, suggesting seminal obstruction or atresia or ejaculatory tract duct obstruction.

Disorders of the seminal vesicles subsequently reduces fructose concentration in semen that results in a reduced motility of sperm. Another condition is polyzoospermia and low motility due to deficiency of fructose. It is important for both qualitative and quantitative estimation of fructose while evaluating patients of male infertility through commercially available reagents.[16]

Reactive Oxygen Species Levels

Oxidative stress (OS) has been shown to be a major contributing cause of male infertility due to numerous medical conditions, including varicocele, leukocytospermia, diabetes mellitus, and obesity. OS negatively affects all sperm functions, including sperm DNA integrity, and thereby the fertilization process and reproductive outcomes. Spermatozoa are particularly susceptible to ROS-induced damage compared to other cells as they have relatively large quantities of polyunsaturated fatty acids in the membrane, and their cytoplasm contains a low concentration of scavenging enzymes.[17]

ROS can be estimated in whole ejaculate using various chemiluminescence methods or by semi-quantitative assays using oxidative indicators. Therefore, seminal OS can be used as a diagnostic parameter to predict sperm fertilizing potential. Personalized lifestyle and antioxidant intervention may potentially improve the fertility of subfertile couples.

Sperm DNA Fragmentation

Sperm DNA undergoes compaction during the process of spermatogenesis. The sperm DNA encircles histone proteins which gradually undergo condensation and substituted by highly basic protamine. Torsional stress is exerted by dsDNA during the process of condensation resulting in nicks and breaks in the DNA. SDF is also caused by oxidative stress, varicocele, infections, inflammation of the male genital tract, drugs, chemotherapy, radiotherapy, cancer, obesity, advanced age, as well as environmental pollutants and toxins **(Fig. 3)**. This testing is a prerequisite for proper embryo development, implantation, and pregnancy.

The 6th edition describes and elaborates on different methods of SDF testing—direct and indirect sperm DNA fragmentation. Direct SDF includes the TUNEL assay, Acridine Orange assay, and Comet assay. Except for the Comet assay, these tests are deemed useful for clinical testing. Indirect testing includes toluidine blue staining, chromomycin A3 staining, and sperm chromatin dispersion assay.[18]

Direct Sperm DNA Fragmentation Tests

- *Terminal deoxynucleotidyl transferase dUTP nick-end labeling (TUNEL):* TUNEL assay is used to identify "nicks," or free ends of DNA by using fluorescent nucleotides. The TUNEL assay was invented by Mitchell et al. The principle uses relaxing the whole chromatin structure before fixation to permit contact with all "nicks". The assay measures the integration of dUTP into dsDNA or ssDNA breaks via an enzymatic reaction. It further creates an indication that is multiplied by the number of DNA breaks. Evaluation of the sample is carried out through a standard fluorescence microscope. The test is

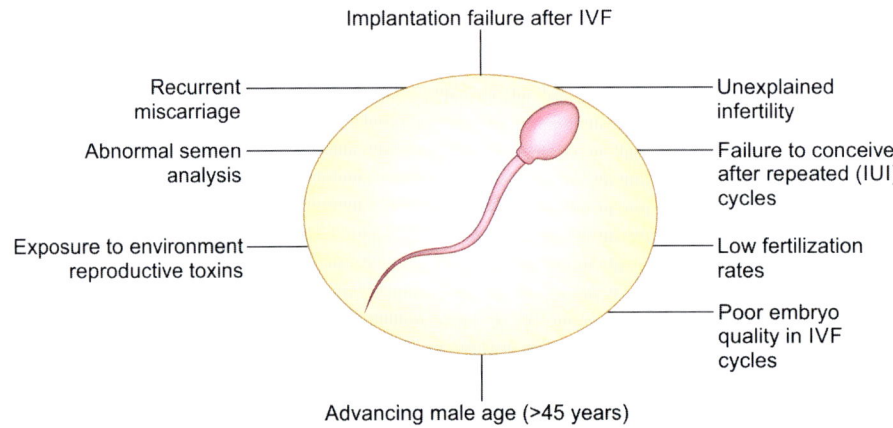

Fig. 3: Indications of sperm DNA fragmentation. (IUI: intrauterine insemination; IVF: in vitro fertilization)

limited by the lack of strict standardization which makes the comparison between laboratories more difficult.

- *Single-cell gel electrophoresis assay (Comet):* Single-cell gel electrophoresis or Comet assay quantifies the aggregate of DNA damage per spermatozoon, as a single cell can be followed on the gel. This test can detect sperm DNA damage at a single-cell level, it can be used for the assessment of cases with severe oligozoospermia. The staining power of the comet test depends on the quantity of migrated DNA, which is an indication of different degrees of SDF. Comet assay can not only detect ss and ds breaks but also identify altered bases. The method is inappropriate for quick diagnosis because of its ability to analyze different kinds of DNA damage in a single cell by utilizing electrophoresis. The information generated in this assay requires highly experienced staff for the analysis of results.

Indirect Sperm DNA Fragmentation Tests

- *Sperm chromatin structure assay (SCSA):* Sperm chromatin structure assay evaluates the susceptibility of sperm DNA to denaturation. The principle underlying SCSA is based on increased susceptibility of abnormal chromatin structure in the sperm DNA to acid or heat denaturation and uses metachromatic characteristics of AO for this purpose. This is a flow cytometry-based assay that assesses a large number of cells quickly and strongly. It has the advantage of a standardized protocol for lowering interlaboratory differences. DNA fragmentation index (DFI) is used in SCSA as the measure of SDF.

- *Sperm chromatin dispersion test (SCD):* The principle underlying the SCD test is that sperm with fragmented DNA fails to produce the characteristic halo of dispersed DNA loops after acid denaturation and removal of nuclear proteins, normally seen in sperms with nonfragmented DNA. The test is also known as Halosperm® test (patented by Halotech). There is no requirement for complex instruments and has limitation by the interobserver variation resulting from its feature of subjective evaluation under the microscope.

The halos of the spermatozoa in the samples can be classified according to the criteria of Fernández et al.:[19]

- *Large:* Halo width is similar to or larger than the minor diameter of the core.
- *Medium:* Halo size is between those with large and with small halo.
- *Small:* Halo width is similar to or smaller than one-third of the minor diameter of the core.
- *Without halo/Without halo-degraded:* Those that show no halo and present a core irregularly or weakly stained. This category is associated with severe damage affecting both DNA and protein compound.

Interpretation of DFI using the halo-sperm tests are:
- <20% DFI = Good fertility potential
- >20 to <30% DFI = Suspicious
- >30% DFI = Clinically significant.

EVIDENCES ON SPERM FUNCTION TESTS IN CLINICAL PRACTICE

The most commonly investigated sperm function tests are AR test, sperm capacitation test, hemi-zona-binding assay, sperm

DNA fragmentation test, seminal ROS test, mitochondrial dysfunction tests, antisperm antibody test, nuclear chromatin decondensation (NCD) test, and hypo-osmotic swelling test. The different advance sperm function tests analyze different aspects of sperm function. Hence, any one test may not be helpful to appropriately predict the male fertility potential. Therefore, a battery of tests may be needed to declare sperms competent that evaluate the AR and binding abilities, besides DNA fragmentation and immune stability. Currently, the unavailability of high-quality clinical data, robust thresholds, complex protocols, high cost, there is no convincing evidence to offer sperm function tests routinely. The above reasons are thus prohibiting the current usage of sperm function tests to evaluate the male partner comprehensively.[20]

Semen parameters were shown to be negatively correlated with sDNA fragment and sperm aneuploidies. As sDNA fragmentation testing and sperm aneuploidy testing were associated with semen abnormalities and male age, it is suggested their inclusion in the routine evaluation of infertile men, thus adding important complementary information about the fertility status **(Flowchart 2)**.[21] A systematic review by Sugihara A, et al. suggest lack of evidence to use sperm DNA fragmentation tests in the routine work-up of couples undergoing IUI.[22] This is in line with the conclusion formulated by the ASRM Opinion Committee[23] which recognizes the value of the research on DNA fragmentation but does not recommend routine testing in the clinical setting.

A major goal of new tests should be the identification of molecular defects in sperm function, allowing rapid development of biochemical tests, with the goal to specifically target therapies toward male subfertility. Tests with high sensitivity, high predictive

Flowchart 2: Algorithm presenting the diagnostic-therapeutic evaluation of sperm function test.

(ICSI: intracytoplasmic sperm injection; IUI: intrauterine insemination; IVF: in vitro fertilization)

value, and low false positive rate are desirable. Sperm function test should not be routine investigations as they are complex, expensive, not rigorously tested, the present sperm function assays are highly predictive of IUI/IVF results. However, the implementation of ICSI has basically eliminated the need for such tests. If patients fail sperm functional testing, then it would eliminate the time, effort, and expense of couples undergoing lower complexity therapies such as IUI and direct them to ICSI without delay.

Future sperm function tests need to accurately predict the success of fertilization in vitro and whether the progeny will be healthy. Multicentric clinical trials are essential for developing robust thresholds to integrate sperm function test especially DNA tests into routine clinical practice as they could predict ART clinical outcome. They must have strong predictive value for pregnancy outcome and have little overlap between fertile and infertile samples Moreover, tests that are simple, cheap, reliable, and repeatable will be effective combined with more robust assessments.

This may include using epigenetics and deep sequencing studies for clinical diagnosis of male infertility to discover spermatozoan epigenetic disorders, spermatozoan small noncoding RNA defects and other subtle genetic abnormalities that may impact fertilizing potential and the outcome of the progeny.[24]

■ CONCLUSION

The medical professionals providing care to infertility patients should focus on providing the best care to the patients and the child yet to be born, without ignoring the health of the sperm. We must also confront the fact that ICSI is overused and the male factor is commonly overlooked. The existing data clearly indicate that sperm DNA damage is associated with reproductive health issues in the male and in the embryo. Thus, the use of sperm DNA testing is evidence-based and should be implemented by ART clinics.

The primary objectives are to improve IUI and ART success, but more importantly, to improve the health of the father and resulting offspring. It is our expectation that advances in molecular biology techniques may allow for the development of simpler assays, may be based on recombinant proteins or analogs, in the form of different assays, leading to simpler, improved, and physiologically oriented sperm–ZP binding and AR assays. These newly developed assays may indeed have a true impact on the implementation of novel diagnostic and therapeutic changes for optimized management of male factor infertility.

■ KEY LEARNING POINTS

- Conventional semen analysis does not reflect fertilization ability of the spermatozoa.
- WHO Manual on Semen, 6th Edition provides a detailed technical aspects of sperm function tests.
- Sperm function focuses on the steps, a spermatozoon must undergo before fertilization occurs.
- Commonly used sperm function tests are: sperm penetration assay, sperm-zona pellucida binding test (hemizona assay), acrosomal reaction test, hyaluronan-binding test, sperm DNA fragmentation, etc.
- Utility of different sperm function tests are assessed based on its fertility predictive value.
- Clinical practice algorithm for improving IUI and ART success.

- Tests with high sensitivity, predictive value, and low false positive rates are desirable in future.

REFERENCES

1. Purkayastha N, Sharma H. Prevalence and potential determinants of primary infertility in India: Evidence from Indian demographic health survey. Clin Epidemiol Global Health. 2021;9:162-70.
2. Alahmar AT, Singh R, Palani A. Sperm DNA fragmentation in reproductive medicine: a review. J Hum Reprod Sci. 2022;15(3):206-18.
3. Boitrelle F, Shah R, Saleh R, Henkel R, Kandil H, Chung E, et al. The Sixth Edition of the WHO Manual for Human Semen Analysis: A Critical Review and SWOT Analysis. Life. 2021;11:1368.
4. Kızılay F, Altay B. Sperm function tests in clinical practice. Turk J Urol. 2017;43(4):393-400.
5. WHO. (2021). WHO laboratory manual for the examination and processing of human semen, 6th Edition, 2021. [online] Available from: https://www.who.int/publications-detail-redirect/9789240030787 [Last accessed January, 2024].
6. Esteves SC, Sharma RK, Thomas AJ, Jr, Agarwal A. Effect of in vitro incubation on spontaneous acrosome reaction in fresh and cryopreserved human spermatozoa. Int J Fertil Women Med. 1997;43:235-42.
7. Rogers BJ, van Campen H, Ueno M, Lambert H, Bronson R, Hale R. Analysis of human spermatozoal fertilizing ability using zona-free ova. Fertil Steril. 1979;32:664-70.
8. Oehninger S, Franken DR, Sayed E, Barroso G, Kolm P. Sperm function assays and their predictive value for fertilization outcome in IVF therapy: a meta-analysis. Hum Reprod Update. 2000;6:160-8.
9. Vogiatzi P, Chrelias C, Cahill DJ, Creatsa M, Vrachnis N, Iliodromiti Z, et al. Hemizona assay and sperm penetration assay in the prediction of IVF outcome: a systematic review. Biomed Res Int. 2013;2013:945825.
10. Oehninger S. Clinical and laboratory management of male infertility: an opinion on its current status. J Androl. 2000;21:814-21.
11. Burkman LJ, Coddington CC, Franken DR, Kruger TF, Rosenwaks Z, Hodgen GD. The hemizona assay (HZA): development of a diagnostic test for the binding of human spermatozoa to the human hemizona pellucida to predict fertilization potential. Fertil Steril. 1988;49:688-97.
12. Arslan M, Morshedi M, Arslan EO, Taylor S, Kanik A, Duran HE, et al. Predictive value of the hemizona assay for pregnancy outcome in patients undergoing controlled ovarian hyperstimulation with intrauterine insemination. Fertil Steril. 2006;85:1697-707.
13. Yanagimachi R. Mammalian fertilization. in: Knobil E, Neill JD (eds). The Physiology of Reproduction, 2nd edition. New York: Raven Press, Ltd.; 1994; pp. 189-317.
14. Oehninger S, Franken DR, Ombelet W. Sperm functional tests. Fertil Steril. 2014; 102(6):1528-33.
15. Parmegiani L, Cognigni GE, Bernardi S, Troilo E, Taraborrelli S, Arnone A, et al. Comparison of two ready-to-use systems designed for sperm–hyaluronic acid binding selection before intracytoplasmic sperm injection: PICSI vs. Sperm Slow: a prospective, randomized trial. Fertil Steril. 2012;98:632-7.
16. Sharma R, Gupta S, Agarwal A, Henkel R, Finelli R, Parekh N, et al. Relevance of leukocytospermia and semen culture and its true place in diagnosing and treating male infertility: review. World J Mens Health. 2022;40(2):191-207.
17. Talwar P, Hayatnagarkar S. Sperm function test. J Hum Reprod Sci. 2015;8:61-9.
18. Henkel R, Kierspel E, Stalf T, Mehnert C, Menkveld R, Tinneberg HR, et al. Effect of reactive oxygen species produced by spermatozoa and leukocytes on sperm functions in non-leukocytospermic patients. Fertil Steril. 2005;83:635-42.
19. Sugihara A, Avermaete F, Roelant E, Punjabi U, Neubourg DD. The role of sperm DNA fragmentation testing in predicting intra-uterine insemination outcome: a systematic review and meta-analysis. Eur J Obstet Gynecol Reprod Biol. 2020;244:8-15.

20. Fernández JL, Muriel L, Goyanes V, Segrelles E, Gosálvez J, Enciso M, et al. Simple determination of human sperm DNA fragmentation with an improved sperm chromatin dispersion test. Fertil Steril. 2005;84(4):833-42.
21. Sanyal D, Arya D, Nishi K, Balasinor N, Singh D. Clinical utility of sperm function tests in predicting male fertility: a systematic review. Reprod Sci. 2023.
22. Maia M, Almeida C, Cunha M, Gonçalves A, Soares SS, Severo M, et al. P-042 Impact of semen parameters, sperm DNA fragmentation and sperm aneuploidy in male infertility. Hum Reprod. 2021;36(1): deab130.041.
23. ASRM. The clinical utility of sperm DNA integrity testing: a guideline. Fertil Steril. 2013;99(3):673-7.
24. Wang C, Swerdloff RS. Limitations of semen analysis as a test of male fertility and anticipated needs from newer tests. Fertil Steril. 2014;102(6):1502-7.

CHAPTER 18

Optimizing Sperm Preparation for Intrauterine Insemination

Keshav Malhotra

OVERVIEW OF THE SPERM PREPARATION PROCESS

Sperm preparation is a crucial step in the intrauterine insemination (IUI) process,[1] aimed at enhancing the quality and concentration of sperm before introducing them into the female reproductive system. This section provides a fundamental understanding of the steps involved in sperm preparation:
- *Collection:* Sperm is typically collected through ejaculation into a sterile container. The collection process can be done at the fertility clinic or at home, depending on the specific requirements of the procedure.
- *Initial processing:* Once collected, the semen undergoes initial processing to remove the seminal fluid. This step helps to concentrate the sperm, providing a more potent sample for insemination.
- *Centrifugation:* The processed semen is subjected to centrifugation, a technique that separates sperm from other components based on their density. This step is pivotal in isolating the most motile and viable sperm for IUI.

SIGNIFICANCE OF SPERM QUALITY IN INTRAUTERINE INSEMINATION SUCCESS

The success of IUI is significantly influenced by the quality of prepared sperm.[1] This subsection highlights the importance of various sperm parameters, including:
- *Motility:* Progressive and rapid sperm motility is crucial for sperm to navigate through the female reproductive tract and reach the egg successfully.
- *Viability:* The percentage of live sperm in the prepared sample is a key determinant of its fertilization potential.
- *Concentration:* Achieving an optimal sperm concentration ensures that an adequate number of sperm are available for successful fertilization.

FACTORS AFFECTING SPERM MOTILITY AND VIABILITY

Understanding the factors that impact sperm motility and viability is essential for effective sperm preparation. This subsection explores various factors such as:
- *Temperature control:* Maintaining an optimal temperature during the sperm preparation process to prevent thermal stress and damage.
- *pH levels:* The importance of maintaining proper pH levels to support sperm function and prevent adverse effects on motility.
- *Oxygen levels:* Managing oxygen levels to avoid oxidative stress, which can negatively impact sperm viability.

In mastering the basics of sperm preparation, clinicians and laboratory staff can lay the foundation for successful IUI outcomes. The subsequent sections will delve deeper into specific techniques and advancements in the field, providing a comprehensive guide for optimizing sperm preparation.

TECHNIQUES FOR SPERM PREPARATION[1-3]

Numerous methods are available for sperm preparation, but they can generally be categorized into three main groups.

Initially, spermatozoa can be chosen based on their swimming ability, a method known as the "swim-up technique". In this procedure, culture medium is layered over liquefied semen, and motile spermatozoa move up into the culture. The upper layer of the medium is then carefully extracted for further use.

A second method involves selecting spermatozoa through density gradients. The semen sample is placed on top of a density column and then subjected to centrifugation. This process separates spermatozoa based on their density, allowing for the selection of motile and morphologically normal spermatozoa in the solution with the highest gradient concentration. This selected solution is aspirated for further use. Density gradient centrifugation has been a standard technique in assisted reproductive techniques, initially using Percoll gradients and later replaced with silica stabilized with covalently bound hydrophilic silane.

The third method combines the conventional wash technique with centrifugation, traditionally employed for diagnostic purposes. In this approach, the semen sample is diluted with a medium, centrifuged, and the resulting pellet is resuspended in a small amount of medium until the time of insemination.

While the swim-up technique is the oldest and most commonly used method, particularly in IUI and in vitro fertilization (IVF) laboratories worldwide, density gradient techniques offer easier standardization and more consistent results. The choice of sperm preparation technique is often guided by the nature of the semen sample. The swim-up technique is frequently employed when semen samples are predominantly considered normal, whereas density gradient techniques may be preferred in cases of male factor infertility due to the greatest total number of recovered motile spermatozoa.

CENTRIFUGATION METHODS

Centrifugation is a fundamental technique in sperm preparation, facilitating the separation of sperm from seminal plasma based on differences in density. This section explores various centrifugation methods employed in the preparation process:

- *Centrifugation:* This method involves spinning the semen sample at different speeds to separate sperm from seminal fluid and debris. It is a traditional yet effective approach.
- *Density gradient centrifugation (DGC):* DGC is a more sophisticated technique that utilizes density gradients, typically composed of colloidal silica or other materials. Sperm are layered on top of the gradient and then centrifuged, allowing for the isolation of highly motile sperm from the gradient.

SWIM-UP TECHNIQUE

The swim-up technique is an alternative to centrifugation, relying on the natural ability of sperm to swim against gravity. This section delves into the swim-up technique:

- *Procedure:* The prepared semen is layered on a medium, and sperm with enhanced

motility swim up into a separate layer over time. This upper layer is then collected for IUI.
- *Advantages:* The swim-up technique is considered gentler on sperm compared to centrifugation, reducing the risk of damage, and maintaining sperm quality.
- *Limitations:* It may yield lower sperm concentrations compared to centrifugation, making it more suitable for cases with higher sperm counts.

COMPARATIVE ANALYSIS OF TECHNIQUES

This section provides a comparative analysis of the various sperm preparation techniques, considering factors such as:
- *Efficacy:* The ability of each technique to achieve optimal sperm concentration and quality.
- *Sperm viability:* Assessing the impact of each technique on sperm viability and motility.
- *Clinical considerations:* Tailoring the choice of technique to specific patient profiles, including sperm count and motility.
- *Cost and resources:* Considering the practicality of each technique in terms of laboratory resources and associated costs.

PROTOCOLS

The nature of the sperm sample and its intended use determine the sperm preparation process. Sperm preparation approaches for assisted reproduction, such as IVF, must produce a sperm population with low DNA damage. An ideal sperm preparation procedure should yield a highly functional sperm population that maintains DNA and does not cause dysfunction due to reactive oxygen species (ROS) generated by sperms and the leukocytes. The recovered sperms from different types of processing should have appropriate morphology and functional motility.

Required Reagents
- HEPES (4-(2-hydroxyethyl)-1-piperazineethanesulfonic acid)/MOPS (3-(N-morpholino)propanesulfonic acid) buffer media
- Density gradient media 90 and 45%
- Sperm washing media/HTF.

Required Equipment
- Laminar air flow hood
- Incubator Heracell
- Compound microscope
- Spermifuge/Centrifuge
- IVF witness system.

Required Disposables
- Conical test tubes
- Round bottom test tubes
- Serological pipette with pump
- Pasteur pipette
- Microscopic glass slides and glass slips.

Discontinuous Density Gradient Technique

It separates spermatozoa based on their density, and each spermatozoon is found at the gradient level that corresponds to its density at the end of each centrifugation. Furthermore, a typically normal morphological spermatozoon has a density of at least 1.10 g/mL, but an aberrant one has a density of 1.06–1.09 g/mL.

This method involves centrifuging sperm through density gradients made of colloidal silica covered with silane, which separate cells only on the basis of density.

Procedure:
1. In the 15 mL conical tube, add 1 mL of lower phase (90 or 80%).

2. Pour 1 mL of the upper phase (45 or 40%) on top of the lower phase without mixing the two gradients.
3. Now, add 2 mL liquefied semen sample and centrifuge at 1,500 rpm for 15–20 minutes.
4. Remove the supernatant from the tube without disturbing the pellet at the bottom.
5. To the pellet add 4 mL of sperm wash media (HTF) and mix.
6. Centrifuge for 10 minutes at 1,000 rpm, discard the supernatant, without disturbing the pellet.
7. Add 0.3 mL of fertilization media to the pellet and allow swim up in the incubator for 10–15 minutes.
8. Post-wash analysis should be done to check the motility and concentration of the sperms.

Simple Wash Technique

If the semen samples are of good quality, this simple washing process provides a high yield of spermatozoa, but it does not remove debris or leukocytes from the semen.

Procedure:
1. Mix the sperm sample thoroughly.
2. To remove seminal plasma, dilute the entire semen sample 1 + 1 (1:2) with medium (MOPS/HEPES).
3. Centrifuge for 5 minutes at 1,000 rpm.
4. Carefully aspirate the supernatant and discard it.
5. Resuspend the sperm pellet, in a volume of medium appropriate for final disposition by means of gentle pipetting.

Direct Swim-up Technique

The capacity of spermatozoa to swim out of seminal plasma and into culture media may be used to select them. Prior to swim-up, the semen should not be diluted or centrifuged, since this can induce peroxidative damage to the sperm membranes.

Procedure:
1. Add 1 mL of sperm wash medium/HEPES in falcon sterile round bottom tube.
2. Allow semen to liquefy before preparing it.
3. Gently underlay liquefied semen sample 1 mL in the sterile tube's bottom.
4. Place the round bottom tube in incubator at 45° for 30–60 minutes with tube firmly capped. The sperm cells that are motile move upward in the sperm wash media.

POSTSPERM PREPARATION STEPS[4-7]

Sperm analysis:
- *Concentration:* The concentration of sperm in the prepared sample is determined to ensure an adequate number for successful fertilization.
- *Motility:* The motility of the sperm is assessed to ensure that they have the capability to navigate the female reproductive tract and reach the egg.
- *Viability:* The percentage of live and healthy sperm in the prepared sample is evaluated.

Quality control checks:
- The laboratory performs quality control checks to ensure that the sperm preparation process was conducted according to established protocols.
- Any deviations or irregularities may prompt additional steps or adjustments.

Timing for IUI procedure:
- The timing of the IUI procedure is crucial and is often synchronized with the woman's ovulation cycle.

- Ultrasound monitoring and hormonal assessments help to determine the optimal time for the IUI, usually within 24–36 hours of ovulation.

Preparation for IUI:
- The prepared sperm sample is loaded into a thin, flexible catheter that is inserted through the cervix into the uterus.
- The woman may be positioned on an examination table, and the IUI procedure is typically performed in a clinical setting.

IUI procedure:
- The insemination procedure involves depositing the prepared sperm directly into the woman's uterus, increasing the chances of sperm reaching the egg for fertilization.
- The procedure is relatively quick and is generally well-tolerated by most patients.

Post-IUI monitoring:
- After the IUI procedure, some clinics may provide postprocedure monitoring, and patients may be advised to rest for a short period before resuming normal activities.

Post-IUI care and follow-up:
- Patients may receive guidance on post-IUI care, including any restrictions or recommendations for activities.
- A follow-up plan may be established to monitor progress, and a pregnancy test is typically scheduled about 10–14 days after the IUI to determine its success.

It is important to note that the entire process, from sperm collection to post-IUI follow-up, is a collaborative effort between the healthcare provider, the laboratory team, and the patient. Detailed instructions and guidance are typically provided to patients at each step of the process. The success of the IUI procedure can be influenced by various factors,[7] including the quality of the prepared sperm, the timing of the procedure, and individual patient factors.

Based on Cochrane review in terms of the quality of evidence, it is unclear whether there exists a distinction in clinical pregnancy rates (CPR) between the swim-up technique and the gradient technique. The odds ratio (OR) was 0.83 with a 95% confidence interval (CI) from 0.51 to 1.35, and there was considerable heterogeneity ($I^2 = 71\%$). Based on four randomized-controlled trials (RCTs) involving 370 participants, the evidence is of very low quality. The findings suggest that assuming a 24% chance of pregnancy with the gradient technique, the likelihood of pregnancy with the swim-up technique falls between 14 and 30%.

Furthermore, uncertainties persist regarding ongoing pregnancy rates per couple. The OR was 0.39 with a 95% CI from 0.19 to 0.82, and heterogeneity was not applicable. This conclusion is based on one RCT involving 223 participants, and the evidence quality is very low.

Examining multiple pregnancy rates (MPR) per couple, there is uncertainty about the differences between the swim-up and gradient techniques, as both methods resulted in an MPR of 0%. This conclusion is based on one RCT with 25 participants, and the evidence quality is very low.

Similarly, uncertainties prevail regarding miscarriage rates (MR) per couple. The OR was 0.85 with a 95% CI from 0.28 to 2.59, and there was heterogeneity ($I^2 = 44\%$). This conclusion is drawn from three RCTs involving 330 participants, and the evidence quality is very low.

It is important to note that no studies provided information on ectopic pregnancy rate, fetal abnormalities, or infection rate in the context of comparing the swim-up and gradient techniques.

CHAPTER 18: Optimizing Sperm Preparation for Intrauterine Insemination

MICROFLUIDIC DEVICES

Overview of Microfluidic Technology

- Principle:
  - Microfluidic devices utilize tiny channels and chambers to manipulate fluids on a microscale.
  - Provide a controlled environment for sperm selection and preparation.

Advantages and Limitations

- Advantages:
  - Improved precision in selecting highly motile and viable sperm.
  - Reduction in processing time compared to traditional methods.
  - Potential for lower sperm sample volumes, minimizing discomfort for the patient.
- Limitations:
  - Initial cost and resource investment for adopting microfluidic technology.
  - Ongoing research to optimize and standardize protocols.

Current Research and Future Prospects

- Current applications:
  - Microfluidic devices are being used for sperm selection in assisted reproductive technologies (ART), including IUI and IVF.
  - Ongoing studies explore the integration of microfluidics into point-of-care fertility diagnostics.
- Future directions:
  - Research is focused on expanding the capabilities of microfluidic devices, potentially incorporating real-time monitoring and analysis.
  - Exploration of personalized microfluidic systems tailored to individual patient profiles.

FACTORS INFLUENCING SPERM QUALITY[5]

Lifestyle and Environmental Factors

Impact of Diet and Nutrition

Balanced diet and sperm health: A well-balanced diet plays a pivotal role in supporting overall health, including reproductive function. Here, we explore the specific ways in which diet and nutrition influence sperm quality.

Essential nutrients for sperm health:

- Zinc:
  - *Role in sperm production:* Zinc is a crucial mineral for the synthesis of DNA and proteins, essential for sperm production (spermatogenesis).
  - *Antioxidant properties:* Acts as an antioxidant, protecting sperm from oxidative damage and supporting overall sperm quality.
  - *Food sources:* Include zinc-rich foods in the diet, such as lean meats, poultry, seafood, nuts, seeds, and dairy products.
- Selenium:
  - *Sperm motility:* Selenium is important for sperm motility, and a deficiency can impact the movement and function of sperm.
  - *Antioxidant action:* Like zinc, selenium functions as an antioxidant, helping to neutralize free radicals that can harm sperm.
  - *Food sources:* Incorporate selenium through foods such as Brazil nuts, fish, poultry, eggs, and whole grains.
- Vitamin C:
  - *Antioxidant support:* Vitamin C is a powerful antioxidant that protects sperm from oxidative stress, helping to maintain sperm viability.

- *Collagen synthesis:* Supports collagen synthesis, crucial for the structural integrity of various reproductive organs.
- *Food sources:* Citrus fruits, strawberries, kiwi, bell peppers, and broccoli are excellent sources of vitamin C.
■ Vitamin D:
- *Regulation of hormones:* Vitamin D plays a role in regulating hormonal balance, which is essential for normal sperm production.
- *Sperm motility:* Adequate vitamin D levels are associated with better sperm motility.
- *Food sources:* While vitamin D is synthesized in the skin through exposure to sunlight, dietary sources include fatty fish, fortified dairy products, and egg yolks.
■ Omega-3 fatty acids:
- *Cell membrane structure:* Omega-3 fatty acids contribute to the structural integrity of sperm cell membranes, affecting sperm motility and viability.
- *Anti-inflammatory properties:* Possess anti-inflammatory properties that may benefit reproductive health.
- *Food sources:* Include fatty fish (salmon and mackerel), flaxseeds, chia seeds, and walnuts in the diet.

Antioxidants and Sperm Protection

■ Importance of antioxidants for sperm health:
- *Neutralizing free radicals:* Antioxidants play a crucial role in neutralizing free radicals, which are reactive molecules that can cause oxidative stress.
- *Preserving sperm viability:* By counteracting oxidative stress, antioxidants help to preserve the viability and function of sperm, including motility and DNA integrity.
■ Common antioxidants in sperm health:
■ Vitamin C:
- *Sperm protection:* Vitamin C is a potent antioxidant that shields sperm from oxidative damage.
- *Collaboration with vitamin E:* Works synergistically with vitamin E to enhance its antioxidant effects.
■ Vitamin E:
- *Membrane protection:* Vitamin E protects the integrity of sperm cell membranes, crucial for maintaining sperm structure and function.
- *Sperm DNA integrity:* Contributes to the preservation of sperm DNA integrity.
■ Selenium:
- *Sperm motility:* Selenium, as an antioxidant, supports sperm motility by preventing oxidative stress-induced damage.
- *Collaboration with enzymes:* Works with selenoproteins, essential antioxidant enzymes, in safeguarding sperm health.

Staff Training and Competency[5]

Continuous Education

■ Provide ongoing training programs for laboratory staff to keep them abreast of the latest techniques and technologies.
■ Ensure that staff is well-trained in advanced sperm preparation methods.

Competency Assessments

■ Conduct regular competency assessments to verify that staff members consistently meet or exceed established standards.
■ Encourage a culture of continuous learning and improvement within the laboratory team.

Quality Assurance for Equipment and Reagents[4,5]

Equipment Calibration and Validation

- Regularly calibrate and validate laboratory equipment to ensure accuracy in measurements and procedures.
- Maintain detailed records of equipment maintenance and calibration.

Quality-controlled Reagents

- Source high-quality reagents and ensure their proper storage.
- Conduct routine quality control checks on reagents to confirm their effectiveness.

CONCLUSION

As technology advances and our understanding of reproductive science deepens, the optimization of sperm preparation for IUI continues to evolve. This chapter provides a comprehensive guide, amalgamating scientific insights, technological innovations, and practical recommendations to empower clinicians, embryologists, and patients in enhancing the success of IUI treatments.

KEY LEARNING POINTS

- Sperm preparation is a crucial step in the intrauterine insemination (IUI) process.
- Understanding the factors that impact sperm motility and viability is essential for effective sperm preparation.
- It is important to note that the entire process, from sperm collection to post-IUI follow-up, is a collaborative effort between the healthcare provider, the laboratory team, and the patient.
- Research is focused on expanding the capabilities of microfluidic devices, potentially incorporating real-time monitoring and analysis.

REFERENCES

1. Carrell DT, Kuneck PH, Peterson CM, Hatasaka HH, Jones KP, Campbell BF. A randomized, prospective analysis of five sperm preparation techniques before intrauterine insemination of husband sperm. Fertil Steril. 1998;69(1):122-6.
2. Dodson WC, Moessner J, Miller J, Legro RS, Gnatuk CL. A randomized comparison of the methods of sperm preparation for intrauterine insemination. Fertil Steril. 1998;70(3):574-5.
3. Abed F, Zadehmodarres S. A comparative study of swim-up and upstream methods for isolating sperm cell for intra uterine insemination. Int J Women's Health Reprod Sci. 2015;3(2):103-6.
4. Lemmens L, Kos S, Beijer C, Braat DDM, Jonker MA, Nelen WLDM, et al. Optimization of laboratory procedures for intrauterine insemination: survey of methods in relation to clinical outcome. Andrology. 2018;6:707-13.
5. Bahadur G, Homburg R, Muneer A, Racich P, Alangaden T, Al-Habib A, et al. First line fertility treatment strategies regarding IUI and IVF require clinical evidence. Hum Reprod. 2016b;31:1141-6.
6. Haagen EC, Nelen WL, Adang EM, Grol RP, Hermens RP, Kremer JA. Guideline adherence is worth the effort: a cost-effectiveness analysis in intrauterine insemination care. Hum Reprod. 2013;28:357-66.
7. Ombelet W. Evidence-based recommendations for IUI in daily practice. Middle East Fert Soc J. 2013;18:4.

CHAPTER 19

Setting Up an Intrauterine Insemination Laboratory

Sonal Vaidya

■ INTRODUCTION

Since many centuries, intrauterine insemination (IUI) has been the first line of treatment in assisted reproductive techniques (ART) for couples facing difficulty in conceiving, to achieve successful pregnancy. It is a minimally invasive and cost-effective treatment which is commonly used for patients with unexplained infertility, cervical factor, immunological factor, ovulatory dysfunction, endometriosis, vaginismus, mild oligoasthenozoospermia, erectile dysfunction to name a few.[1] As a result, the need for developing a basic laboratory catering to the Andrology services is much in demand. The IUI process includes collection of the semen sample either from the male partner or from a donor[2] followed by "washing" of the semen and insertion of concentrated motile sperm fraction in the uterus of the female partner. The IUI procedure can be done either as a natural cycle or may be combined together with mild ovarian stimulation; in any which case, the IUI procedure is performed following the follicle rupture to maximize the chances of achieving pregnancy. Seemingly simple job, the success rate of an IUI cycle can range from as high as 45% (cumulative pregnancy rates when all influencing factors such as age of the female partner, indication and duration of infertility, final post wash count and motility over the threshold value of 5 million/mL, are all conducive) to as low as 5% where multiple factors are involved in the couple.

■ ASSISTED REPRODUCTIVE TECHNOLOGY ACT, 2021[2,3]

The gazetted notification by Ministry of Law and Justice of India (Legislative Department) has published on 20th December 2021—The Assisted Reproductive Technology (Regulation) Act, 2021 (No. 42 of 2021). This ART Act, 2021 has been enforced on all ART Clinics and ART Banks across India since 25th January 2022. The detailed information was further published in gazetted notification dated 7th June 2022. Under the provisions of the ART Act, 2021, it is mandated that the laboratories performing IUI procedures should perform following duties:

1. *"Must register with the National Registry as ART Clinic Level-1:* Format and manner of an application for registration is to be directed to the appropriate authority by submitting duly filled Form-1. Every application is to be accompanied with a fee of: Rs. 50,000/- for Level 1 ART Clinic. *Certificate of Registration:* The appropriate authority shall, after making such enquiry and after satisfying itself that the applicant has complied with all the requirements, grant a certificate of registration in Form 3 to the applicant. One copy of the certificate of registration shall be displayed by the

registered ART clinic at a conspicuous place at its place of business.
2. *Staff requirements:* As per Schedule 1 Part 1 (Rule 4): Minimum 01 gynecologist is mandated.

   Qualification of the gynecologists is stated as medical postgraduate in gynecology and obstetrics.
3. *Minimum requirement of Equipment for ART Clinics Level-1:*
   (i) Microscope, (ii) Centrifuge, and (iii) Refrigerator
4. *Eligibility criteria:* The ART Clinics are directed to offer their services to the Commissioning couple (infertile married couple with woman above the age of 21 years and below 50 years and the man above the age of 21 years and below the age of 55 years). The ART services can also be offered to single women above the age of 21 years and below 50 years, with the use of donor semen sample procured through Registered ART Bank only.
5. The ART Clinics shall procure donor semen samples through the Registered ART Bank. Furthermore, the sperm donor should be aged between 21 years and 55 years both inclusive, should be recruited, screened by the Registered ART Bank and the donor can donate only once in the lifetime.
6. The ART Clinics must ensure that a woman shall not be treated with gametes or embryos derived from more than one man or woman during any one treatment cycle; a clinic shall never mix semen from two individuals for the procedures specified under this Act.
7. The Consent form for IUI using husband's sperms and the Consent form for IUI using donor's sperms are to be maintained in the prescribed format.
8. Clause 29 enlists Restriction on sale, etc., of human gametes, zygotes, and embryos. The sale, transfer or use of gametes, zygotes and embryos, or any part thereof or information related thereto, directly or indirectly to any party within or outside India shall be prohibited except in the case of transfer of own gametes and embryos for personal use with the permission of the National Board.

   As a result, gamete transport, i.e., transport of processed semen sample from IUI laboratory to the Clinician's OPD or to the referral clinic, i.e., functioning of Satellite IUI laboratories is strictly prohibited.
9. Clause 30: Research on human gametes—(i) The use of any human gametes or their transfer to any country outside India for research shall be absolutely prohibited. (ii) The research on human gamete within India shall be performed in such manner as may be prescribed.
10. Clause 31: Rights of child born through assisted reproductive technology.—(i) The child born through ART shall be deemed to be a biological child of the commissioning couple and the said child shall be entitled to all the rights and privileges available to a natural child only from the commissioning couple under any law for the time being in force. (ii) A donor shall relinquish all parental rights over the child or children which may be born from his or her gamete".

ADDITIONAL REGISTRATIONS

- *Preconception and prenatal diagnostic techniques (PCPNDT):*[4] The PCPNDT License comes under the Prenatal Diagnostic Techniques (Registration and Prevention of Misuse) Act, 1994 and has been enacted by the Government of State to provide for Registration and Regulation

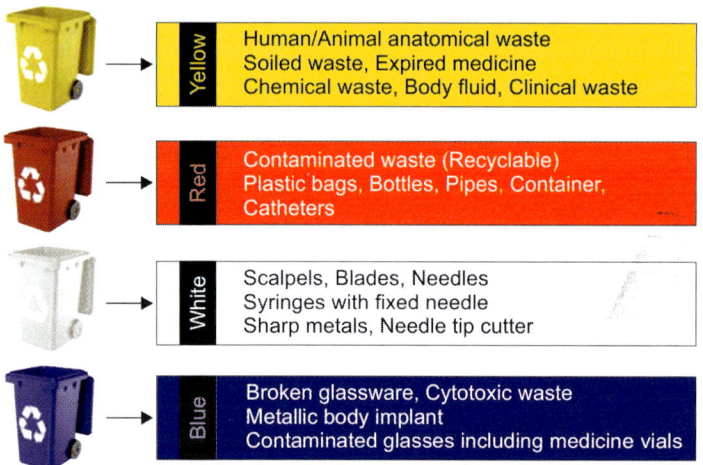

Fig. 1: Four categories of biomedical waste.

of all Clinical Establishments that have USG equipment in the state.

- *Biomedical waste management:*[5] The biomedical waste management registration is compulsory for all persons who generate, collect, receive, store, transport, treat, dispose, or handle biomedical waste in any form. Every registered center is required to submit an annual report to the prescribed authority by 30th of June every year. There are four categories of biomedical waste as follows **(Fig. 1)**:
- *Clinical establishment Act:*[6] An Act to provide for the registration and regulation of clinical establishments in the country and for matters connected therewith or incidental thereto.

It is noteworthy that as per the ART Act, 2021 7th June 2022 notification, the Registration form for ART Clinics Level-1 as well as ART Clinics Level-2 is the same and only two registered Acts of Authorities are mentioned in the form—the Medical Termination of Pregnancy (MTP) Act and the Preconception and Prenatal Diagnostic Techniques (PCPNDT) Act. The applicant is to state whether the said clinic is registered or not with the above-mentioned Acts.

SERVICES OFFERED AND EQUIPMENT LIST

As is evident, the ART Act, 2021 enlists the minimal requirements of equipment as: (i) Microscope, (ii) Centrifuge, and (iii) Refrigerator. However, the andrology services offered by the ART Clinic Level-1 would largely dictate not only the additional equipment required, but also the space to be allotted as well as designing of the given space. Generally, andrology services offered include semen analysis (Manual and/or computer-aided), viability assessment, sperm processing, sperm DNA fragmentation test and semen freezing—thawing (for long distance married couples or when husband is not in town on the scheduled day of IUI procedure or for pooling of suboptimal semen samples), storage of donor semen sample received from a Registered ART Bank till the time where IUI for an assigned couple is scheduled.

The factors affecting the success of an IUI cycle is not limited to the infertility indications for the couple, for example, age of the woman, semen parameters, rupture of follicle/s, non-traumatic insemination, luteal phase support etc.; but also includes factors such as: sterile precautions, semen collection methods, culture media conditions, duration between semen collection and processing,[7] duration between semen processing and insemination,[8] etc.

Keeping in mind the inherently low success rates of the IUI procedure, absolute regulation of the equipment, media storage and its use, consumables and disposables and the standardization of the protocols form the basis of a good laboratory.

■ SPACE[9,10]

The laboratory should be located from 2nd floor and above to avoid traffic, dust, pollution. The basement area should be strictly avoided as it is prone to moisture.

The ART Clinic Level-1 must have clear areas specified as "sterile" and "nonsterile" zones.

Nonsterile zone will include waiting area or reception. Dedicated record keeping room is essential as the ART Act, 2021 mandates that the ART Clinics have to maintain data for 10 years, following which period, the records need to be shifted to the National Registry. Additionally, Consulting Room with USG machine, Procedure Room, Semen collection room (with attached toilet, adjacent to semen processing laboratory and a pass-window) are prerequisites.

The sterile zone must include the scrub area, the IUI laboratory. This area should ideally have a positive pressure with a dedicated air-handling unit (AHU) ensuring controlled temperature and HEPA filtered clean air inflow.

The IUI laboratory should be a clean space with restricted entry. The IUI laboratory should be designed as per the workload with a little room for expansion in the future. The space should be at least 100 square feet for proper placing of the equipment. Power points should be installed with respect to the number and placing of equipment with the provision of extras. The space should not be overcrowded, therefore, all necessary equipment can be termed as "Critical equipment" and must have a UPS back-up.

Additionally, generator back-up is also mandatory. Stainless steel furniture with granite tops are the best materials for furniture and counter-tops as these materials are durable, easy to maintain and disinfect. The lights should be concealed, but easy to replace.

The IUI laboratory must have a well-defined scrub area with no water drainage within the laboratory in order to avoid fungal infections, seepage, and pests.

■ EQUIPMENT PREFERRED

- Laminar air flow (LAF) or a biosafety cabinet (BSC)
- High resolution compound microscope: Eyepieces—10X or 20X, Objectives: 10X, 20X, 40X, 100X... Could be trinocular (optional).
- CASA (optional)
- Refrigerator
- Makler counting chamber
- Heating block (37°C) for liquefaction of the semen sample
- Centrifuge (till 3,000 rpm)
- CO_2 incubator with CO_2 cylinders (optional) OR temperature controlled dry incubator
- Cryocans (Storage and Transport cans—optional) with cryoaccessories.

The equipment must be kept clean, maintained, and serviced regularly to ensure optimal functioning **(Figs. 2 to 4)**.

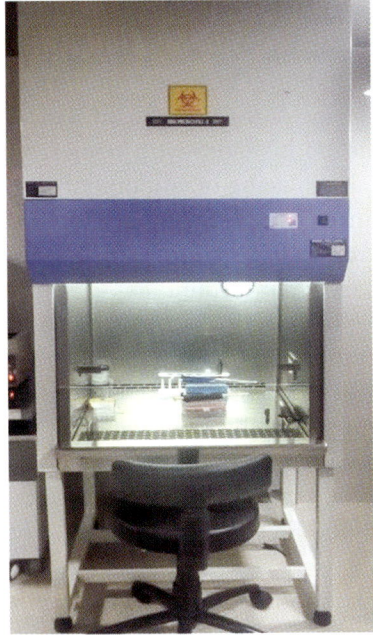

Fig. 2: Biosafety cabinet

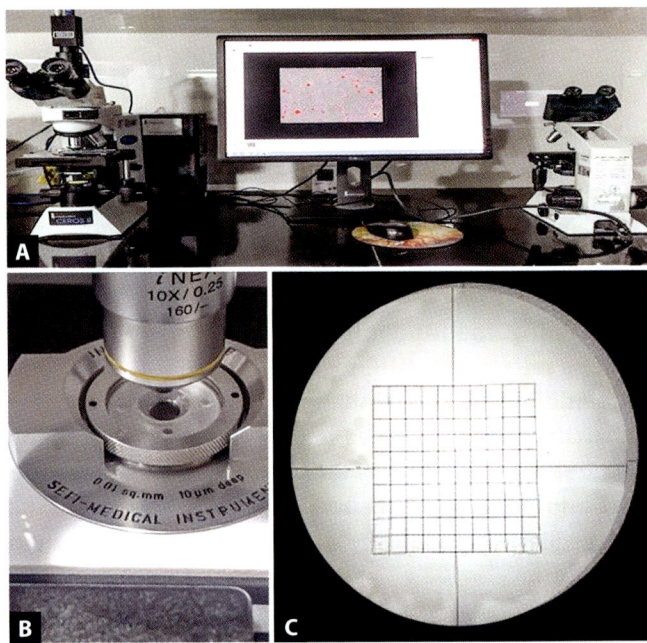

Figs. 3A to C: (A) CASA and compound microscopes; (B and C) Makler's chamber.

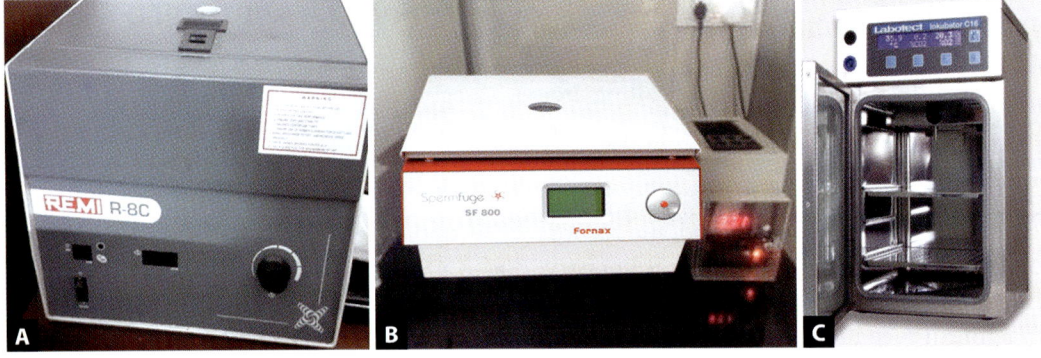

Figs. 4A to C: (A and B) Centrifuges and heating block; (C) Incubator.

CONSUMABLES AND DISPOSABLES

The sterile, non-toxic and single-use plastic-ware disposables are to be used. The disposables should be gamma-radiated sterile. Catheters usually are ETO sterilized due to practical reasons, but the catheters usually undergo rounds of washing and drying before they are released by the manufacturer **(Figs. 5A and B)**.

- Sterile filtered tips (volume specific)
- Volume adjustable micro-pipettes (100–1,000 µL, 40–200 µL, and 5–40 µL)
- Slides and coverslips
- Stains: Eosin and Negrosin
- Seliwanoff reagent
- Prestained morphology slides

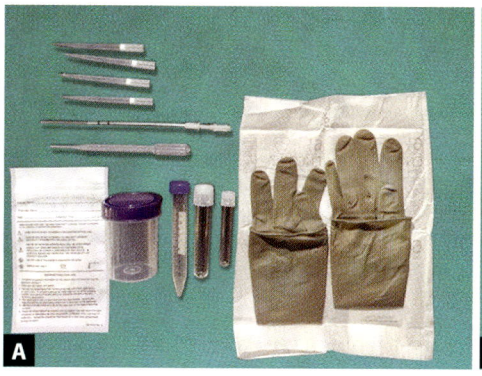 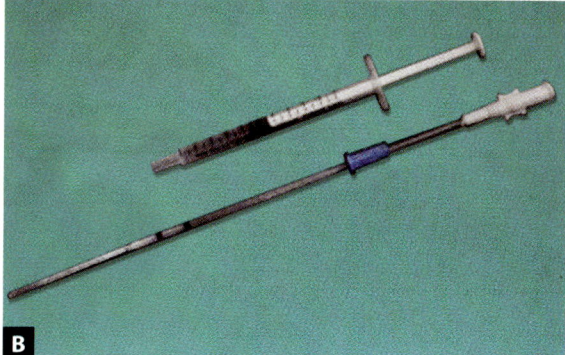

Figs. 5A and B: Disposables—tips, pipettes, test tubes, collection jar, catheter, syringe, and gloves.

- DFI kits
- Glass beakers
- Distilled water
- Isopropyl alcohol
- Permanent markers
- Sterile tissues
- Semen collection jar
- Test tubes: Round bottom (14 mL and 5 mL), Conical tubes
- IUI catheters
- Nonspermicidal condoms
- Sterile and nonpowdered gloves
- Dustbins and sharp disposals
- Stationery.

■ SEMEN COLLECTION[11-14]

The method and ways with which semen is collected plays the basic yet much important part of an IUI outcome. The collection jar needs to be gamma-radiated sterile. The semen must be preferably collected by masturbation for avoiding loss of first part of the semen sample as well as to avoid affecting sperm motility adversely due to acidic pH of the vagina. In case the male partner insists on coitus interruptus as the method, use of nonspermicidal condoms to collect the semen is preferred.

Before collection, clear verbal and written instructions like voiding the urine, cleaning, and drying of hands and private parts, avoiding lubricants, prelabeling sterile containers with identifying double markers and filling the form with personal details (full name, date of birth, contact information, and spouse name), abstinence, time of collection, and consents with eligibility proof must be clearly explained to avoid interference with the protocols.

■ CULTURE MEDIA

The sperm processing/freezing media is readily available. Particular attention needs to be given to the buffers used in the media. The media can either be HEPES/MOPS buffered, requiring 4–5 hours of equilibration at 37°C prior to its use or it can be bicarbonate buffer, requiring overnight equilibration in CO_2 incubator with cap loose at 37°C prior to its use.[12] The sole factor that decides the need of CO_2 incubator for a laboratory is the buffering system used in the media. Generally, while centrifugation, the media used is HEPES/MOPS buffered while the final sperm suspension is in the bicarbonate buffer.[13]

The cold-chain maintenance of the media prior to its use, inventory status, its shelf-life, turbidity, pH needs to be tightly regulated. The media contents include glucose, calcium chloride, antibiotics, antioxidants, and may be

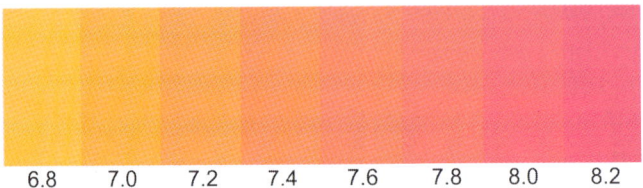

Fig. 6: Calculated colors for pH from 6.8 to 8.2 (absorbance multipliers = 1.3)

supplemented with human serum albumen (HSA). Certain media may include phenol red as a pH indicator thereby appearing pink in color. Change in the color is an indication of proper media equilibration prior to use **(Fig. 6)**.

Elevated temperatures or prolonged exposure of culture media to CO_2 causes degradation of proteins, carbohydrates and even vitamins. On the other hand, frozen media results in increased concentration of solutes making media inhomogeneous and also degrades the proteins. Therefore, media must be stored at 2–8°C prior to use. It is also advisable to use media within 7 days of its aliquoting irrespective of its shelf life.

Therefore, smaller size culture media bottles are preferred to avoid wastage.

Good laboratory practices[14] must be followed while handling media and the semen samples.

STANDARD OPERATING PROCEDURES

Standard operating procedures (SOPs) form the backbone of any IUI laboratory. These are defined to ensure reproducibility and standardization of the protocols. These must include the technical protocols, responsibilities of personnel for procuring consent forms, cleaning schedule, schedule for AMC of equipment, trouble-shooting, record keeping, and quality control. SOPs are usually in the form of paperwork.

TRAINED PROFESSIONALS

Although the ART Act 2021 does not specify the qualifications and experience of Andrology technician, it is one of the most crucial aspects in terms of the outcome of an IUI cycle. The personnel handling the semen samples must be trained in the techniques, aseptic precautions, equipment handling and troubleshooting, documentation and record keeping, QC procedures, etc.

Special training and emphasis must be imparted on proper handling of the semen samples and ensuring correct identification and traceability to avoid erroneous semen sample mix-ups, leading to catastrophic outcomes. The witnessing protocol can be either manual or electronic. Sample identifying markers must include patient's full name, spouse's name, and respective date of births. An accidental error of using the same micro-tip/disposable for more than one patient's sample or in the sperm processing media can lead to a disaster and hence it is advisable to process one sample at a time and to clear the work bench before proceeding with the next sample. The sample traceability will begin from the time the semen collection jar enters the IUI laboratory, and will continue till the IUI procedure is done. From the time of collection of semen sample to its journey through the IUI laboratory and finally till the sample is used for insemination, the sample is shifted between many hands and, therefore, every personnel including husband, technician, nurse, and doctor will ensure that at each and every step, identifying markers are verified by the stage specific relevant operator. Before final insemination, couple's name, identification of final sperm suspension and consent is verified by the doctor and the assisting nurse.

Monitoring of the working conditions using simple logical/visual analysis for temperatures of the heated surfaces, assessing clarity/turbidity of the processing media, condensation on incubator doors/cryocans, etc. should be encouraged.

Safety of the personnel is ensured by screening the patients for human immunodeficiency virus (HIV), hepatitis B surface antigen (HBsAg), and hepatitis C virus (HCV). Special protocols must be followed in case of seropositive patients. Moreover, the personnel must be vaccinated against hepatitis B and other viral diseases and proper SOPs must be in place to safeguard the personnel in case of needle-stick injury or cryoburns.

QUALITY CONTROL[15]

The quality analysis (QA)/quality control (QC) of an IUI laboratory needs to be in place in order to establish standardization and to ensure optimization.[9,10] QC is a continuous and extensive process. All protocols, personnel, equipment functioning and breakdown, sterility assessment, and key performance indicators (KPIs) like final yield of the sample and the outcome have to be regularly documented and reviewed. These include:
- *Daily checks:* Temperatures of heated stages/blocks and incubators, equipment functioning, yield calculations.
- *Weekly checks:* LN2 refilling in cryocans.
- *Monthly checks:* Culture reports from work benches, incubators, cleaning of incubators.
- *Quarterly checks:* Outcome assessment and sperm survival tests (SSTs).
- *Biannual checks:* Pipettes, servicing and calibration of equipment, and cleaning of refrigerators.
- Disposables, consumables, media, and reagents to be checked for receiving conditions, expiry dates, lot numbers, storage conditions, and sterility certificates.

All the above checks are to be maintained either in the form of log-books/registers.

YIELD CALCULATION

The semen parameters are largely affected by abstinence, frequency of ejaculation, personal habits such as smoking, alcohol consumption, etc. The final sperm suspension thus is a reflection of combined factors like the volume of semen used to process the sample, the prewash seminal parameters such as count, motility, and morphology and the final volume of re-suspension/overlay. Thus, for every semen sample collected, the final yield will differ. The performance assessment of the personnel cannot be made by pregnancy outcomes as innumerable factors as mentioned earlier have a role to play. Hence, performance assessment can be based on calculation of the yield by using the following formula:

$$\text{Expected yield} = \frac{(\text{Sperm prewash count} \times \text{Ejaculate volume} \times \text{Total motility})}{100}$$

So, for example, if the prewash count is 30 million/mL, sample volume is 3.0 mL and motility is 50%, the yield is calculated as:

$$\text{Expected yield} = \frac{(30 \times 10^6 \times 3 \times 50)}{100}$$
$$= 45 \times 10^6 = 45 \text{ million sperms}$$

Alternatively, relative yield[16] can also be determined with prewash and postwash count, volume, and percentage of motile sperms as known values.

SPERM SURVIVAL TEST[17,18]

Sperm survival test is usually performed to check the toxicity of media, and disposables. This test can be performed easily due to availability of semen samples, as the test is inexpensive and reliable contact bioassay.

Processed semen samples are placed for 24 hours in incubation. The benchmark is considered as 50% survival after 24 hours. Usually, semen samples with normal seminal parameters are used for this test. Only one "test" item to be reviewed for QC is altered (termed as variable) and the results are compared the "control" wherein all the items are standard (nonvariable). The test allows to determine the difference in the survivability of the sperms.

CONCLUSION

The requisites for setting up an IUI laboratory are manyfold. The complexities of the influencing factors and the limited success rates warrant the need to establish a well-planned laboratory setup. Clearly, as was advertised by certain companies, IUI itself is not just an office procedure. Attention to details is the central theme. The implementation of the ART Act, 2021 has initiated the process of regularization of all ART Clinics across India and although a lot more clarity and standardizations are awaited in the amendments that are expected in the future, ART Act can be considered as the first step toward achieving the goal to provide quality services. All new set-ups need registrations as ART Clinic Level-1 before the IUI laboratory can start functioning, and no registrations will be granted unless the State Board inspects the premises. It is important to note that registrations will be issued with the validity of 5 years.

Additionally, variations in the semen samples, possibilities of mix-up errors, and regulatory bodies demand a proper set-up and thus adds layers of complexity to the setting up of an IUI laboratory. Compromises in the quality of services would be translated to suboptimal outcomes and may lead to potential disasters. Therefore, an IUI laboratory can be considered a "mini IVF laboratory" requiring dedicated team of professionals to handle the daily routine. The expenses for registrations and running of an ART Level-1 Clinic are high. Moreover, the procedural cost incurred on the couple for the treatment has to be competitively priced and hence, needless to say, before venturing into this project, the turnover needs to be carefully and realistically calculated for an IUI laboratory to be a viable project.

Considering all these practical issues, establishment of an IUI set-up can be overbearing. Proper planning and strategizing before starting an IUI laboratory are the key points. The first part of the project must include identifying the minimal and crucial requirements with respect to the infrastructure, personnel, equipment, manual witnessing protocol, acquiring mandatory registrations, and the documentation as mandated by the ART Act, 2021.

Since the success of this project is result dependent, expansion, and improvement plans as a part of continuous development of the IUI laboratory can be enforced as a next step in an existing IUI set-up to avoid financial burdens.

KEY LEARNING POINTS

- Laboratory regulations and licenses.
- Requisite space and equipment.
- Factors contributing to successful outcome.
- Importance of identification and traceability of samples.
- Documentation and record keeping.

REFERENCES

1. Zippl AL, Wachter A, Rockenschaub P, Toth B, Seeber B. Predicting success of intrauterine insemination using a clinically based scoring system. Arch gynecol obstet. 2022;306(5):1777-86.
2. Gazette of India. (2022). Ministry of Law and Justice (Legislative D). The Assisted Reproductive Technology (Regulation) Act, 2021 (No. 42 of 2021.) [online] Available from https://thc.nic.in/Central%20 Governmental%20Rules/Assisted%20 Reproductive%20Technology%20 (Regulation)%20Rules,%202022,%20%20.pdf [Last accessed January, 2024].
3. Gazette of India. Ministry of Law and Justice (Legislative D). The Assisted Reproductive Technology (Regulation) Act, 2021 (7th June notification). [online] Available fromhttps://thc.nic.in/Central%20Governmental%20 Rules/Assisted%20Reproductive%20 Technology%20(Regulation)%20Rules,%20 2022,%20%20.pdf [Last accessed January, 2024].
4. Professionals. Pre-Conception and Pre-Natal (PCPNDT) Act, 1994 as amended by Diagnostic Techniques Rules 2020 bare Act. Delhi: Professional Book Publishers; 2020.
5. Gazette of India. Ministry of Environment, Forest and Climate Change Notification, New Delhi, the 16th March, 2018 Bio-Medical Waste Management Rules, 2016 (amendments).
6. Gazette of India. Ministry of Health and Family Welfare. The Clinical Establishments (Registration and Regulation) Act, 2010.
7. Punjabi UVan Mulders H, Van de Velde L, Goovaerts I, Peeters K, Cassauwers W, et al. Time intervals between semen production, initiation of analysis, and IUI significantly influence clinical pregnancies and live births. J Assist Reprod Genet. 2021;38(2):421-8.
8. Statema-Lohmeijer CH, Schats R, Lissenberg-Witte BI, Kostelijk EH, Lambalk CB, Vergouw CG. A short versus a long-time interval between semen collection and intrauterine insemination: a randomized controlled clinical trial. Hum Reprod. 2023;38(5):811-9.
9. Mortimer D, Cohen J, Mortimer ST, Fawzy M, McCulloh DH, Morbeck DE, et al. Cairo consensus on the IVF laboratory environment and air quality: report of an expert meeting. Reprod BioMed Online. 2018;36(6): 658-74.
10. Malhotra J, Malhotra K, Talwar P, Kannan P, Singh P, Kumar Y, et al. ISAR consensus guidelines on safety and ethical practices in in vitro fertilization clinics. J Hum Reprod Sci. 2021;14:S48-68.
11. World Health Organization. WHO Laboratory Manual for the Examination and Processing of Human Semen, 6th edition. Geneva, Switzerland: WHO Press; 2021.
12. Will M, Clark N, Swain J. Biological pH buffers in IVF: help or hindrance to success. J Assist Reprod Genet. 2011;28(8):711-24.
13. Peirce KL, Roberts P, Ali J, Matson P. The preparation and culture of washed human sperm: A comparison of a suite of protein-free media with media containing human serum albumin. Asian Pacific J Reprod. 2015;4(3):222-7.
14. Magli MC, Van den Abbeel E, Lundin K, Royere D, Van der Elst J, Gianaroli L, Committee of the Special Interest Group on Embryology. Revised guidelines for good practice in IVF laboratories. Hum reprod (Oxford, England). 2008;23(6):1253-62.
15. Agarwal A, Sharma R, Gupta S, Finelli R, Parekh N, Selvam MKP, et al. Standardized Laboratory Procedures, Quality Control and Quality Assurance Are Key Requirements for Accurate Semen Analysis in the Evaluation of Infertile Male. world j men's health. 2022;40(1):52-65.
16. Mortimer D. Sperm preparation methods. J androl. 2000;21(3):357-66.
17. Meintjes M. Sperm Survival Assay for Quality Control in the IVF Laboratory. In: Montag MHM, Morbeck DE (eds). Principles of IVF Laboratory Practice: Optimizing Performance and Outcomes. Cambridge: Cambridge University Press; 2017. pp. 73-8.
18. de Jonge CJ, Centola GM, Reed ML, Shabanowitz RB, Simon SD, Quinn P. Andrology Lab Corner: Human Sperm Survival Assay as a Bioassay for the Assisted Reproductive Technologies Laboratory. J Androl. 2003;24:16-8.

CHAPTER 20

Assisted Reproductive Technology Act 2022: Level 1 Clinic

Ashwini Yelikar Kale, Ashish Kale

◼ INTRODUCTION

The notification came in force by, Ministry of Health and Family Welfare (Department of Health Research) *Notification, New Delhi, the 7th June, 2022 G.S.R. 419(E).—In exercise of the powers conferred by section 42 of the Assisted Reproductive Technology (ART) (Regulation) Act, 2021 (42 of 2021), the Central Government hereby makes the following rules, for setting up of level 1 and 2 ART clinics.*

Level 1 ART clinics, where only intrauterine insemination (IUI) procedure is carried out as part of treatment.

An application for registration shall be made by the ART clinics or any such health facility which is carrying out procedures related to the ART, as defined in the Act, to the appropriate authority in Form-1 (with fees of Rupees 50,000/- for Level 1 ART clinic for 5 years).

Provided that if an application for registration of any ART clinic has been rejected by the appropriate authority, no fee shall be required to be paid on re-submission of the application by the applicant for the same clinic and the application fees once paid shall not be refunded:

Certificate of Registration

The appropriate authority shall, after making such enquiry and after satisfying itself that the applicant has complied with all the requirements, grant a certificate of registration in *Form 3* to the applicant. One copy of the certificate of registration shall be displayed by the registered ART clinic at a conspicuous place at its place of business.

Grievance redressal: Every clinic and every bank shall maintain a grievance cell in respect of matters relating to such clinics and banks and the manner of making a compliant before such grievance cell be as specified in *Form 5*.

◼ MAINTAIN THE FOLLOWING CONSENT FORMS

- Consent for IUI with husband's semen or sperm as specified in *Form 7*
- Consent for IUI with donor semen as specified in *Form 8*.

Every ART clinic shall allow inspection of their place, equipment, and records by the National Board, National Registry, State Board, or appropriate authority or any officer authorized in this behalf. Such inspection of an already registered clinic may take place without any notice. The authorities on inspection shall ensure that entry and search procedure does not place at risk the gametes or embryos stored in the facility.

The staff requirements and qualifications of the staff in the ART clinics:
(a) ART Level 1 clinic: Minimum 01 gynecologist

Qualification: The gynecologist shall be a medical postgraduate in gynecology and obstetrics.

No mention about size of sterile and non-sterile zone.

The minimum equipment in ART clinics:
(i) Microscope, (ii) Centrifuge, and (iii) Refrigerator.

Attached are the Forms to be filled:
1. Form 7
2. Form 8
3. Form 3: Certificate of registration.

FORM-3
[See rule 8]
Certificate of Registration
ART clinic (Level 1/Level 2)/ART bank (To be issued in duplicate)
Certificate No.: _____

1. In exercise of the powers conferred under Section 16 (1) of the Assisted Reproductive Technology (Regulation) Act, 2021, the Appropriate Authority _____ hereby grants registration to the ART Clinic named below for purposes of carrying out Assisted Reproductive Technology procedures as per the aforesaid Act, for a period of _____ ending on _____
   (a) Name and address of the ART Clinic;
   (b) Type of institution (Government or Private) and
   (c) Type of facility: Level 1 or Level 2.

OR

   The ART Bank named below for purposes of carrying out activities and procedures as per the aforesaid Act, for a period of _____ ending on _____
   (a) Name and address of the ART Bank;
   (b) Type of institution (Govt./Private)

2. This registration is granted subject to the aforesaid Act and Rules thereunder and any contravention there of shall result in suspension or cancellation of this certificate of registration before the expiry of the said period of five years.
3. Registration No. allotted
4. For renewed Certificate of Registration only:
   Period of validity of earlier Certificate of Registration from _____ to _____

Date: _____
Place: _____

Signature
Name and Designation of the Appropriate Authority

SEAL

Display one copy of this certificate at a conspicuous place at the place of business.
*Strike out whichever is not applicable or necessary.

FORM-7

[See rule 13(f) (ii)]

Consent for IUI with Husband's Semen/Sperm

_____ and _____
_____, being husband and wife and both of legal age, authorize Dr _____ to inseminate the wife intrauterine with the semen/sperm of the husband for achieving conception.

We understand that even though the insemination may be repeated as often as recommended by the doctor, there is no guarantee or assurance that pregnancy or a live birth will result.

We have also been told that the outcome of pregnancy may not be the same as those of the general pregnant population, for example, in respect of abortion, multiple pregnancies, anomalies or complications of pregnancy or delivery.

The procedure carried out does neither ensure a positive result nor does it guarantee a mentally and physically normal child. This consent holds good for all the cycles performed at the clinic.

Signature of intending couple

Husband:

Wife:

Endorsement by the ART Clinic

I/We have personally explained to _____ and _____ the details and implications of his/her/their signing this consent/approval form, and made sure to the extent humanly possible that he/she/they understand these details and implications.

Name, Address, and Signature of the Witness from the clinic

Signed: _____ (Husband)

_____ (Wife)

Name and Signature of the Doctor:

Name and Address of the ART Clinic:

Dated:

FORM-8
[See rule 13 (f) (iii)]
Consent for Intrauterine Insemination with Donor Semen

I/We, _____ being of legal age, authorize Dr _____ to inseminate me intrauterine with semen/sperm of a donor Aadhar no. _____ (ART Bank's no. _____; obtained from ART bank with valid registration no) for achieving conception.

I/We understand that even though the insemination may be repeated as often as recommended by the doctor, there is no guarantee or assurance that pregnancy or a live birth will result.

I/We have also been told that the outcome of pregnancy may not be the same as those of the general pregnant population, for example, in respect of abortion, multiple pregnancies, anomalies or complications of pregnancy or delivery.

I/We declare that we shall not attempt to find out the identity of the donor.

I, the husband, also declare that should my wife bear any child or children as a result of such insemination(s), such child or children shall be as my own and shall be my legal heir(s). (if applicable).

The procedure carried out does neither ensure a positive result nor does it guarantee a mentally and physically normal body. This consent holds good for all the cycles performed at the clinic.

Signature of intending couple/intending woman

Endorsement by the ART Clinic

I/We have personally explained to _____ and the details and implications of his/her/their signing this consent/approval form, and made sure to the extent humanly possible that he/she/they understand these details and implications.

Name, Address and Signature of the
Witness from the Clinic

Signed: _____ (Husband)

_____ (Wife)

Name and Signature of the Doctor:

Name and Address of the ART Clinic:

Dated: _____

Note: An appropriate modification of this form may be used for Artificial Insemination or Intrauterine Insemination of a single woman with donor semen.

SECTION 7: Andrology and Laboratory Aspect

Till date 35 gazettes have been published ART REGULATION ACT 2021—got published on 20th December 2021. All provisions of both ART and Surrogacy Regulation Act will come into force on 25th January 2022.

I.11019/07/2024-HR (RTI)
भारत सरकार/Government of India
स्वास्थ्य और परिवार कल्याण मंत्रालय/ Ministry of Health & Family Welfare
स्वास्थ्यअनुसंधानविभाग/ Department of Health Research
(समन्वयअनुभाग/ Co ordination Section)
***

IRCS Building, Red Cross Road
New Delhi- 110001,
Dated: 18 January, 2024.

To,
Sh. Arunmuthuvel
13, 1st main road, kasthuribai nagar,
Adyar-600020
Email: arunmuthuvel@gmail.com

Subject: RTI application dated 09/01/2024 registration no. DOHRE/R/E/24/00012 under Right to Information Act, 2005.

Sir,

I am directed to refer to your RTI application dated 09/01/2024 and to say that as per guidelines in accordance with DoPT O.M. No. 1/69/2007-IR, dated the 27th February, 2008, (para 8), the CPIO is not supposed to create information; or to interpret information; or to solve the problems raised by the Applicants; or to furnish replies to hypothetical questions. However, the following information is provided for your assistance:

Ques 1. Can level 1 clinics do ovarian stimulation for IVF and do the IVF at level 2 clinic?

Reply: As per Para 3 (i) of the Assisted Reproductive Technology Rules, 2022, Level 1 ART Clinics can carry out only intrauterine insemination (IUI) procedure as part of treatment. Ovum stimulation can only be done in Level 2 clinic as per Para 3 (ii) the Assisted Reproductive Technology Rules, 2022.

Ques 2. Can level 1 clinics do IUI as well as ovarian stimulation?

Reply: The query stands replied to in Question no.1 above.

2. Smt. Richa Khoda, Joint Secretary, Department of Health Research, 2nd Floor IRCS Building, Red Cross Road, New Delhi- 110001, is the appellate Authority.

3. This disposes of the RTI Application mentioned above.

Yours faithfully

(S.N. Jasra)
Director & CPIO
Tele: - 23736218

Copy to: RTI Cell, RTI Portal

SECTION 8: Techniques

21. **Procedure of Intrauterine Insemination**
    Sunita Tandulwadkar, Darshan SM

CHAPTER 21

Procedure of Intrauterine Insemination

Sunita Tandulwadkar, Darshan SM

■ INTRODUCTION

The intrauterine insemination (IUI) procedure can roughly be separated into three steps:
1. Diagnosis and indication
2. Cycle preparation
3. Technical stage.

The third step, including the whole process between semen collection and insemination, is barely included in the guidelines. Only the World Health Organization (WHO) laboratory manual attempted to describe the process but this description is incomplete, because parts of the pre- and postlaboratory stages are missing.

The available literature on the following procedures or variables of IUI will be reviewed: ejaculatory abstinence (EA), semen collection place, time intervals, semen preparation methods, centrifugation medium, centrifugation and storage temperature, timing of IUI, use of different disposables (e.g., catheters), and duration of bed rest after IUI.

■ EJACULATORY ABSTINENCE

The WHO recommends an EA period of 2–7 days before semen collection both for diagnostics and semen preparation. A certain level of reactive oxygen species (ROS) is required for the maturation of epididymal spermatozoa. Excessive ROS, however, can induce oxidative damage which negatively affects the fertilization potential of spermatozoa. The exposure time of spermatozoa to ROS is influenced in an EA time-dependent manner, thereby influencing the incidence of sperm DNA fragmentation, especially in infertile men.[1] As a consequence, a shorter period of EA will result in higher pregnancy rates (PR) both in natural and IUI cycles, especially in subfertile men.

■ TIME INTERVAL

The time intervals between semen collection to processing, processing to insemination, and semen collection to insemination have impact on IUI PRs.

■ SAMPLE COLLECTION ROOM

Preferably take place in a private room near the clinical laboratory, but when collection at home is preferred, the semen should be delivered to the laboratory within 1 hour after collection (while protected from extremes of temperature).

■ STORAGE TIME AFTER PROCESSING

It is the time interval between processing and insemination. A shorter time interval was related to a lower proportion of premature sperm chromatin decondensation, to less sperm DNA fragmentation, and to a higher PR due to the storage time-dependent spontaneous acrosome reaction. In practice, however, no consensus was shown in reported ideal time intervals. PRs were comparable when IUI was performed <30 minutes or 31–60 minutes of storage, but decreased >60 minutes, only in human menopausal gonadotropins (hMG)-treated women.

SEMEN PREPARATION METHODS

After semen production and liquefaction, it is necessary to separate sperm from the seminal plasma, thereby preventing uterine cramps, extended ROS formation and inhibition of fertilization. According to the WHO, the choice of semen preparation technique should be based on the nature of the semen sample (WHO, 2020). It is recommended to use swim-up in cases of normozoospermia, while density gradients should be the method of choice in other cases. There is consensus that the swim-up technique resulted in lower recovery rates compared to density gradient centrifugation, making it suitable only in cases of normozoospermia. As swim-up selects spermatozoa based on their motility, one would expect that it would result in a high fraction of motile spermatozoa.

pH BUFFER OF WASHING AND STORAGE MEDIUM

To maintain an optimal pH level, the WHO recommends to select a buffer medium based on the used incubator: Zwitterion-buffered medium HEPES (4-(2-hydroxyethyl)-1-piperazineethanesulfonic acid), and MOPS3- (N-morpholino)propanesulfonic acid) if the incubator contains atmospheric air and a bicarbonate-based medium if the incubator contains an atmosphere of 5% CO_2 (and if gas exchange is allowed). Meanwhile, most commercially available sperm wash media contain zwitter ions for pH buffering, although a certain level of bicarbonate is present as key capacitating agent for sperms. Although these media are effective, there are concerns that zwitter ion buffers may interfere with some important processes in different cell types, consequently, have negative effects on gametes and embryos.

TRANSVAGINAL SONOGRAPHY ON THE DAY OF INTRAUTERINE INSEMINATION

- Use nontoxic sterile probe cover.
- Check for ovulation: Collapsed follicles with irregular crenated margins, free fluid in the pouch of Douglas (POD) or periovarian fluid.
- Reconfirm position of uterus: Anteverted or retroverted.
- Assess endometrial lining.

INTRAUTERINE INSEMINATION CANNULA

Nontoxic, atraumatic, sterile, and disposable cannula should be used. In difficult inseminations, use more rigid cannulas.

IMPORTANT PRECAUTIONS

- Use nonpowdered and nontoxic gloves.
- Expose cervix—do not hold.
- Preparation of vagina with normal saline—avoid any antiseptics.
- Inseminate just above the internal os.
- Inseminate slowly over 3 minutes.
- Wait for a few seconds: prevent efflux.
- Withdraw slowly.
- Withdraw speculum, lay patient supine for 10 minutes.
- Atraumatic transfer.

INFLUENCE OF SPERM QUALITY ON INTRAUTERINE INSEMINATION OUTCOME

It is not possible to define clear lower cut-off of pre- or postwash sperm parameters below which IUI should be withheld. Total motile sperm count (TMSC) >1 million and a morphology >4% are of possible prognostic value. In such a case, below these cut-off levels IUI should be withheld. Van Weert et al. found the postwash TMSC to be predictive for nonpregnancy but the lower cut-off levels varied between 0.8 and 5 million.

THE BEST TIMING OF INSEMINATION

The timing of insemination comprises two variables: (1) the detection/induction of ovulation and (2) the time interval from this point to insemination. The WHO guideline provides no recommendations for one timing method over the other. Providers can determine the method of triggering in IUI stimulated with gonadotropins as there is no evidence to recommend for or against a method.[2] One can determine the method of timing IUI in natural cycles as there is no evidence to recommend for or against a method. If human chorionic gonadotropin (HCG) injection is used, single IUI can be performed any time between 24 and 40 hours after HCG injection without compromising pregnancy rates. IUI in a natural cycle should be performed 1 day after luteinizing hormone (LH) rise.

NUMBER OF INSEMINATIONS

In both unexplained and male infertility there is insufficient evidence that the intervention, a double IUI, within the same cycle will lead to better pregnancy rates than a single IUI within a cycle. Women undergoing IUI should be offered a single insemination per cycle.[3]

INTRAUTERINE INSEMINATION DEVICES

The most important devices of influence on IUI results are laboratory and clinical disposables and media, like semen containers, wash media, and catheters. Two possible impacts of these products can be distinguished: (1) Function and (2) toxicity. With respect to function, the type of catheter and ultrasound guidance can be of influence. A soft-tip catheter was found to cause less trauma to the endometrium compared to a hard-tip catheter, but was not superior in PR in a Cochrane review (van der Poel et al. 2010). Ultrasound guidance during insemination makes it possible to visualize the movement of the catheter inside the endometrial cavity and could so avoid endometrial trauma and uterine contractions.

BED REST AFTER INTRAUTERINE INSEMINATION

The WHO guideline provides no recommendations for bed rest after IUI (WHO, 2020). The rationale for a short period of supine positioning after insemination is that the spermatozoa may reach the tubes within 10 minutes. Immediate mobilization might counteract this movement due to gravity.

PREVENTION OF MULTIPLE PREGNANCIES AND OVARIAN HYPERSTIMULATION SYNDROME IN AN INTRAUTERINE INSEMINATION PROGRAM

To reduce multiple pregnancy rate (MPR) in IUI–OS, IUI should be withheld when more than two dominant follicles (DF) >15 mm or more than five follicles >10 mm at the time of HCG injection or LH surge are present. When gonadotropins are used in IUI, regimens with 75 IU or lower should be used because higher doses have similar pregnancy rates but increased MPR.

- Clomiphene citrate (CC) and/or tamoxifen are acceptable alternatives to

low-dose gonadotropins for low MPR and with lesser costs, although at a lower live birth rate than with gonadotropins.
- Addition of gonadotropin-releasing hormone (GnRH) agonist to gonadotropins in IUI–OS is not recommended because there is no increase in pregnancy rate despite increased MPR and increased costs.[4]
- *Good practice point:* As an alternative to cycle cancellation, aspiration of excess follicles at the time of HCG injection or LH surge might be additional option for reducing the risk of MPR in IUI–OS.[5]

CONSENT

- "Consent form" to be signed by the Couple/woman as specified in Form 12.
- Consent for Intrauterine Insemination with Husband's Semen/Sperm as specified in Form 13.
- Consent for Intrauterine Insemination with Donor Semen as specified in Form 14.
- Record of use of Donor Gametes as specified in Form 19, 19A, and 19B.
- Results of screening of Semen Donors/Oocyte Donor as specified in Form 20.
- Consent Form for the Donor of Sperm as specified in Form 22.

CONCLUSION

Most of the current evidence if of modern quality. IUI with or without ovarian induction/stimulation still remains the first line of management for many couple in India. Care to be taken to prevent infections.

KEY LEARNING POINTS

- Success rate of IUI does not vary profoundly with different IUI methodology and procedure.
- A more number of large placebo controlled trials of IUI is required determining the optimal length, duration and procedure.

REFERENCES

1. World Health Organization. Laboratory Manual for the Examination and Processing of Human Semen, 5th edition. Geneva: World Health Organization; 2010.
2. van Weert JM, Repping S, Van Voorhis BJ, van der Veen F, Bossuyt PMM, Mol BWJ. Performance of the postwash total motile sperm count as a predictor of pregnancy at the time of intrauterine insemination: a meta-analysis. Fertil Steril. 2004;82:612-20.
3. van der Poel N, Farquhar C, Abou-Setta AM, Benschop L, Heineman MJ. Soft versus firm catheters for intrauterine insemination. Cochrane Database Syst Rev. 2010.
4. National Institute for Health and Clinical Excellence. Fertility: Assessment and Treatment for People with Fertility Problems. London: Royal College of Obstetricians and Gynaecologists; 2013.
5. Bahadur G, Homburg R, Muneer A, Racich P, Alangaden T, Al-Habib A, et al. First line fertility treatment strategies regarding IUI and IVF require clinical evidence. Hum Reprod. 2016c;31:1141-6.

SECTION 9

Luteal Phase Support

22. Luteal Phase Support
Pratap Kumar, Prashanth K Adiga

CHAPTER 22

Luteal Phase Support

Pratap Kumar, Prashanth K Adiga

■ INTRODUCTION

Luteal phase is the time period after ovulation and the onset of menstruation or establishment of pregnancy.[1] The corpus luteum (CL) has the important function of maintaining the luteal phase by secreting hormones, i.e., progesterone and estrogen. For successful implantation, there must be sustained coordination between the receptive endometrium and competent embryo. Assisted reproduction practices often use intrauterine insemination (IUI) in conjunction with controlled ovarian stimulation (OS).[2] In in-vitro fertilization (IVF) treatment, luteal phase defect is well known, but its role in OS—IUI cycles are debatable.

■ PHYSIOLOGY OF LUTEAL PHASE

The menstrual cycle has two phases: (1) follicular and (2) luteal phase. These phases are separated by ovulation and ends when the patient menstruates. Estrogen dominates the follicular phase and the luteal phase is dominated by progesterone. Estrogen causes endometrial proliferation while progesterone inhibits endometrial proliferation and determines the endometrial receptivity. After ovulation, the CL is formed, which is an important organ which secretes hormones. Low-level of luteinizing hormone (LH) stimulation helps the luteal cells produce progesterone, which is dependent on the availability of its circulating cholesterol substrate.[3]

The life span of the CL ranges from 11 to 17 days. It appears that each individual CL has a predetermined lifespan that is unaffected by LH production. Rapidly increasing human chorionic gonadotropin (HCG) produced by the trophoblast in early pregnancy can save CL from luteolysis and allow it to continue producing progesterone. The survival of the CL depends on an early pregnancy, but the survival of an early pregnancy also depends on a functioning CL.

■ LUTEAL PHASE DEFICIENCY

Deficiency of progesterone exposure to sustain a healthy secretory endometrium and permit healthy embryo implantation and growth is called luteal phase deficiency (LPD).[4] Manifestation of luteal phase defect may be in the form of (a) short luteal phase (<9 days from the time of ovulation till the onset of menses)[5] (b) spotting, days before the onset of menstruation, in the absence of infection or structural cause.[6] Implications of LPD includes (1) irregular menstrual cycle, (2) infertility, and (3) recurrent pregnancy loss.

Why does luteal phase deficiency occur?
It is to be noted that the occurrence of LPD in ovulation induction (OI) with IUI is debatable.

The occurrence of LPD in IVF cycles has been well established. LPD is reasonably common in in-vitro fertilization (IVF) cycles. The reasons for LPD in IVF cycles have been due to (a) impaired CL deficiency and (b) abnormal endometrial response to progesterone.

Impaired CL deficiency is probably due to (a) abnormally high levels of steroids in the serum, often seen during cycles of stimulation, negatively impact the release of LH, which is necessary for the creation and upkeep of CL[7] and (b) ovulation triggering agents used for final oocyte maturation before oocyte pick-up,[8] and (c) supraphysiologic steroid hormones released during the early LP of an IVF cycle by the various CLs.[9]

Another factor contributing to the clinical picture of LPD is endometrial progesterone resistance, or an aberrant endometrial response to normal progesterone levels. The primary reason of endometrial resistance to progesterone appears to be the predominant expression of a less active progesterone receptor isoform in the endometrial stromal and epithelial cells.[10]

Does ovarian stimulation with intrauterine insemination need luteal phase support?

The commonly used drugs for OS are (1) clomiphene citrate, (2) letrozole, and (3) gonadotropins, which are clubbed with IUI. There has been debate concerning the role of exogenous progesterone support during the luteal phase of IUI cycles.

■ CLOMIPHENE CITRATE CYCLES

Clomiphene citrate increases the LH levels when compared with gonadotropins, which causes a decrease in LH concentration. By competing with estrogen receptors in the hypothalamus, clomiphene citrate can promote ovulation. The blockade of the estrogen receptors causes increase in the release of follicle-stimulating hormone (FSH) and LH. In a study by Kyrou et al., luteal phase support with vaginal progesterone was given to normo-ovulatory patients stimulated with clomiphene citrate for IUI, the rate of continuing pregnancies was not higher than in patients who did not receive vaginal progesterone treatment.[11] The meta-analysis by Green et al. demonstrated that patients receiving clomiphene citrate for OI did not benefit from progesterone support.[12] The same study also concluded that there is no enough data to support the use of progesterone support in clomiphene plus gonadotropin OI-IUI cycles.[12]

■ LETROZOLE-INDUCED CYCLES

It has been suggested that women with polycystic ovarian syndrome (PCOS) who are resistant to clomiphene citrate could benefit from therapy with letrozole.[13] The role of luteal phase support in patients who have been induced with letrozole, in PCOS patients is controversial. The study by Monteville et al. showed that utilizing intravaginal progesterone support increased the clinical pregnancy rates among PCOS women who used letrozole for OI.[14] On the contrary, in the study by Dilday et al., luteal support with vaginal progesterone does not significantly increase clinical pregnancy rate (CPR) in women where OS was done using letrozole.[15] In letrozole plus gonadotropin OI-IUI cycles, there is no enough data to assess the impact of progesterone for luteal support.[12]

■ GONADOTROPIN CYCLES

The effect of gonadotropin stimulation on hormone levels during IUI may be similar to those of IVF cycles. The reported incidence of a short luteal phase in cycles stimulated by gonadotropins is about 20%. When gonadotropins are administered for OI, supplementing the luteal phase with vaginal progesterone improved live birth rates.[16] In patients undergoing gonadotropin OI and IUI, exogenous progesterone administered during the luteal phase enhances the clinical pregnancy and live birth rates (level I evidence).[12]

CHOICE OF PROGESTERONE

It has been proved that luteal phase support by supplementing with exogenous progesterone improves the outcomes, especially in those cycles where gonadotropins have been used.[12] Progesterone may be supplemented by (1) vaginally with a progesterone gel or in capsules of naturally micronized progesterone, (2) oral micronized progesterone, (3) subcutaneous injections of progesterone, (4) intramuscular injections of progesterone in oil, and (5) dydrogesterone.

Oral formulations of natural progesterone have poor bioavailability, making them less useful. Vaginal preparations have an inherent problem of discomfort and discharge, however, by avoiding the first-pass metabolism, they produce high-serum concentrations, resulting in sufficient endometrial transformation and continuous circulating levels for 24 hours.[17]

Progesterone based on oil administered intramuscularly produces high quantities of progesterone in circulation, however, there is pain and discomfort associated with the injections. In contrast to intramuscular preparations, a novel aqueous progesterone preparation is used subcutaneously, potentially producing comparable progesterone levels with less discomfort.[18]

Dydrogesterone: Compared to vaginal progesterone, dydrogesterone (6-dehydro-retroprogesterone) has a greater oral absorption and tolerance and is chemically and pharmacologically identical to natural progesterone.[19]

COMPARISON BETWEEN MICRONIZED PROGESTERONE VERSUS DYDROGESTERONE

Dydrogesterone and micronized vaginal progesterone are equally effective as a luteal phase support. The study by Khosravi et al. concluded that for luteal-phase support in women undergoing IUI cycles, oral dydrogesterone is as effective as vaginal progesterone.[20] In comparison to the micronized progesterone group, the dydrogesterone group had greater mean serum progesterone levels.[20] Oral dydrogesterone may be recommended for luteal phase support in IUI due to its ease of administration, safety concerns, and improved patient tolerability.[21]

DOSE OF MICRONIZED VAGINAL PROGESTERONE

In both IVF and controlled ovarian hyperstimulation (COH)–IUI cycles, the dosage of micronized vaginal progesterone typically ranges between 300 and 600 mg. The study by Biberoglu et al. demonstrated that 300 mg of micronized vaginal progesterone was sufficient instead of 600 mg in IUI cycles. The success rates of continued pregnancies were comparable for both doses. In COH–IUI cycles, luteal phase support can produce an acceptable pregnancy rate with a maximum daily dose of 300 mg of intravaginal micronized progesterone.[22]

CONCLUSION

Luteal phase is the time period after ovulation, where the corpus luteum (CL) has the important function of maintaining the luteal phase by secreting hormones, i.e., progesterone and estrogen. Luteal phase deficiency (LPD) is well established in IVF cycles but its role OS—IUI cycle is controversial.

There is no role for progesterone supplementation as luteal phase support when oral ovulogens are used. Progesterone supplementation in patients undergoing gonadotropin OI and IUI, is useful as it enhances the clinical pregnancy and live birth rates.

Dydrogesterone and micronized vaginal progesterone are equally effective as a luteal phase support. The safety profile and improved tolerability of dydrogesterone scores over micronized vaginal progesterone as luteal phase support.

■ KEY LEARNING POINTS

- The existence of luteal phase defect in patients undergoing OI with IUI cycles is debatable.
- Patients receiving clomiphene citrate for OI with IUI do not benefit from progesterone support, as a luteal phase support.
- There is insufficient data to support the use of progesterone support in clomiphene plus gonadotropin OI-IUI cycles.
- In letrozole plus gonadotropin OI-IUI cycles, there is no enough data to assess the impact of progesterone as luteal support.
- In patients undergoing gonadotropin OI and IUI, exogenous progesterone administered during the luteal phase enhances the clinical pregnancy and live birth rates (level I evidence).
- Maximum dose of micronized vaginal progesterone for luteal phase support in IUI cycles is 300 mg.

■ REFERENCES

1. Fatemi HM, Popovic-Todorovic B, Papanikolaou E, Donoso P, Devroey P. An update of luteal phase support in stimulated IVF cycles. Hum Reprod Update. 2007;13(6): 581-90.
2. Gün İ, Özdamar Ö, Yılmaz A. Luteal phase support in intrauterine insemination cycles. Turkish J Obstet Gynecol. 2016;13(2):90.
3. Barbieri RL. The endocrinology of the menstrual cycle. Methods Mol Biol. 2014; 1154:145-69.
4. Practice Committee of the American Society for Reproductive Medicine. Current clinical irrelevance of luteal phase deficiency: a committee opinion. Fertil Steril. 2015;103(4):e27-32.
5. Schliep KC, Mumford SL, Hammoud AO, Stanford JB, Kissell KA, Sjaarda LA, et al. Luteal phase deficiency in regularly menstruating women: prevalence and overlap in identification based on clinical and biochemical diagnostic criteria. J Clinical Endocrinol Metabol. 2014;99(6):E1007-14.
6. Mesen TB, Young SL. Progesterone and the luteal phase: a requisite to reproduction. Obstet Gynecol Clin. 2015;42(1):135-51.
7. Tavaniotou A, Albano C, Smitz J, Devroey P. Impact of ovarian stimulation on corpus luteum function and embryonic implantation. J Reproductive immunol. 2002; 55(1-2):123-30.
8. Beckers NG, Macklon NS, Eijkemans MJ, Ludwig M, Felberbaum RE, Diedrich K, et al. Nonsupplemented luteal phase characteristics after the administration of recombinant human chorionic gonadotropin, recombinant luteinizing hormone, or gonadotropin-releasing hormone (GnRH) agonist to induce final oocyte maturation in in vitro fertilization patients after ovarian stimulation with recombinant follicle-stimulating hormone and GnRH antagonist cotreatment. J Clin Endocrinol Metabol. 2003;88(9):4186-92.
9. Fatemi HM. The luteal phase after 3 decades of IVF: what do we know? Reprod biomed online. 2009;19:1-3.

10. Hu M, Li J, Zhang Y, Li X, Brännström M, Shao LR, et al. Endometrial progesterone receptor isoforms in women with polycystic ovary syndrome. Am J Translat Res. 2018; 10(8):2696.
11. Kyrou D, Fatemi HM, Tournaye H, Devroey P. Luteal phase support in normo-ovulatory women stimulated with clomiphene citrate for intrauterine insemination: need or habit? Hum Reprod. 2010;25(10):2501-6.
12. Green KA, Zolton JR, Schermerhorn SM, Lewis TD, Healy MW, Terry N, et al. Progesterone luteal support after ovulation induction and intrauterine insemination: an updated systematic review and meta-analysis. Fertil Steril. 2017;107(4):924-33.
13. Mitwally MF, Casper RF. Use of an aromatase inhibitor for induction of ovulation in patients with an inadequate response to clomiphene citrate. Fertil steril. 2001; 75(2):305-9.
14. Montville CP, Khabbaz M, Aubuchon M, Williams DB, Thomas MA. Luteal support with intravaginal progesterone increases clinical pregnancy rates in women with polycystic ovary syndrome using letrozole for ovulation induction. Fertil steril. 2010; 94(2):678-83.
15. Dilday E, Gigg M, Hoyos L, Quinn M, Markovic D, Kroener L. Luteal phase support with progesterone does not improve pregnancy rates in patients undergoing ovarian stimulation with letrozole. Reprod BioMed Online. 2023;46(1):123-8.
16. Miralpeix E, González-Comadran M, Solà I, Manau D, Carreras R, Checa MA. Efficacy of luteal phase support with vaginal progesterone in intrauterine insemination: a systematic review and meta-analysis. J Assist Reprod Genet. 2014;31:89-100.
17. Blake EJ, Norris PM, Dorfman SF, Longstreth J, Yankov VI. Single and multidose pharmacokinetic study of a vaginal micronized progesterone insert (Endometrin) compared with vaginal gel in healthy reproductive-aged female subjects. Fertil steril. 2010;94(4):1296-301.
18. Sator M, Radicioni M, Cometti B, Loprete L, Leuratti C, Schmidl D, et al. Pharmacokinetics and safety profile of a novel progesterone aqueous formulation administered by the sc route. Gynecol Endocrinol. 2013; 29(3):205-8.
19. Barbosa MW, Silva LR, Navarro PA, Ferriani RA, Nastri CO, Martins WD. Dydrogesterone vs progesterone for luteal-phase support: systematic review and meta-analysis of randomized controlled trials. Ultrasound Obstet Gynecol. 2016;48(2):161-70.
20. Khosravi D, Taheripanah R, Taheripanah A, Monfared VT, Hosseini-Zijoud SM. Comparison of oral dydrogesterone with vaginal progesteronefor luteal support in IUI cycles: a randomized clinical trial. Iran J Reprod Med.. 2015;13(7):433-8.
21. Taş M, Uludag SZ, Aygen ME, Sahin Y. Comparison of oral dydrogesterone and vaginal micronized progesterone for luteal phase support in intrauterine insemination. Gynecol Endocrinol. 2020;36(1):77-80.
22. Biberoglu EH, Tanrıkulu F, Erdem M, Erdem A, Biberoglu KO. Luteal phase support in intrauterine insemination cycles: a prospective randomized study of 300 mg versus 600 mg intravaginal progesterone tablet. Gynecol Endocrinol. 2016;32(1):55-7.

SECTION 10

Analyzing Results

23. **Intrauterine Insemination Results and Coping with Failure**
    N Sanjeeva Reddy, Radha Vembu

CHAPTER 23: Intrauterine Insemination Results and Coping with Failure

N Sanjeeva Reddy, Radha Vembu

INTRODUCTION

Infertility is defined as the inability to conceive after 12 months of regular and unprotected intercourse. Although 60–75% conceive within 6 months and 85–90% by 12 months, still 48.5 million couples are affected by infertility worldwide.[1] So, it is a global problem affecting 8–12% of couples worldwide.[2] Male factor contributes up to 50% and is solely responsible in 20–30% of overall infertility.

Intrauterine insemination (IUI) is a simple and minimal invasive procedure which is performed with less expensive infrastructure, with minimal risks if appropriately monitored,[3] and the clinical pregnancy varies from 10 to 20% per cycle. But, the main drawback is low delivery rate of 8% per cycle according to the European Society of Human Reproduction and Embryology (ESHRE).[4] So, to improve the clinical outcome of IUI, indications must be refined in addition to adequate ovarian stimulation (OS), semen processing and timing with ovulation.

IUI is the first line of treatment for various causes of infertility such as cervical factor, ovulation dysfunction, mild-to-moderate male factors, and unexplained infertility. There are many factors influencing the outcome of IUI cycle namely patient's age, ovarian function, oocyte quality, duration of infertility, ovarian stimulation, endometrial thickness, number of inseminations, and time duration between semen collection and insemination.

FACTORS INFLUENCING THE INTRAUTERINE INSEMINATION OUTCOME

Female Factor

Maternal Age

As the age advances, there is progressive follicular depletion, decline in granulosa function, poor oocyte quality (both nuclear and cytoplasmic), compromised endometrial receptivity, chromosomal abnormalities, higher anovulatory cycles, and aging of reproductive tract.[5]

Duration of Infertility

It is one of the significant predictors of success which is better with short duration of infertility and those with longer duration should be counseled for in-vitro fertilization (IVF) or intracytoplasmic sperm injection (ICSI). Studies have shown that the treatment outcomes worsen with increasing duration of infertility.[6]

Ovarian Reserve

Decreased ovarian reserve is commonly seen in advanced maternal age and very low ovarian reserve is a limiting factor for IUI success. Among all the markers, antral follicle count (AFC) and anti-Müllerian hormone (AMH) have shown promising results and hence are commonly measured. The patients with elevated basal luteinizing hormone (LH) levels can have significantly low conceptions in all modalities of treatment as they are less likely to respond to OS.[7]

Lifestyle

A body mass index (BMI) between 25 and 29.99 kg/m^2 or ≥30 kg/m^2 does not appear to have a negative effect on live birth after IUI. But, obesity may be associated with a higher risk of biochemical pregnancy after IUI.[8] Conversely, some authors could not find an association between BMI and IUI success.[9]

A high BMI (>45 kg/m^2) is known to compromise the success of IUI.[7] This can be due to poor oocyte quality, hostile intrauterine environment, and deranged insulin and androgen sensitivity.

Smoking has a detrimental effect on IUI outcome by increasing the gonadotropin dose requirement for OS, lower estradiol levels with decreased fertilization rates, implantation rates and hence LBRs. So, lifestyle modification might improve the success of IUI.

Drugs for Ovarian Stimulation

Clinical pregnancy is optimal when there is development of two to three follicles. So, drugs for ovulation induction (in cases of anovulation and OS in already ovulatory patients) is performed to overcome subtle ovulatory defects which remain undiagnosed. Clomiphene citrate, letrozole, and gonadotropins are more commonly used drugs. Even though the success rate of IUI is more with gonadotropins, there is increased risk of multifollicular development and multiple pregnancy.

Poor Oocyte Quality

It is difficult to assess the oocyte quality in IUI cycles unlike IVF/ICSI cycles. However, the indirect markers which can indicate the poor oocyte quality include:
- Poor follicular development assessed by folliculometry as seen in endometriosis with standard OS
- Development of empty follicles
- Too slow or too rapid growth of follicles
- The follicles with ill-defined margins and hazy look of follicles also indicate poor oocyte quality and lower success rate with IUI.

Timing of Intrauterine Insemination

IUI can be planned from 24 to 72 hours posttrigger. But, the success rate is more when it is timed 36–42 hours of ovulation trigger. There is no improvement in success rate with double IUI.[10] However, it is preferred in donor IUI cycles and cycles with variable ovulation time.

Male Factor

There is good evidence in literature that IUI is a most cost-effective procedure for male factor infertility. However, it is difficult to identify individual semen parameters predicting the likelihood of pregnancy after IUI. This might be due to lack of standardization of semen analysis, patient selection, type of OS, number of IUI cycles, number of insemination per cycle and sperm preparation technique. The sperm morphology and the inseminating motile sperm count after preparation are the two most important semen parameters which determine the success of IUI cycle. Even though a universal threshold level above which IUI can be performed has not been determined, success of IUI is impaired when <4% normal morphology sperms and inseminating motile sperm concentration <1 million/mL is inseminated.

Advanced Paternal Age

There are controversial results in literature suggesting advanced paternal age (>40 years) decrease fertility and increase the pregnancy complications.[11] However, some of the studies have shown no effect on the outcome.[12]

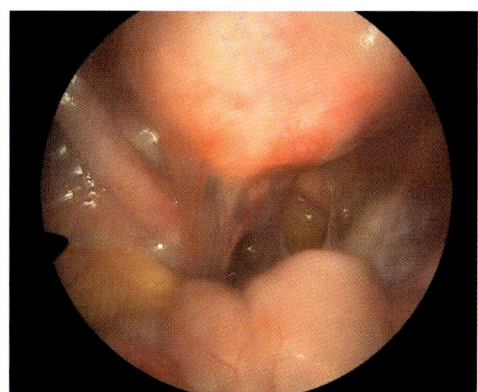

Fig. 1: Adhesions in pouch of Douglas (POD).

EVALUATION AFTER FAILED INTRAUTERINE INSEMINATION CYCLES AND FURTHER MANAGEMENT

Hysterolaparoscopy

This gives a broad view of the pelvic reproductive anatomy and magnified view of peritoneal surfaces. There might be certain abnormalities which may not be picked up during routine investigations for infertility which might affect the IUI outcome. The main advantage of this procedure is, "see and treat approach" in the same sitting and hence can improve the reproductive outcome.

The abnormal findings seen during laparoscopy include endometriosis, pelvic adhesions, peritubal adhesions distorting the tubo-ovarian relationship, adnexal mass, hydrosalpinx and other features of pelvic inflammatory disease and pelvic tuberculosis.

The minor tubal defects noticed in unexplained infertility during laparoscopy are:
- Tubal kinks due to serosal adhesions
- Stretched tubes toward iliac fossae can shorten the infundibulo-pelvic ligament.
- Fimbrial pathologies like fimbrial eversion and agglutination.

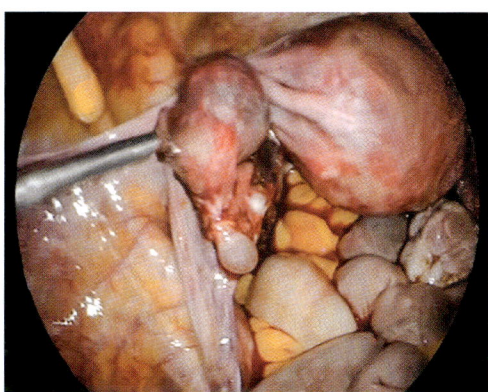

Fig. 2: Fimbrial cyst.

- Peritubal adhesions interfering with tubal motility, adhesions in pouch of Douglas (POD) causing hindrance to reservoir function and egg pick up **(Fig. 1)**.
- Cornual or terminal tubal block developed between previous hysterosalpingography (HSG) and present laparoscopy.
- Pedunculated fimbrial cysts **(Fig. 2)**, blocking the fimbrial opening of tubes like a ball–valve causing temporary tubal block.[13]

During hysteroscopy, there can be minimal intrauterine adhesions, small endometrial polyps, septate uterus, submucous fibroid, and features suggestive of chronic endometritis **(Figs. 3A and B)**.

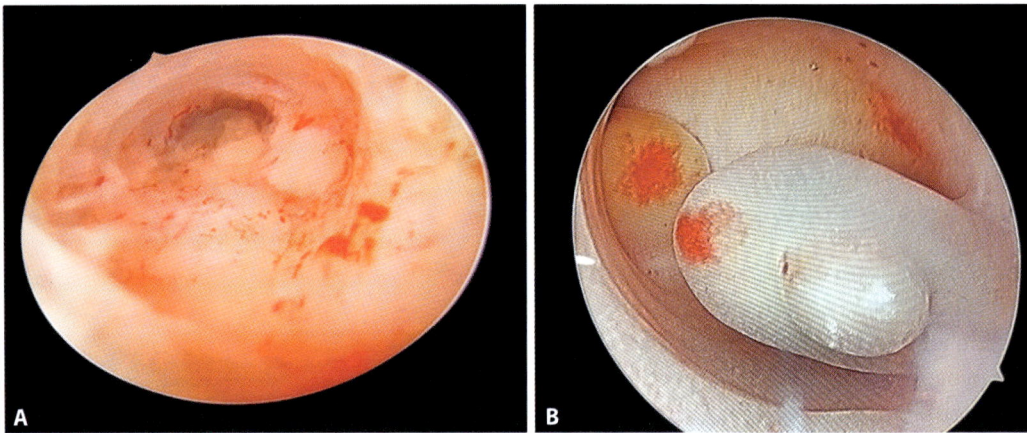

Figs. 3A and B: Hysteroscopic images. (A) Tuberculosis and (B) Endometrial polyp.

Endometrial Scratching

The role of endometrial scratching is controversial after IUI failure. However, in a recent systematic review and meta-analysis,[14] endometrial scratch significantly improved the biochemical, clinical pregnancy, and LBR.[15] In a study, three cycles of OS-IUI was compared with expectant management (EM) in unexplained infertility with Hunault score <30%. They observed 10% LBR/IUI cycle and 31% cumulative LBR in IUI cycle versus 9% in EM. So, one cycle of IUI with OS had similar LBR when compared to three cycles of EM and three cycles of OS with IUI are comparable to one cycle of IVF with single embryo transfer.

■ SEMEN ANALYSIS

Semen analysis done in a standard laboratory forms the cornerstone of male infertility evaluation. Recently, it has provided updated sampling and laboratory guidelines.[16] However, there remains several limitations with conventional semen analysis. This has led to the need for advanced sperm function tests and seminal fluid quality assessments like oxidative stress, sperm DNA fragmentation.

Morphologically abnormal sperms have multiple defects either in the head, middle piece, or tail and are associated with a series of genetic defects affecting the sperm function.

■ SPERM DNA FRAGMENTATION

Sperm DNA fragmentation (SDF) is one of the most common disturbances affecting the genetic material either as single- or double-strand breaks. Although fertilization capacity of sperms and SDF may not be impaired, it may affect embryo development, implantation, and pregnancies in both natural and assisted reproduction. It is prevalent more commonly among men with abnormal semen parameters and it is also seen in normozoospermic men. As SDF is only partially related to semen quality, it is one of the promising markers in andrology.

In a recent study analyzing SDF and clinical outcomes in 1,500 IUI cycles, normal sperm DNA fragmentation index (DFI) group had a higher biochemical pregnancy rate, clinical pregnancy rate, delivery rate and live birth rate (LBR) than the abnormal sperm DFI group, but there were no significant statistical differences. So, this study concluded that SDF had no impact on clinical outcomes of IUI.[17]

GENETIC ABNORMALITIES

Over a period of years, there is significant number of genetic or genomic abnormalities with an increase in the awareness about gene mutations. There are only few laboratories performing genetic testing and the methodology is not specific for semen related defects.

Among unselected infertile men, there is 10-fold increase in the incidence of sperm chromosomal aneuploidy even with normal karyotype.

Aneuploid oocytes are more common with maternal aging and results in aneuploid embryos and loss. Similarly, Robertsonian translocations are one of the well-known causes for increase in aneuploid sperms. These aneuploid sperms are more common in men with spermatogenic failure, oligozoospermia, oligoasthenozoospermia and among normozoospermic men with couple having recurrent pregnancy loss. This can be detected more commonly by fluorescence in situ hybridization (FISH).

TIMING OF INSEMINATION FROM PREPARATION

Studies have shown that the time interval between the semen preparation and IUI have shown to impact the pregnancy rate. It is found that clinical pregnancy is better if the time interval is between 40 and 80 minutes, with a maximum clinical pregnancy at 60 minutes. If IUI is performed too soon (<40 minutes), the reduced results may be seen due to lower proportion of uncondensed chromatin of sperms. This incubation period is required to enhance the phenomenon of sperm chromatin decondensation involved in fertilization. Earlier studies have shown that no fertilization occurs when the decondensation was <70%.[18] For IUI, if duration was >80 minutes, there is decrease in clinical pregnancy due to harmful effects of in vitro conditions and/or time incubation on sperm.

SPERM ACROSOME REACTION

Sperm acrosome reaction is a requisite for natural fertilization and the ICSI. This reaction should happen only on contact with the oocyte. If spontaneous acrosome reaction occurs in culture medium, it can lower the success rate of IUI.[19]

IN VITRO FERTILIZATION/ INTRACYTOPLASMIC SPERM INJECTION

Over the past 2 decades, IVF/ICSI has become an effective treatment for all causes of infertility. However, it is more invasive and costly. Following three cycles of OS and IUI, if the women does not conceive, then IVF will be a suitable option to reduce emotional and physical burden and hence expediate treatment. It is also recommended in women with advanced age ≥38 years.

The success of IUI in unexplained infertility is substantially lower probably linked to fertilization disorder.[20] So, many advise ICSI after three IUI failures.[21] According to the American Society for Reproductive Medicine (ASRM), the best initial therapy for unexplained infertility is a course of OS with oral medications and IUI followed by IVF.[22]

CONCLUSION

The outcome of IUI cycle is low and is influenced by various factors. The decision for IVF/ICSI is individualized by patient characteristics such as age, duration of infertility, previous treatment, and previous pregnancy.

KEY LEARNING POINTS

- IUI is one of the cost effective options for infertile couple with a clear indication.
- The couple should be evaluated further if they do not conceive after three cycles of ovarian stimulation (OS) and IUI.
- The most important evaluation for a female will be transvaginal ultrasound and hysterolaparoscopy, for male a good semen analysis in a standard laboratory and sperm DNA fragmentation helps in deciding for line of management.

REFERENCES

1. Agarwal A, Parekh N, Panner Selvam MK, Henkel R, Shah R, Homa ST, et al. Male oxidative stress infertility (MOSI): proposed terminology and clinical practice guidelines for management of idiopathic male infertility. World J Men's Health. 2019;37(3):296-312.
2. Kumar N, Singh AK. Trends of male factor infertility, an important cause of infertility: a review of literature. J Hum Reprod Sci. 2015;8:191-6.
3. Kandavel V, Cheong Y. Does intra-uterine insemination have a place in modern ART practice? Best Pract Res Clin Obstet Gynaecol. 2018;53:3-10.
4. De Geyter C, Calhaz-Jorge C, Kupka MS, Wyns C, Mocanu E, Motrenko T, et al. ART in Europe, 2015: Results Generated from European Registries by ESHRE. Hum Reprod Open. 2020;hoz038.
5. Yousefi B, Azargon A. Predictive factors of intrauterine insemination success of women with infertility over 10 years. J Pak Med Assoc. 2011;61(2):165-8.
6. Ejzenberg D, Gomes TJO, Monteleone PAA, Serafini PC, Baracat JMSEC. Prognostic factors for pregnancy after intrauterine Insemination. Int J Gynecol Obstet. 2019; 147:65-72.
7. Garcia-Grau E, Oliveira M, Amengual MJ, Rodriguez-Sanchez E, Veraguas-Imbernon A, Costa L, et al. An algorithm to predict the lack of pregnancy after intrauterine insemination in infertile patients. J Clin Med. 2023;12:3225.
8. Whynott RM, Summers KM, Van Voorhis BJ, Mejia RB. Effect of body mass index on intrauterine insemination cycle success. Fertil Steril. 2021;115(1):221-8.
9. Isa AM, Abu-Rafea B, Alasiri SA, Binsaleh S, Ismail KH, Vilos GA. Age, body mass index, and number of previous trials: are they prognosticators of intra-uterine-insemination for infertility treatment? Int J Fertil Steril. 2014;8:255-60.
10. Wg Cdr Arunav S, Wg Cdr Mustajib A, Col Rajesh S. Outcome of single and double intrauterine insemination techniques in infertility cases. J Marine Med Soc. 2023; 25(2):193-7.
11. Horta F, Vollenhoven B, Healey M, Busija L, Catt S. Male ageing is negatively associated with the chance of live birth in IVF/ICSI cycles for idiopathic infertility. Hum Reprod. 2019;34:2523-32.
12. Belloc S, Hazout A, Zini A, Merviel P, Cabry R, Chahine H, et al. How to overcome male infertility after 40: influence of paternal age on fertility. Maturitas. 2014;78:22-9.
13. Chatterjee S, Bagchi B, Chatterjee A. Intrauterine insemination—can we make it more successful? Int J Surg Med. 2020; 6(5):42-6.
14. Baradwan S, Alshahrani MS, AlSghan R, Alkhamis WH, Alsharif SA, Alanazi GA, et al. The effect of endometrial scratch on pregnancy rate in women with previous intrauterine insemination failure: a systematic review and meta-analysis of randomized controlled trials. Reprod Sci. 2023;30(5):1399-407.
15. Farquhar CM, Liu E, Armstrong S, Arroll N, Lensen S, Brown J. Intrauterine insemination with ovarian stimulation versus expectant management for unexplained infertility (TUI): a pragmatic, open-label, randomised, controlled, two-centre trial. Lancet. 2018; 391:441-50.
16. Boitrelle F, Shah R, Saleh R, Henkel R, Kandil H, Chung E, et al. The sixth edition of the WHO manual for human semen analysis: a critical

review and SWOT analysis. Life (Basel). 2021;11(12):1368.
17. Zhu C, Zhang S, Chen F, She H, Ju Y, Wen X, et al. Correlations between elevated basal sperm DNA fragmentation and the clinical outcomes in women undergoing IUI. Front Endocrinol. 2022;13:987812.
18. Gopalkrishnan K, Hinduja IN, Kumar TC. In vitro decondensation of nuclear chromatin of human spermatozoa: assessing fertilizing potential. Arch Androl. 1991;27:43-50.
19. Fauque P, Lehert P, Lamotte M, Bettahar-Lebugle K, Bailly A, Diligent C, et al. Clinical success of intrauterine insemination cycles is affected by the sperm preparation time. Fertil Steril. 2014;101(6):1618-23.e1-3.
20. Bungum L, Bungum M, Humaidan P, Andersen CY. A strategy for treatment of couples with unexplained infertility who failed to conceive after intrauterine insemination. Reprod Biomed Online. 2004;8:584-9.
21. Aboulghar M, Mansour R, Serour G, Abdrazek A, Amin Y, Rhodes C. Controlled ovarian hyperstimulation and intrauterine insemination for treatment of unexplained infertility should be limited to a maximum of three trials. Fertil Steril. 2001;75:88-91.
22. Penzias A, Bendikson K, Falcone T, Hansen K, Hill M, Jindal S, et al. Evidence-based treatments for couples with unexplained infertility: a guideline. Fertil Steril. 2020;113(2):305-22.

SECTION 11
Intrauterine Insemination in Special Situations

24. **Intrauterine Insemination in Female Subfertility**
    Fessy Louis T, Mounika Jampala

25. **Intrauterine Insemination in Endometriosis**
    Kuldeep Jain, Maansi Jain

26. **Intrauterine Insemination in Polycystic Ovarian Syndrome**
    Devika Gunasheela, Ashwini M, Akhila MV

27. **Intrauterine Insemination in Human Immunodeficiency Virus Serodiscordant Couples**
    Noushin Abdul Majid, Subhashini S

28. **Intrauterine Insemination in Unexplained Infertility**
    Sandeep Talwar, Rohit Gutgutia, Sonia Malik

29. **Cost-effective Intrauterine Insemination**
    Rita Bakshi, Riva Kiran KC

CHAPTER 24

Intrauterine Insemination in Female Subfertility

Fessy Louis T, Mounika Jampala

INTRODUCTION

Infertility is a major health concern on the rise with an estimated prevalence of nearly 10–15%.[1] As per the global data collected by the World Health Organization (WHO) between 1990 and 2021, approximately one in six adults might have experienced infertility once in their lifetime.[2]

INFERTILITY, SUBFERTILITY, AND STERILTIY: IS THERE ANY DIFFERENCE?

Infertility is defined as a disease characterized by the failure to establish a clinical pregnancy after 12 months of regular, unprotected sexual intercourse or due to an impairment of a person's capacity to reproduce, either as an individual or with his/her partner. Many clinicians use the term subfertility interchangeably with infertility. Subfertility is defined as any form or grade of reduced fertility in couples unsuccessfully trying to conceive within 6–12 months considering the maximum chances of fecundability during the initial six cycles; while sterility is a permanent state of infertility with no time restriction for being called sterile unlike infertility.[3,4]

The fecundity in humans is considered to be around 20% per cycle within 1 year of having regular unprotected intercourse provided all male and female factors being normal. This fecundity rate is considered to decline to 2–3% with each passing year thereby considering the time period of one year to diagnose a couple as infertile. The treatment modalities for infertility aim at increasing this fecundity to 20% once the couple starts their journey to achieve pregnancy. In vitro fertilization (IVF) is considered to have a higher success rate of approximately 50% among all infertility treatments owing to the selection of gametes and embryos used for the purpose of achieving pregnancy.[5] Intrauterine insemination (IUI) is considered as a first-line procedure amongst other ART techniques owing to its low cost, simplistic procedure, ease of management, and lesser incidence of complications in selected patients.

The efficacy of IUI treatment lies in increasing the number of gametes (ovarian stimulation in females and sperm wash techniques increase sperm concentration and motility) and increasing the number of gametes present in the female genital tract around the time of ovulation.[6]

Important prognostic indicators predicting the success of an IUI cycle are:[7]
- Age of the patient (with advanced maternal age fecundity begins to decrease with subfertility being more pronounced after 35 years).[8]
- Duration of infertility
- Cause of infertility

- Patency of the tube (at least one tube to be patent)
- Ovarian stimulation protocol
- Number of cycles of IUI performed
- Number of preovulatory follicles on the day of trigger
- Sperm preparation techniques
- Processed motile sperm count and inseminated sperm count
- Timing of insemination.

The indications for IUI could be either male or female factors, most commonly being:
- Cervical factor
- Ovulatory dysfunction
- Minimal to mild endometriosis
- Mild to moderate male factor
- Ejaculatory dysfunction
- Unexplained infertility.

This chapter will specifically deal with the female factor contributing to infertility and the prerequisites required for a female subfertile patient undergoing IUI.

■ CERVICAL FACTOR

Cervical factor infertility includes anatomical abnormality due to primary cervical stenosis/secondary to cervical scarring and abnormal cervical mucus. Cervical mucus has a critical physiological role to play in fertility. Cervical mucus is hormonal dependent during the cycle and it enables sperm survival and transport. Under estrogenic influence, the cervical mucus enables the duration of fertile window in normal fertile females to be around 6 days including the day of ovulation. Vaginal secretions are hostile to sperm and in the absence of fertile cervical mucus, the sperm would not last more than a few hours. It also serves as a biological valve enabling the entry of the sperm only during the fertile period which is subjected to estrogenic and progestogenic influence.[9]

The most recommended method for diagnosis of cervical factor infertility was post coital test (PCT).[10] Postintercourse (before ovulation) cervical mucus at the external os is evaluated for PH, cellularity, viscosity (stretchability of cervical mucus under estrogenic influence), clarity, salinity (crystallization of cervical mucus when dried on a glass slide), and number and motility of the surviving sperms. It is recommended to do the PCT 2 days prior to the luteinizing hormone (LH) surge; however, the test results may not be accurate due to poor test timing. With the advent of IUI, cervical factor testing with PCT is no longer recommended as PCT results do not change the clinical management. The approach to cervical factor infertility is not to evaluate the patient for cervical factor but to avoid evaluation and proceed with IUI or IVF.[9] Pregnancy rates were seen to be higher with IUI compared with expectant management (51 vs. 33%) in those with abnormal postcoital tests with normal semen parameters.[11]

■ OVULATORY DISORDERS

Ovulatory disorders are common in reproductive-age women and constitute nearly 25% cases of female infertility. It is important to understand that the term "ovulatory disorder" is not synonymous with the term "anovulation." The ovulatory disorder is considered secondary to either episodic or chronic dysfunction of hypothalamic–pituitary–ovarian (HPO) axis eventually causing anovulation. The most common cause of anovulation is polycystic ovarian syndrome (PCOS), which affects nearly 70% of the women with anovulation.[12]

Ovulation typically occurs 14 days prior to ovulation and a cycle length of 21–35 days [latest International Federation of

TABLE 1: Ovulatory disorders categorized by World Health Organization.		
Group 1	*Group 2*	*Group 3*
Hypothalamic/pituitary failure (Hypogonadotropic hypogonadism)	Hypothalamic/pituitary dysfunction (Eugonadotropic hypogonadism)	End-organ failure (Hypergonadotropic hypogonadism)
Examples: • Kallmann syndrome • Sheehan's syndrome • Idiopathic GnRH deficiency • Stress or exercise-induced amenorrhea • Pituitary tumors	*Examples:* • Polycystic ovary syndrome	*Examples:* • Primary ovarian insufficiency (formerly called *premature ovarian failure*) • Gonadal dysgenesis (Turner syndrome) • Fragile X premutation carriers
(GnRH: gonadotropin-releasing hormone)		

Gynecology and Obstetrics (FIGO) consensus says 24–34 days] is considered normal. When the menstrual history is unclear, serum progesterone levels (value >3 ng/mL) 1 week prior to the expected menses may be diagnostic of ovulation.[13]

Earlier WHO categorized ovulatory disorders into three groups that are enumerated in **Table 1**.[14]

International Federation of Gynecology and Obstetrics in August 2022 came up with a newer classification of ovulatory disorders constituting four groups:
1. Type I: Hypothalamic
2. Type II: Pituitary
3. Type III: Ovarian
4. Type IV: PCOS

Referred by the acronym "HyPO-P," where P is separated from the other categories as it does not confine to a single anatomical location. Subcategories for each group can be referred by the acronym "GAIN-FIT-PIE (**Fig. 1**)."[15]

Patients with ovulatory disorders may exist in a spectrum ranging between occasional ovulatory dysfunction to chronic anovulation (**Fig. 2**). Most of the patients also have existing menstrual irregularities, hence

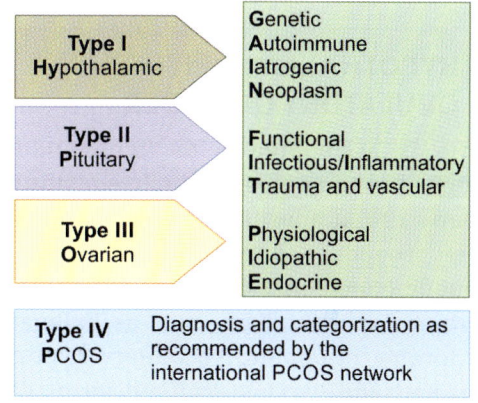

Fig. 1: FIGO ovulatory disorders classification (HyPO-P). (FIGO: International Federation of Gynecology and; PCOS: polycystic ovarian syndrome)

thorough history regarding the present and past menstrual cycles is extremely important while evaluating a patient of infertility.

Intrauterine insemination remains the first choice of treatment for couples with ovulatory dysfunction with a pregnancy rate of nearly 10–15% per cycle.[16] Accepted stimulation regimens for different causes of ovulatory disorders and infertility vary from using oral ovulogens [such as letrozole (LE) and clomiphene citrate (CC)], gonadotropins (Gn), or a combination of these.

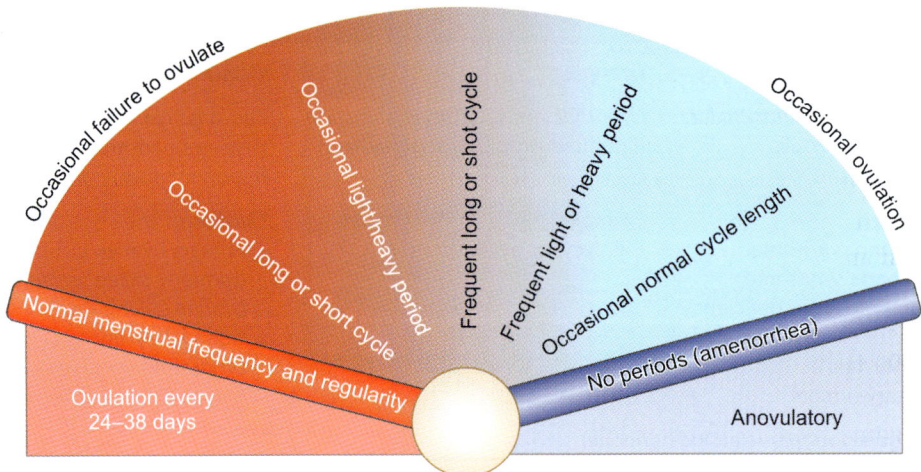

Fig. 2: Disorders of ovulation exist on a spectrum that ranges from occasional failure to ovulate to chronic anovulation.

HYPOTHALAMIC/PITUITARY OVULATORY DISORDER

This is associated with hypogonadotropic hypogonadism, which constitutes nearly 10% of anovulatory women. Usually seen secondary to various causes such as genetic (congenital causes of hypogonadotropic hypogonadism, such as Kallmann syndrome/idiopathic secondary hypogonadism) and various acquired forms that occur after sexual maturation. The condition results from a deficient secretion of episodic gonadotropin-releasing hormone (GnRH)/pituitary gonadotropin secretion, and thereby causing delayed puberty and infertility with diminished ovarian function. Depending upon the onset of the condition, basal levels of follicle-stimulating hormone (FSH), LH, E2, androstenedione, and prolactin are significantly lower in these patients. Due to long-term gonadotropin deficiency, they may have features of hypoestrogenism, uterine hypoplasia, ovulation inefficiency, and amenorrhea. Thorough investigations to rule out the cause of hypogonadism should be carried out before embarking on fertility treatment.

The principal target of treatment is supplying exogenous gonadotropins depending on the timing, and aims of treatment being either pubertal induction, infertility, or general health. Hormone replacement therapy (HRT) with estrogen and progesterone (at least three cycles) in patients with hypoplastic uterus is applied for uterine development. If the size of the uterus is normal, ovarian stimulation with gonadotropins (both FSH and LH)/pulsatile GnRH should be used to induce follicular development.[17] Pulsatile GnRH can be given in hypothalamic amenorrhea/idiopathic hypogonadotropic hypogonadism but not in hypopituitarism. This is more physiological and enables monofollicular development and thereby helps in restoring ovarian function.[18,19] However, for the availability and ease of administration, gonadotropins are more commonly used in clinical practice. Patients with hypopituitarism might have low adrenocorticotropic hormone (ACTH), growth hormone (GH), and thyroid-stimulating hormone (TSH) levels which need to be replaced along with FSH and LH.

Due to very low levels of LH in these patients, only FSH stimulation in them can lead to inadequate follicular growth, inadequate oocyte maturation, low E2 levels, and low endometrial thickness thereby decreasing their pregnancy rates.[20]

Human menopausal gonadotropin or recombinant FSH with rec LH combination should be used for stimulation in these patients. Ovulation triggers either 5,000 or 10,000 IU of human chorionic gonadotropin or 250 µg recombinant HCG (choriogonadotropin alfa) should be used in these patients.

Ovulation induction (OI) with gonadotropins is associated with more nonphysiological stimulation, risk of ovarian hyperstimulation, multiple pregnancies, and high cycle cancellation rates. A pregnancy rate of 12.7% per cycle has been reported with gonadotropin stimulation followed by IUI in patients with hypogonadotropic hypogonadism.[17] The other end of the spectrum is the possibility of cycle cancellation due to poor ovarian response in these patients due to failure of prediction of ovarian response with ovarian volume, antral follicle count, and anti-Müllerian hormone (AMH) levels. Ovarian reserve markers may not be representative of ovarian response in these patients.[21]

POLYCYSTIC OVARY SYNDROME (HYPOTHALAMIC/PITUITARY DYSFUNCTION)

Polycystic ovarian syndrome is the most common ovulatory disorder in reproductive-age women characterized by oligoovulation/anovulation, clinical or biochemical hyperandrogenism, and the presence of polycystic ovarian morphology. It accounts nearly to 8–19% of cases of infertility in reproductive-age group and 80% of anovulatory infertility. The presence of two out of three criteria diagnoses a case of polycystic ovary (PCO). As per the latest 2023 International evidence-based guidelines for the assessment and management of PCOS, serum AMH has been included in the diagnosis of PCO to define polycystic ovary morphology (PCOM) morphology. Either serum AMH or ultrasound [follicle number per ovary (FNPO) ≥20, follicle number per section (FNPS) ≥10, or ovarian volume ≥10 mL) can be used for diagnosis of PCOM.[13]

In 2016, the WHO global guidance management recommendation proposed the use of oral ovulogens like CC for six to nine cycles for the management of PCOS-associated infertility.[22] Australian National Health and Medical Research Council (NHMRC) in 2018 and the International 2023 PCOS consensus recommend LE as first-line pharmacological treatment agent for anovulatory PCOS. The use of LE is still off-label in many countries including India as it has not been approved by the USFDA for this purpose. Letrozole should be considered over CC to improve ovulation rate, clinical pregnancy, and live birth rates. When clomiphene is used, combination of clomiphene with metformin is recommended over either of the drugs alone to improve ovulation and clinical pregnancy rates. Gonadotropins are the second-line pharmacological agents of choice in those who failed to respond to oral ovulogens (CC failure or resistance).[13]

In recent years several randomized controlled trials have focused on IUI as a less invasive treatment for patients with PCOS-related infertility. Biochemical and clinical pregnancy rates were found to be higher in those patients undergoing IUI after OI with clomiphene than timed intercourse after OI with PCOS.[23]

Letrozole in Polycystic Ovary Syndrome

Classification of aromatase inhibitors is enumerated in **Table 2**.

Letrozole is a third-generation reversible competitive nonsteroidal aromatase inhibitor (AI) with a short half-life of 45 hours. Hence it has a lesser antiestrogenic effect on the endometrium and cervix compared to selective estrogen receptor modulators (SERMs) like clomiphene. It is because of this shorter half-life it is known to be completely eliminated out of the system before implantation occurs. It was first used by Mitwally and Casper for OI who were resistant to CC and who had persistent thin endometrium with SERM.[24] It is recommended as the first-line pharmacological agent in anovulatory PCOS with no other fertility factors.[13,25] Aromatase is a cytochrome 450 hemoprotein-containing enzyme (P450arom) that catalyzes the rate limiting step in the conversion of androstenedione and testosterone into estrone and estradiol respectively inhibits the enzyme aromatase thereby causing a reduction in E2 levels by 97–99%.[26] It is started from day 2 or 3 of menses for a period of 5 days and is given in a dose of 2.5–7.5 mg/day depending on the body mass index (BMI). Letrozole is considered to have a conception rate of 41.2% and live birth rate of 27.5% when used as a first-line agent for anovulatory PCOS.[27,28]

Patients with a higher LH/FSH ratio (≥1.83), higher AMH levels (≥9.78 ng/mL), a higher [free androgen index (FAI) ≥5.99] require a higher dose of LE than the lowest dose of 2.5mg/day to induce ovulation.[29]

Letrozole is usually administered as a multiple fixed dose regimen starting with 2.5 mg/day for 5 days increasing to a maximum of 7.5 mg/day depending on the individual ovarian response. A novel protocol with multifollicular development has been proposed with LE, a step-up protocol where it is administered in dose of one to four tablets on 2–5 days of the menstrual cycle respectively. The suppression effect on E2 levels causes a feedback increase in endogenous gonadotropins. This leads to the proliferation of granulosa cells and thereby increased aromatase expression and breakthrough estrogen production. This rise in E2 may cause endogenous gonadotropin suppression. The incremental dose of LE administration increases the window of elevated endogenous gonadotropins, and thereby causing multi-follicular development. A higher clinical pregnancy rate per treatment cycle of 27.3 versus 11.8 with step-up LE has been observed compared to clomiphene.[30]

Extended LE is another OI protocol where AI is administered for a period of 10 days in a dose of 2.5 mg/day. It has been proposed as a novel protocol in PCOS patients with LE resistance being who failed to ovulate after 5-day regimen of 5 mg LE/day at least in one OI cycle. In a study by Zhu, et al.[31] They have administered LE as a two-step

TABLE 2: Classification of aromatase inhibitors.

Generation	Type I Steroidal inhibitor	Type II Nonsteroidal inhibitor
First	None	Aminoglutethimide
Second	Formestane	• Fadrozole • Rogletimide
Third	Exemestane (Aromasin)	• Anastrozole (Arimidex) • Letrozole (Femara) • Orozole (Rivizor)

regimen. Initially, 5 mg was given for 7 days and those who did not ovulate were given an extended LE regimen for 10 days. They documented a ovulation rate of 92.75% after a two-step extended LE regimen with a cumulative clinical pregnancy rate of 31.88% and cumulative live birth rate of 24.63%. This is a feasible method of OI in PCOS patients with LE resistance.

Recently single dose LE of 25 mg on day 3 instead of traditional dosing for 5 days has been proposed to be equivalent peak E2 levels, number of follicles recruited, and pregnancy rates. However, further studies are warranted to follow this in routine practice.[32]

Clomiphene in Polycystic Ovary Syndrome

Clomiphene has been the first-line OI drug in this population for a long time. It is a nonsteroidal triphenylethylene derivative and acts as SERM similar to tamoxifen and raloxifene. They act as competitive inhibitors to estrogen at the receptor level and can have agonist or antagonistic activity depending on the target tissue. The commercially available form is a stereoisomeric mixture of zuclomiphene and enclomiphene with the latter being a more potent form with greater antiestrogenic activity and that which enables follicular growth.[33] It binds to estrogenic receptors at various levels including the hypothalamus, pituitary, ovary, and endometrium. Its binding effect on the hypothalamus causes a feedback increase in hypothalamic GnRH pulse frequency and an increase in the concentration of pituitary gonadotropins. Usually started in a dose of 50 mg/day for a period of 5 days and a maximum of up to 150 mg/day is used [United States Food and Drug Administration (USFDA) approved].

An ovulatory rate of 80% has been documented in anovulatory PCOS. The risk of ovarian hyperstimulation syndrome (OHSS) is <1% with a multiple pregnancy rate of 7%.[28] Approximately 15% of PCOS patients do not respond to the highest dose of this medication and is considered to be resistant. Clomiphene resistance is defined as failure to ovulate in at least three cycles after receiving 150 mg of CC/day for a period of 5 days. Hyperandrogenism, obesity, and insulin resistance are the most common reasons for CC resistance. The use of insulin-sensitizing agents like metformin as an adjunct to OI is useful in patients who are resistant to clomiphene.[34] Gonadotropins also can be added in these patients as second-line pharmacological agents for OI.[35]

Stair-step protocol has been advised for patients who failed to respond to the traditional CC protocol. Here 50 mg of CC is given from day 3 of the menstrual cycle. Folliculometry is done on day 7 and if there is no follicle >10 mm, 100 mg CC is given for another 5 days. Follicular scan is performed 7 days after the initial scan and dose increased till 200 mg (maximum dose)/day for 5 days with follicular scan being done 7 days after the previous scan. This stair-step protocol claims to have a higher cumulative ovulation rate of 7.43% versus 55.68% with the traditional protocol. A traditional protocol with a higher cumulative dose of 750 and 1,250 mg would yield an ovulation rate of 20.45 and 11.36% versus 34.52 and 23.81% with stair-step protocol. The cumulative pregnancy rate is significantly higher in the stair-step group compared to the traditional group (45.24% vs. 30.68%).[36] This protocol aids in knowing the sensitivity and resistance of patient with PCOS in a shorter duration of time compared to traditional protocol which might take multiple cycles and enables to decide on alternative modalities for the treatment of infertility.

Combined CC and LE regimen has been proposed to be superior to LE alone in inducing ovulation in PCOS and infertility. The peripheral mechanism of action of LE and the central action of CC are supposed to cause a synergistic effect on ovulation rates. Letrozole 2.5 mg/day along with CC 50 mg/day was given from days 3–7 of menses.[37]

Advantages of Letrozole over Clomiphene in Polycystic Ovary Syndrome

- LE induces a high rate of monofollicular development thereby reducing the multiple pregnancy rates.
- A shorter half-life (45 hours compared to 2 weeks) and absence of peripheral estrogen receptor blocking action enables lesser antiestrogenic side effects with fewer adverse effects on the endometrium and cervix.
- Lesser E2 levels are especially useful in patients of estrogen-dependent tumors undergoing ovarian stimulation.
- According to the PPCOS II (Pregnancy in Polycystic Ovary Syndrome II) trial, LE is associated with higher live birth rates and cumulative ovulation rates than CC[28] and those with PCOS associated with obesity.

Gonadotropins in Polycystic Ovary Syndrome

Several combinations and stimulation protocols of oral ovulogens have been proposed to induce ovulation without the use of gonadotropins to reduce the cost of treatment. They remain the second-line pharmacological agents who fail to respond to oral ovulogens even at a higher cumulative dose.[13] Owing to the cost of this therapeutic modality tubal patency is recommended before starting gonadotropins and IUI is chosen over timed intercourse when gonadotropins are used. Gonadotropin therapy produces an ovulatory rate of 70–72% in anovulatory PCOS and a 15–30% pregnancy rate per cycle.

There are several gonadotropin protocols used for OI in IUI:

- Step-up protocol uses 75–150 IU/day of gonadotropins for 2–4 days starting from day 2 or 3 of the menstrual cycle.[10] Following this transvaginal ultrasound and serum E2 levels are measured to look for any follicular recruitment. The dose is gradually increased until an appropriate response is seen. Though this protocol is used in hypogonadotropic hypogonadism patients who require higher doses of gonadotropins as they have never been exposed to, use in PCOS may lead to OHSS and increase in multiple pregnancy rate.
- In a low dose step-up protocol, 37.5–75 IU/day of gonadotropin is started between days 3 and 5 of menses, and ovarian response is monitored for 14 days of administration. In the absence of ovarian response, the dose is increased by 37.5 IU/day and response is monitored every week thereafter. A maximum dose of 225 IU/day, and the dose is maintained when a dominant follicle is seen. This protocol claims to improve ovulation rates and clinical pregnancy rates due to a low dose of gonadotropin used and also the lesser incidence of multifollicular development. Body mass index is a significant factor that affects the outcome of this protocol.[38]
- Combined therapy with oral ovulogens is also another viable option to reduce the overall cost of treatment by reducing the number of injections required for

dominant follicle growth. Gonadotropins alone or in combination with oral ovulogens like CC have a higher clinical pregnancy rate and lower miscarriage rate with an increased risk of multiple pregnancies compared to oral ovulogens alone.[39]

There have been comparable pregnancy rates between different gonadotropins and no significant difference has been observed on the mode of administration of gonadotropins emphasizing on the individualization of the treatment protocols. Cycle cancellation or conversion to IVF cycles is usually done when more than four follicles of 15 mm are seen on folliculometry to reduce the risk of OHSS.

MINIMAL/MILD ENDOMETRIOSIS

Controlled ovarian stimulation with IUI has been proposed in early cases of endometriosis and surgically corrected cases with normal pelvic anatomy. Comparable clinical pregnancy rates have been reported in minimal/mild endometriosis and unexplained infertility with controlled ovarian hyperstimulation (COH)-IUI. Cumulative live birth rates were comparable in the first three to four cycles of COH-IUI in these patients. Clinical pregnancy rate per cycle was found to be lower with or without COH-IUI in surgically untreated minimal/mild endometriosis compared to unexplained infertility.[40] Intrauterine insemination yields poor pregnancy rates in minimal/mild endometriosis with normal semen parameters and patent fallopian tubes with abnormal uterotubal transport on hysterosalpingography (HSG).[41] The European Society of Human Reproduction and Embryology (ESHRE) 2022 guidelines on endometriosis recommend using ovarian stimulation with IUI instead of IUI or expectant management alone in revised American Society for Reproductive Medicine (rASRM) stage I/II endometriosis, as it increases the pregnancy rates. They also recommend considering OI with IUI in rASRM stage III/IV with tubal patency for a short period, though its value is uncertain to improve pregnancy rates.[42]

UNEXPLAINED INFERTILITY

The ESHRE 2023 guidelines on unexplained infertility recommend OI with IUI as first-line management option in couples with unexplained infertility. Low-dose gonadotropin regimen is recommended to alleviate the risk of OHSS.[43] Earlier FASTT (Fast Track And Standard Treatment) trial suggested fast forwarding the treatment to IVF if the patient fails to conceive with three cycles of OI with CC and IUI rather than introducing gonadotropins with IUI as they found no additional advantage in terms of pregnancy rates and time to pregnancy.[44]

ROLE OF INTRAUTERINE INSEMINATION IN ADVANCED MATERNAL AGE

For women >40 years IVF becomes the treatment of choice for achieving a live birth rate. However, OI/IUI may be considered in this population to those not willing /not affording IVF for a maximum of four cycles.[45]

Step-down protocol is of particular use in this subgroup of women as they have less number of primordial follicular pools and require a higher dose of gonadotropins to evoke an ovarian response. Though exact protocols differ, a higher dose of 150 IU/day is started and continued until a follicle response of >10 mm is seen. The dose is serially reduced 5 days apart (112.5 and 75 IU) until the dominant follicle is seen to trigger ovulation.[10]

Though stimulated cycle IUI is preferred in women <35 years, natural cycle IUI is preferred in women ≥35 years. The clinical pregnancy rates and abortion rates were similar in older women who underwent stimulated IUI and natural cycle IUI.[46]

ROLE OF DOUBLE INTRAUTERINE INSEMINATION IN FEMALE SUBFERTILITY

Double IUI is performing IUI twice in the same cycle in order to improve the timing of IUI around ovulation. The rationale behind increasing the frequency of IUI being increasing the chance that semen is inseminated around the optimal moment around ovulation. 2010 Cochrane Review on double IUI tells higher pregnancy rates compared to single IUI; however, it was low-quality evidence. Double IUI is ideally performed first around 12–14 hours after the HCG trigger and second around 36–40 hours after the HCG trigger. A significantly higher pregnancy rate was found when IUI was performed at 12 and 34 hours after HCG than at 34 and 60 hours after HCG.[47,48]

2021 Cochrane Review on double IUI in female subfertility showed low-quality evidence that double IUI improves live births and reduces miscarriage compared to a single IUI. The chance of live births following a single IUI is considered to be 16%, while that following a double IUI is between 12 and 27%. The review stated the chance of multiple pregnancies following a single IUI is 0.7% and that following a double IUI is between 0.7 and 3.2%.[49]

CONCLUSION

- In spite of higher success rates with IVF-ICSI treatment, it would be a cost-effective and feasible option to consider IUI for subfertile couples who have a possibility of natural conception but lack the fecundability rate per cycle.
- According to randomized controlled trials (considering live birth rates than pregnancy rates) initial treatment option in idiopathic infertility should be IUI as opposed to IVF accounting to its efficacy, complications especially multiple pregnancy rates and patient compliance.[50]
- Controlled ovarian stimulation with oral ovulogens or/and gonadotropins and follicular monitoring to document ovulation and to time the IUI.
- Follicular monitoring enables cycle cancellation and avoids complications like OHSS in the presence of more number of follicles. Also, it provides a medium to counsel the patients about the possibility of multiple pregnancies.
- OI with gonadotropins and IUI is a feasible option and relatively cost-effective option in patients with hypogonadotropic hypogonadism with reasonable pregnancy rates per cycle and per patient.
- In limited technology facilities, IUI is the first-line conception enhancing technique especially in women <35 years, with mild to moderate male factor, patent functioning tubes and with shorter duration of infertility with more couple compliance (less dropout rates).
- A maximum of four to six cycles may be considered before thinking of alternative treatment options.
- OI plus IUI is a preferred modality of treatment compared to natural cycle IUI or timed intercourse in the said set of patients.

KEY LEARNING POINTS

- Patient selection is important criteria to determine the success of IUI.

- IUI with ovarian stimulation is the first line management option proposed for patients with unexplained infertility and those with ASRM I/II endometriosis instead of expectant management or IUI alone.
- Number of cycles of doing IUI should be individualized for every patient considering maternal age and other fertility factors before embarking on higher treatment options.
- TVS guided documentation of ovulation followed by IUI is a good practice point.
- Double IUI should not be routinely advocated to all patients owing to limited evidence on improvement in pregnancy rates.
- Proper documentation of ovarian stimulation drugs used, follicular scan, pre- and postwash semen count, difficulty in performing IUI should be done.
- After each failed cycle couple has to be re-evaluated thoroughly.

REFERENCES

1. Hansen KR, He AL, Styer AK, Wild RA, Butts S, Engmann L, et al. Predictors of pregnancy and live-birth in couples with unexplained infertility after ovarian stimulation-intrauterine insemination. Fertil Steril. 2016; 105(6):1575-83.e2.
2. World Health Organization. (2023). Infertility Prevalence Estimates, 1990-2021. [online] Available from: https://www.who.int/publications/i/item/978920068315 [Last accessed January, 2023].
3. Zegers-Hochschild F, Adamson GD, Dyer S, Racowsky C, de Mouzon J, Sokol R, et al. The international glossary on infertility and fertility care, 2017. Fertil Steril. 2017; 108(3):393-406.
4. Reproductive Medicine & Infertility Associates. (2021). Subfertility Or Infertility: Is It Time To Consider IVF?" [online] Available from: https://www.rmia.com/fertility-treatments/subfertility-or-infertility-is-it-time-to-consider-ivf/[Last accessed January, 2023].
5. Eskew AM, Jungheim ES. A history of developments to improve in vitro fertilization. Mo Med. 2017;114(3):156-9.
6. Kop PA, Mochtar MH, O'Brien PA, Van der Veen F, van Wely M. Intrauterine insemination versus intracervical insemination in donor sperm treatment. Cochrane Database Syst Rev. 2018;2018(1):CD000317.
7. Allahbadia GN. Intrauterine Insemination: Fundamentals Revisited. J Obstet Gynaecol India. 2017;67(6):385-92.
8. American College of Obstetricians and Gynecologists Committee on Gynecologic Practice and Practice Committee. Female age-related fertility decline. Committee Opinion No. 589. Fertil Steril. 2014;101(3): 633-4.
9. Keefe CE, Mirkes R, Yeung P Jr. The evaluation and treatment of cervical factor infertility a medical-moral analysis. Linacre Q. 2012;79(4):409-25.
10. Fritz MA, Speroff L. Clinical Gynecologic Endocrinology and Infertility, 8th edition. Philadelphia: Lippincott Williams & Wilkins; 2011. pp. 1168.
11. Steures P, van der Steeg JW, Verhoeve HR, van Dop PA, Hompes PG, Bossuyt PM, et al. Does ovarian hyperstimulation in intrauterine insemination for cervical factor subfertility improve pregnancy rates? Hum Reprod. 2004;19(10):2263-6.
12. Sirmans SM, Pate KA. Epidemiology, diagnosis, and management of polycystic ovary syndrome. Clin Epidemiol. 2013;6:1-13.
13. Teede HJ, Tay CT, Laven JJE, Dokras A, Moran LJ, Piltonen TT, et al. Recommendations From the 2023 International Evidence-based Guideline for the Assessment and Management of Polycystic Ovary Syndrome. J Clin Endocrinol Metab. 2023; 108(10):2447-69.
14. Advances in methods of fertility regulation: report of a WHO scientific group. World Health Organ Tech Rep Ser. 1973;527:1-42.

15. Munro MG, Balen AH, Cho SH, Critchley HOD, Díaz I, et al. The FIGO ovulatory disorders classification system. Int J Gynecol Obstet. 2022;159(1):1-20.
16. Custers IM, Steures P, Hompes P, Flierman P, van Kasteren Y, van Dop PA, et al. Intrauterine insemination: how many cycles should we perform? Hum Reprod. 2008;23(4):885-8.
17. Huseyin K, Berk B, Tolga K, Eser O, Ali G, Murat A. Management of ovulation induction and intrauterine insemination in infertile patients with hypogonadotropic hypogonadism. J Gynecol Obstet Hum Reprod. 2019;48(10):833-8.
18. Gill S, Taylor AE, Martin KA, Welt CK, Adams JM, Hall JE. Specific factors predict the response to pulsatile gonadotropin-releasing hormone therapy in polycystic ovarian syndrome. J Clin Endocrinol Metab. 2001;86(6):2428-36.
19. Yasmin E, Davies M, Conway G, Balen AH; British Fertility Society. Ovulation induction in WHO Type 1 anovulation: Guidelines for practice'. Produced on behalf of the BFS Policy and Practice Committee. Hum Fertil (Camb). 2013;16(4):228-34.
20. Couzinet B, Lestrat N, Brailly S, Forest M, Schaison G. Stimulation of ovarian follicular maturation with pure follicle-stimulating hormone in women with gonadotropin deficiency. J Clin Endocrinol Metab. 1988;66(3):552-6.
21. Chan C, Liu K. Clinical pregnancy in a woman with idiopathic hypogonadotropic hypogonadism and low AMH: utility of ovarian reserve markers in IHH. J Assist Reprod Genet. 2014;31(10):1317-21.
22. Balen AH, Morley LC, Misso M, Franks S, Legro RS, Wijeyaratne CN, et al. The management of anovulatory infertility in women with polycystic ovary syndrome: an analysis of the evidence to support the development of global who guidance. Hum Reprod Update. 2016;22(6):687-708.
23. Atalay E, Ozaksit MG, Tokmak A, Engin-Ustun Y. Intrauterine insemination versus timed intercourse in ovulation induction cycles with clomiphene citrate for polycystic ovary syndrome: a retrospective cohort study. J Gynecol Obstet Hum Reprod. 2019; 48(10):805-9.
24. Mitwally MF, Casper RF. Aromatase inhibitors in ovulation induction. Semin Reprod Med. 2004;22(1):61-78.
25. Franik S, Eltrop SM, Kremer JA, Kiesel L, Farquhar C. Aromatase inhibitors (letrozole) for subfertile women with polycystic ovary syndrome. Cochrane Database Syst Rev. 2018;5(5):CD010287.
26. Pavone ME, Bulun SE. Clinical review: the use of aromatase inhibitors for ovulation induction and superovulation. J Clin Endocrinol Metab. 2013;98(5):1838-44.
27. Lee VC, Ledger W. Aromatase inhibitors for ovulation induction and ovarian stimulation. Clin Endocrinol. 2011;74(5):537-46.
28. Legro RS, Brzyski RG, Diamond MP, Coutifaris C, Schlaff WD, Casson P, et al. Letrozole versus clomiphene for infertility in the polycystic ovary syndrome. N Engl J Med. 2014;371(2):119-29.
29. Guo Z, Chen S, Chen Z, Hu P, Hao Y, Yu Q. Predictors of response to ovulation induction using letrozole in women with polycystic ovary syndrome. BMC Endocr Disord. 2003;23(1):90.
30. Mitwally MF, Said T, Galal A, Chan S, Cohen M, Casper RF, et al. Letrozole Step-Up Protocol: a Successful Superovulation Protocol. 2008;89(4):S23-4.
31. Zhu X, Fu Y. Extending letrozole treatment duration is effective in inducing ovulation in women with polycystic ovary syndrome and letrozole resistance. Fertil Steril. 2023; 119(1):107-113.
32. Martin CE. Novel letrozole dosing: is a single dose of letrozole equivalent to traditional 5-day dosing? F S Rep. 2020;1(3):170.
33. Glasier AF, Irvine DS, Wickings EJ, Hillier SG, Baird DT. A comparison of the effects on follicular development between clomiphene citrate, its two separate isomers and spontaneous cycles. Hum Reprod. 1989; 4(3):252-6.
34. Brown J, Farquhar C. Clomiphene and other antioestrogens for ovulation induction in

35. Costello MF, Garad RM, Hart R, Homer H, Johnson L, Jordan C, et al. A Review of second- and third-line infertility treatments and supporting evidence in women with polycystic ovary syndrome. Med Sci (Basel). 2019;7(7):75.
36. Abd El Kader, Dawood AS, Morsy AT, Salem HA. Clomiphene stair-step protocol versus traditional protocol for ovulation induction in polycystic ovarian syndrome patients. J Advance Med Medic Res. 2021;33(18):1-12.
37. Mejia RB, Summers KM, Kresowik JD, Van Voorhis BJ. A randomized controlled trial of combination letrozole and clomiphene citrate or letrozole alone for ovulation induction in women with polycystic ovary syndrome. Fertil Steril. 2019;111(3):571-8.e1.
38. Yarali H, Basaran M, Yigit N, Bukulmez O, Bildirici I. Gonadotropin treatment using the low-dose step-up protocol in patients with clomiphene citrate (CC) resistant polycystic ovary syndrome (PCOS): factors affecting outcome. Fertil Steril. 2001;76(3):S207-8.
39. Banker M, Patel A, Deshmukh A, Shah S. Comparison of effectiveness of different protocols used for controlled ovarian hyperstimulation in intrauterine insemination cycle. J Obstet Gynaecol India. 2018;68(1):65-9.
40. Werbrouck E, Spiessens C, Meuleman C, D'Hooghe T. No difference in cycle pregnancy rate and in cumulative live-birth rate between women with surgically treated minimal to mild endometriosis and women with unexplained infertility after controlled ovarian hyperstimulation and intrauterine insemination. Fertil Steril. 2006;86(3):566-71.
41. Kissler S, Hamscho N, Zangos S, Gätje R, Müller A, Rody A, et al. Diminished pregnancy rates in endometriosis due to impaired uterotubal transport assessed by hysterosalpingoscintigraphy. BJOG. 2005;112(10):1391-6.
42. Becker CM, Bokor A, Heikinheimo O, Horne A, Jansen F, Kiesel L, et al. ESHRE guideline: endometriosis. Hum Reprod Open. 2022;2022(2):hoac009.
43. Romualdi D, Ata B, Bhattacharya S, Bosch E, Costello M, Gersak K, et al. Evidence-based guideline: unexplained infertility†. Hum Reprod. 2023;38(10):1881-90.
44. Reindollar RH, Regan MM, Neumann PJ, Levine BS, Thornton KL, Alper MM, et al. A randomized clinical trial to evaluate optimal treatment for unexplained infertility: the fast track and standard treatment (FASTT) trial. Fertil Steril. 2010;94(3):888-99.
45. Nesbit CB, Blanchette-Porter M, Esfandiari N. Ovulation induction and intrauterine insemination in women of advanced reproductive age: a systematic review of the literature. J Assist Reprod Genet. 2022;39(7):1445-91.
46. Chen L, Liu Q. Natural cycle versus ovulation induction cycle in intrauterine insemination. Zhonghua Nan Ke Xue. 2009;15(12):1112-5.
47. Ghanem ME, Bakre NI, Emam MA, Al Boghdady LA, Helal AS, Elmetwally AG, et al. The effects of timing of intrauterine insemination in relation to ovulation and the number of inseminations on cycle pregnancy rate in common infertility etiologies. Hum Reprod. 2011;26(3):576-83.
48. Cantineau AEP, Cohlen BJ, Heineman MJ. Ovarian stimulation protocols (anti-oestrogens, gonadotrophins with and without GnRH agonists/antagonists) for intrauterine insemination (IUI) in women with subfertility. Cochrane Database Syst Rev. 2007;2:CD005356.
49. Rakic L, Kostova E, Cohlen BJ, Cantineau AE. Double versus single intrauterine insemination (IUI) in stimulated cycles for subfertile couples. Cochrane Database Syst Rev. 2021;7(7):CD003854.
50. Homburg R. The case for initial treatment with intrauterine insemination as opposed to in vitro fertilization for idiopathic infertility. Hum Fertil (Camb). 2003;6(3):122-4.

CHAPTER 25

Intrauterine Insemination in Endometriosis

Kuldeep Jain, Maansi Jain

INTRODUCTION

Intrauterine insemination (IUI) is a simple procedure offered to infertile couples who fail to conceive on their own with or without ovulation induction in spite of patent tubes. It is the deposition of processed highly motile, morphologically normal sperms, washed free of seminal plasma and other cells, directly into the uterus at the anticipated time of ovulation. Anatomically and functionally, normal tubes, normal tubo-ovarian relation, normal and receptive endometrium and reasonable ovarian function are important prerequisites for successful outcome of IUI. Endometriosis is a complex disorder which affects reproduction potential at all stages depending on grading and severity of disease. Loss of tubo-ovarian relationship is inherent to endometriosis as a result of repeated intraperitoneal bleeding resulting into adhesion formation and nonfunctional tubes in spite of their patency. pregnancy rates are always compromised in endometriosis when compared to other etiologies because of multiple restrictions in endometriosis. Moreover, a lot of controversies and debates are associated with management of infertility in endometriosis. IUI is one of the management strategies in endometriosis especially in cases of minimal and mild endometriosis which has been suggested by both the European Society of Human Reproduction and Embryology (ESHRE) and the American Society for Reproductive Medicine (ASRM).[1,2]

When considering IUI for endometriosis-related infertility, one needs to consider and account for following points:

- Should all patients with endometriosis be offered IUI?
- What are the selection criteria?
- What are the prerequisites?
- Should IUI be done before surgery?
- Should surgery be offered even in absence of endometrioma?
- What is the ideal protocol in endometriosis?
- How many cycles are of IUI?
- What is the evidence and recommendation?
- Should all patients with endometriosis be offered IUI? To answer this question, it is important to understand the rationale and prerequisites of IUI.

Prerequisites for IUI are:
- At least one tube patent with normal tubo-ovarian relationship
- Usable ovarian reserve
- Normal endometrial cavity
- Usable seminal parameters for insemination.

Rationale of IUI is to increase chances of conception by increasing the number of eggs and depositing highly motile fraction of good quality sperm near the site of fertilization at the time of ovulation.

In endometriosis, depending on severity of endometriosis, there is compromised ovarian reserve as well as distorted tubo-ovarian relationship due to adhesion formation because of repeated menstruation in the peritoneal cavity and around the adnexa. this hinders the ovulation process as well as picks up of released egg into the tube, thus, decreasing the chance of conception. This means that grades 1 and 2 with minimal adhesions and maintained tubo-ovarian relationship are the right candidates for IUI and may be advised to undergo the procedure for three to four cycles. while grades 3 and 4 are to be reserved for more advanced procedure like in vitro fertilization.

- Selection criteria for IUI in endometriosis: Prerequisites for IUI should be fulfilled including the maintained tubo-ovarian relationship, young age, good reserve, and normal or mild male factor are the best candidates for IUI and can get equal result when compared to unexplained infertility. Patients with endometrioma grades 3 and 4, endometriosis with other factors such as poor ovarian reserve, moderate/severe male factor, advanced endometriosis, and old age may not be benefitted with IUI or might have minimal chances of conception with IUI.

Patients with endometriosis with or without endometrioma have better chances after surgery when compared to expectant management. fecundity in cases of endometriosis is known to have inverse relationship with severity of disease. minimal and mild endometriosis have better chances of conception with IUI and it can be further enhanced after surgical adhesiolysis/endometriosis fulguration. conception rates decreases sharply in moderate and severe endometriosis even after an extensive adhesiolysis and cystectomy in these cases and IUI may not be very helpful in such cases. Use of endometriosis fertility index (EFI) may be used full in counseling and decision making and is recommended in endometriosis surgery especially moderate and severe endometriosis as it provides an objective assessment of probability of conception with IUI after extensive surgery.[3]

Should IUI be done before surgery? This question remains debatable, especially in cases of minimal and mild endometriosis. it is understood that in mild and minimal endometriosis, tubo-ovarian relations are maintained and there is minimal alteration in anatomy, so these patients behave like unexplained infertility. thus, appealing that logic, IUI may be offered to these patients without going for surgery. However, there are reports of improved fecundity after surgery even in cases of minimal/mild endometriosis.

In moderate endometriosis with or without endometrioma, there is clear-cut advantage of surgery prior to IUI as it corrects the tubo-ovarian relationships, improves tubal functioning score, and decreases the disease burden. There is enough evidence and recommendation of surgery before IUI for improved outcome.[4,5]

Another question regarding surgery needs further clarification, whether cystectomy should be preferred over fulguration. As far as fertility is concerned, there is no significant difference between two groups, but recurrence rates are significantly higher in fulguration group, thus, it is always prefeed and recommended to perform cystectomy if technically possible. Other interventions like surgical drainage only or ultrasound-guided drainage prior to IUI are not having any benefit and should not be performed because of high-recurrence rate and higher infection rates.

Another important point is the time interval between surgery and IUI. Should it be immediate after surgery or after few months of expectant management. As endometriosis is a progressive disease and requires an aggressive management to get maximum benefit of surgery, it is logical to offer IUI immediately after surgery for an improved fecundity postsurgery. expectant management does not give any advantage and may be counterproductive in many cases due to recurrence of disease. ESHRE recommends three cycles of IUI postsurgery for a significantly improved outcome.

Postoperative medical management also does not provide any benefit as far as fertility is concerned and should not be prescribed except in cases of incomplete surgery to avoid recurrence and as a part of ultra long protocol for IVF stimulation.

- *What is the ideal protocol for IUI in endometriosis patients?* Aim of stimulation in IUI is to get at least two mature follicles so as to optimize the outcome. There is no specific protocol for endometriosis patients and both oral ovulogens like aromatase inhibitors and clomiphene or gonadotropins may be used as per the previous response of the patients. fecundity is better with gonadotropin as also seen with nonendometriosis group. Use of gonadotropin-releasing hormone (gnrh) agonist/antagonist does not provide an added advantage for IUI outcome and not to be used routinely. Combined protocol with letrozole/gonadotropin may help in reducing the total gonadotropin use significantly without compromising the outcome and is worth trying for endometriosis patients.

Ovarian response may be compromised and total dose of gonadotropin used is slightly higher when compared to nonendometriotic patients. However, younger patients do respond normally even in presence of endometrioma.

- *How many cycles of IUI should be offered?* Every cycle of IUI needs to be utilized to get maximum benefit of the procedure. However, patients need to be counseled regarding the overall low fecundity in endometriosis. four good cycles with at least two follicles and nonmale factor is good enough to provide maximum cumulative pregnancy rates.[6] Offering more than three cycles do not give any added advantage and should be avoided and failed IUI patients should be counseled and referred for IVF at the earliest because of the associated low reserve and progressive nature of disease.
- *Evidence and recommendations:* there are conflicting reports as far as efficacy of IUI in endometriosis is concerned. In a recent retrospective study, comparing outcome of IUI in endometriosis-associated infertility and unexplained infertility, lower cumulative pregnancy rate was seen in endometrioma group (14.3 vs. 28.9%); however, pregnancy rates were comparable. Study concluded that IUI may be offered to endometriosis patient but suggested more randomized-controlled trial (RCT)[7] while other studies found no difference in mild endometriosis group when compared to unexplained infertility.[8,9]

In a recent systemic review comparing the efficacy of IUI for various indications, IUI for grades 3 and 4 was least productive and it was concluded that IUI is not the treatment of choice in these cases.[6]

Recent ESHRE guidelines on endometriosis 2022 provide a week recommendation for clinician to offer IUI instead of expectant management in women with rASRM stage I/II endometriosis with ovarian stimulation to increase pregnancy rate. It also provides a week recommendation for IUI in stage III/IV though value of this treatment is uncertain in this group.[10]

CONCLUSION

Endometriosis is an enigmatic disease. It is progressive and devilitating. IUI is a simple procedure and can be used in mild disease where tubo-ovarian relationship is maintained. It can also be used post cystectomy in moderate disease if tubo-ovarian relationship is maintained. Use of IUI is not recommended in severe disease and should not be offered. Endometriosis patients should be counselled in detail about the limitation of procedure and maximum 3–4 cycle may give a reasonable fecundity specially in mild disease.

KEY LEARNING POINTS

- Prerequisites and rationale to be kept in mind when offering IUI in endometriosis patients.
- Endometriosis fertility index is a useful predictor of outcome in IUI in endometriosis and should be used in decision making and counseling of patients.
- Surgery is not mandatory in all cases before offering IUI in endometriosis in absence of endometrioma; however, conception rate may be better if endometrioma is removed and tubo-ovarian relations are restored.
- Use of gnRH agonist or antagonist does not provide any additional benefit in IUI outcome and is not recommended however recurrence rates can be minimized with the use of agonists after surgery.
- More than three cycles do not give any benefit and maximal four cycles of IUI are sufficient to give optimal outcome in endometriosis patients.

REFERENCES

1. Kennedy S, Bergqvist A, Chapron C, D'Hooghe T, Dunselman G, Greb R, et al. ESHRE Special Interest Group for Endometriosis and Endometrium Guideline Development Group. ESHRE guideline for the diagnosis and treatment of endometriosis. Hum Reprod. 2005;20(10): 2698-704.
2. Practice Committee of the American Society for Reproductive Medicine. Endometriosis and infertility: a committee opinion. Fertil Steril. 2012;98(3):591-8.
3. Cook AS, Adamson GD. The Role of the Endometriosis Fertility Index (EFI) and Endometriosis Scoring Systems in Predicting Infertility Outcomes. Curr Obstet Gynecol Rep. 2013;2:186-94.
4. Fadhlaoui A, Bouquet de la Jolinière J, Feki A. Endometriosis and infertility: how and when to treat? Front Surg. 2014;1:24.
5. Filip L, Duică F, Prădatu A, Crețoiu D, Suciu N, Crețoiu SM, et al. Endometriosis associated infertility: a critical review and analysis on etiopathogenesis and therapeutic approaches. Medicina. 2020;56:460.
6. Sarkar S, Joseph T, Yadav B, Kamath MS, Kunjummen AT. Comparison of treatment outcomes following ovarian stimulation with intrauterine insemination in minimal or mild endometriosis versus unexplained infertility: a retrospective cohort study. J Hum Reprod Sci. 2022;15(3):272-7.
7. Cai H, Xie J, Shi J, Wang H. Efficacy of intrauterine insemination in women with endometrioma associated infertility: analysis using propensity score matching. BMC Pregnancy Childbirth. 2022;22(1):12.
8. Starosta A, Gordon CE, Hornstein MD. Predictive factors for intrauterine

insemination outcomes: a review. Fertil Res pract. 2020;:6(1):23.
9. Werbrouck E, Spiessens C, Meuleman C, D'Hooghe T. No difference in cycle pregnancy rate and in cumulative live-birth rate between women with surgically treated minimal to mild endometriosis and women with unexplained infertility after controlled ovarian hyperstimulation and intrauterine insemination. Fertil Steril. 2006; 86(3):566-71.
10. Becker CM, Bokor A, Heikinheimo O, Horne A, Jansen F, Kiesel L, et al. ESHRE Endometriosis Guideline Group. ESHRE guideline: endometriosis. Hum Reprod Open. 2022;2022(2):hoac009.

CHAPTER 26

Intrauterine Insemination in Polycystic Ovarian Syndrome

Devika Gunasheela, Ashwini M, Akhila MV

■ INTRODUCTION

Polycystic ovarian syndrome (PCOS) is currently the most common cause of ovulatory dysfunction [World Health Organization (WHO) classification group II] among women of reproductive age group, accounting for about 80% in this category.[1] It has a worldwide prevalence of 6–21% depending on the diagnostic criteria.[2]

The hallmark features of PCOS are hyperandrogenism, oligo/anovulation, and polycystic ovary (PCO) morphology on ultrasound (USG). Several studies have pinpointed the independent role of insulin resistance in PCOS irrespective of obesity.[3] All these factors play a significant role in contributing to the pathophysiology of PCOS and are associated with the development of obesity, dyslipidemia, increased cardiovascular disease risk, obstructive sleep apnea, type 2 diabetes mellitus (T2DM), behavioral problems, and reproductive dysfunction by various mechanisms.[2] The hormonal disturbances include raised luteinizing hormone (LH) levels, decreased follicle-stimulating hormone (FSH) levels, (resulting in an increased LH/FSH ratio), raised anti-müllerian hormone (AMH) levels and elevated estrone levels. These hormonal changes result in abnormal follicular growth, follicular arrest and anovulation, all resulting in menstrual disturbances and subfertility[4] **(Flowchart 1)**.[5]

Management of infertility in PCOS should involve a stepwise approach starting with lifestyle modifications, basic evaluation of male and female fertility status and proceeding with ovulation induction with medications, adjuvants, intrauterine insemination (IUI) and finally in vitro fertilization (IVF) as the last resort if none of the other treatments succeed.

ROLE OF INTRAUTERINE INSEMINATION IN POLYCYSTIC OVARIAN SYNDROME

Intrauterine insemination is the most popular method of assisted reproduction as it is a simple, inexpensive, and noninvasive procedure. It requires minimal expertise, can be performed without expensive infrastructure and can be done in low-resource settings. It is also safe and has minimal risk to patient when monitored carefully with strict cancellation criteria.

According to the WHO and PCOS consensus guidelines 2023, ovulation induction (OI) is recommended as a first-line therapy for anovulatory PCOS.[6,7] Many of these couples face failures with repeated cycles of OI and timed intercourse. OI with IUI can be the next treatment option in such

Flowchart 1: Relationship between insulin resistance/hyperinsulinemia and PCOS.[5]

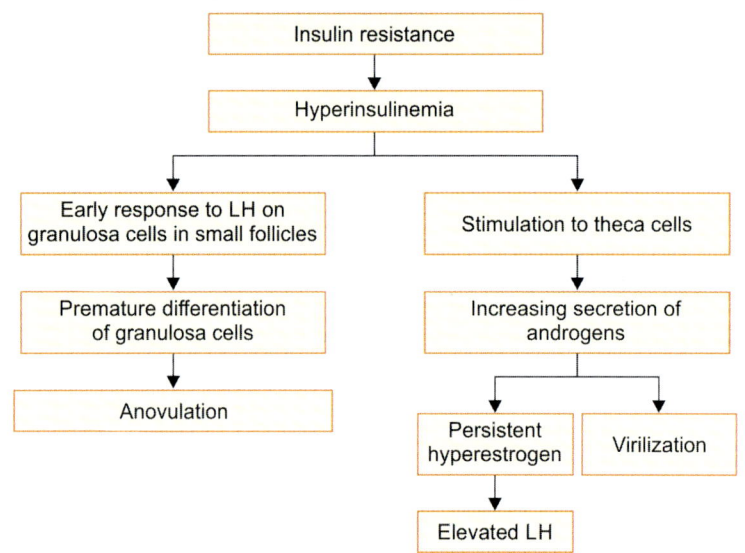

(LH: luteinizing hormone; PCOS: polycystic ovarian syndrome)

women and couples with coexisting mild male-factor infertility.

A study by Gao et al. included 1,868 IUI cycles comprising 1,086 women with PCOS. Women were classified into three groups accordingly: *Group 1:* Patients with no previous OI cycles, *Group 2:* Patients with 1–2 previous failed OI cycles, and *Group 3:* Patients with three or more failed OI cycles. The results of the study showed that clinical pregnancy rates were 21.14% (141/667) in group 1, 21.95% (90/410) in group 2, and 23.64% (187/791) in group 3. As seen above, the number of previous OI attempts did not significantly affect IUI outcomes and the clinical pregnancy rates were significantly higher in comparison to women undergoing OI and timed intercourse.[8]

In the same study, most pregnancies occurred within the first three cycles of IUI. Hence, they recommended three attempts of IUI for PCOS women before switching to IVF/ICSI (intracytoplasmic sperm injection).

PREREQUISITES FOR INTRAUTERINE INSEMINATION IN POLYCYSTIC OVARIAN SYNDROME

The tubal factor evaluation is a must in all patients undergoing IUI. Hysterosalpingo-contrast-sonography (hyCoSy) and hysterosalpingography (HSG) are valid tests for tubal patency. Both are comparable in diagnostic capacity and the selection of the technique depends on the preference of the clinician and the patient.[9] As per the National Institute for Health and Care Excellence (NICE) guidelines, in women with no comorbidities (such as pelvic inflammatory disease, previous ectopic pregnancy, or endometriosis) HSG should be offered to screen for tubal occlusion as it is reliable, less invasive, and makes more efficient use of resources. HyCoSy can be used in cases where appropriate expertise is available and is an effective alternative to HSG. In patients with earlier mentioned comorbidities and in women requiring ovarian drilling, laparoscopy should be offered as both tubal and pelvic pathology can be assessed and treated in the same sitting.[10]

The semen parameters to be considered for an IUI cycle should include total motile sperm count (TMSC), rapid progressive motility, and morphology before and after semen processing.[11] The processed total motile sperm count >10 million and insemination count >1 million with >4% normal spermatozoa are the important prognostic indicators of successful IUI.[12]

The contraindications for IUI include PCOS with severe male factor infertility, bilateral tubal pathology and PCOS associated with severe endometriosis (distorting the normal tubo-ovarian anatomy). These couples will benefit from a direct referral to the IVF/ICSI unit.

OVULATION INDUCTION IN INTRAUTERINE INSEMINATION

Drugs used for OI in IUI are given in **Boxes 1 and 2**.

Letrozole

Letrozole is an aromatase inhibitor that decreases the levels of peripheral estrogen, thus causing a compensatory increase in the pituitary gonadotropin secretion leading to the development of ovarian follicles **(Fig. 1)**.[13] It has a short half-life of 45 hours, an ovulation rate of 60–70%, a pregnancy rate of 27–30%, and a multiple pregnancy rate of 3–3.5%.[14] As per recent 2023 PCOS consensus guidelines,[7] letrozole is recommended as the first-line drug for OI in women with anovulatory PCOS. The American College of Obstetricians and Gynecologists (ACOG) 2018 consensus also suggests letrozole as first-line therapy for OI in obese PCOS women because of the increased live birth rate in comparison to clomiphene citrate (CC).[15]

Letrozole has unique advantages over CC in terms of monofollicular growth, increased ovulation rates, minimal negative effect on endometrial thickness, low ovarian hyperstimulation syndrome (OHSS), and multiple pregnancy rates.

Clomiphene Citrate

Clomiphene citrate is a selective estrogen receptor–modulator (SERM), which blocks the central estrogen receptors in the hypothalamus and impairs the accurate interpretation of circulating estrogen levels, stimulating gonadotropin release and driving ovarian follicular development. CC has an ovulation rate of 50–80%, cumulative pregnancy rate of 55–73%, live birth rate of 23.4%, multiple gestation rate of 8%, and OHSS rate of 1%.[16,17] The side effects from clomiphene treatment are rare and include vasomotor symptoms (20%), nausea (3%), headache (1%), and very rarely blurred vision or scotomata.[3] The main risk factor to consider while OI is the risk of multifetal pregnancy (7–10%) due to multifollicular development. About 15–40% women experience CC resistance/failure to standard CC treatment. Predictors of CC resistance include age,

> **BOX 1:** Oral ovulogens used for ovulation induction.
>
> - *Aromatase inhibitors:* Letrozole
> - *Selective estrogen receptor modulator (SERM):* Clomiphene citrate
> - *Adjuvants:* Metformin, glucocorticoids, myoinositol (MI): D-chiroinositol (DCI) (40:1)

> **BOX 2:** Injectable drugs for ovulation induction.
>
> - *Urinary gonadotropins:* Human menopausal gonadotropins (hMG), highly purified (HP)-hMG, follicle-stimulating hormone (FSH)
> - Recombinant gonadotropin

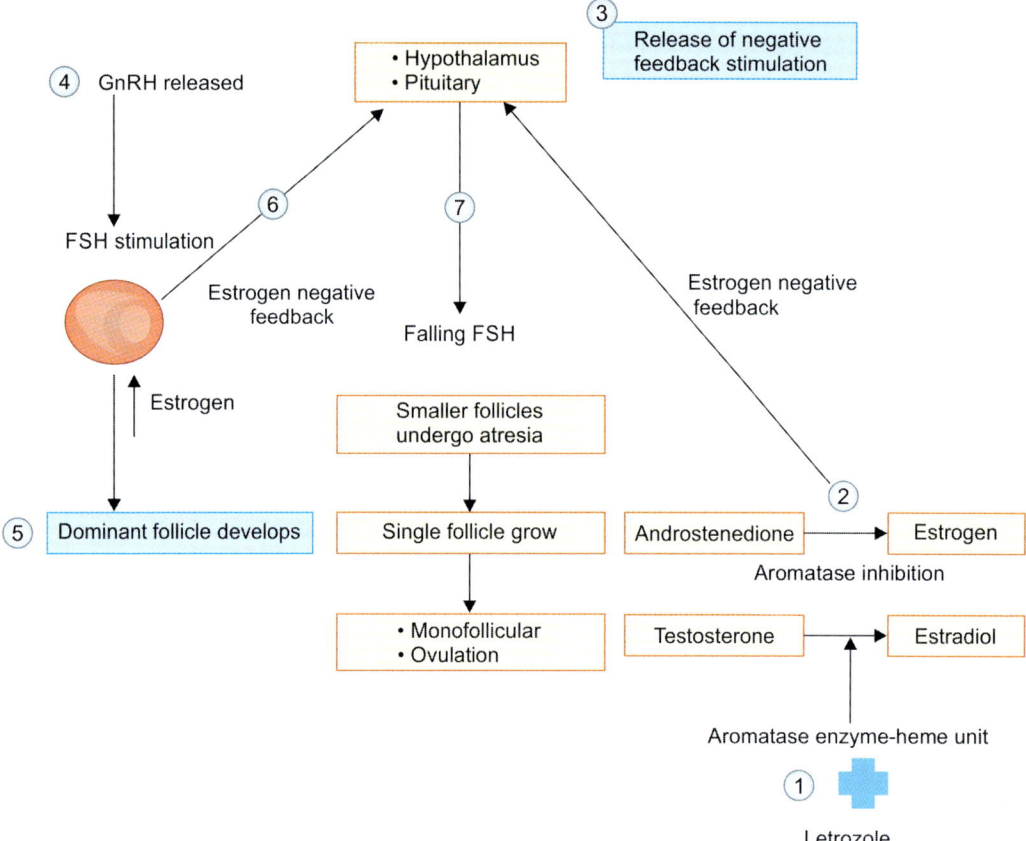

Fig. 1: Mechanism of action of letrozole.[13] (FSH: follicle-stimulating hormone; GnRH: gonadotropin hormone-releasing hormone)

obesity, hyperandrogenemia, higher fasting insulin, and leptin.[18] The treatment options in such cases include combined treatment with adjuvants such as CC with metformin, CC with glucocorticoids, CC with gonadotropins, or the use of letrozole.[3]

Gonadotropins

Gonadotropins are considered as a second-line pharmacological therapy for anovulatory PCOS women.[7] The commonly used gonadotropins subtypes include urinary gonadotropins [human menopausal gonadotropins (hMG) and highly purified (HP)-hMG] and recombinant gonadotropins. It is associated with an ovulation rate of 70–72%, a live birth rate of 15–30% per cycle and a multiple gestation rate of 5–36%.[16]

Gonadotropins can be considered in CC-resistant women as they have a higher live birth rate compared to a combination of CC and metformin. This may be considered after careful counseling about the requirement of regular follicular monitoring by ultrasound, cost factor, and higher multiple pregnancy rates.[7] A Cochrane meta-analysis in 2019 compared the use of different gonadotropin preparations for OI in CC-resistant PCOS women and concluded that there was no significant difference in live birth rate, clinical pregnancy rate, multiple pregnancy rates, or miscarriage rate between urinary-derived gonadotropins and recombinant FSH.[19]

ROLE OF ADJUVANTS IN OVULATION INDUCTION

Metformin

Metformin is a biguanide which reduces hepatic gluconeogenesis, decreases intestinal glucose absorption, increases peripheral glucose uptake and utilization and reduces circulating insulin levels. CC combined with metformin could be used rather than CC alone in women with PCOS with anovulatory infertility to improve ovulation and clinical pregnancy rates but it does not improve the live birth rate.[7] It is started with 500 mg with increments done 1–2 weekly up to a maximum daily dose of 2.5 g in adults.[7] A recent Cochrane meta-analysis including 4,552 women and 41 trials compared metformin with placebo, CC, letrozole, and laparoscopic ovarian drilling (LOD). The conclusions showed uncertain evidence that metformin with CC improves live birth rate compared to CC alone and gastrointestinal side effects were higher with combination medications.[20]

Glucocorticoids

In PCOS women, there is enhanced androgen production from both the ovaries and the adrenal glands (50–70% increase in adrenal androgen synthesis). Glucocorticoids act by inhibiting adrenocorticotropic hormone (ACTH) production, thus causing a reduction in adrenal androgen secretion, reduced total circulating dehydroepiandrosterone (DHEA), and total and free testosterone. This leads to reduced LH levels, LH/FSH ratio and results in improved folliculogenesis. A study by Darwish et al. showed a significant rise in ovulation rates and improved endometrial thickness and midluteal progesterone levels on supplementation with dexamethasone in the dose of 2 mg/day starting from day 3 of the cycle for a period of 10 days.[21]

Myoinositol

Myoinositol (MI) is the most abundant inositol in the body and stimulates aromatase synthesis, thus converting androgens to estrogens. It also reduces LH/FSH ratio in plasma and improves insulin sensitivity in cells. All these changes improve folliculogenesis. Specific types, doses or combinations of inositol cannot be recommended in adults with PCOS due to a lack of quality evidence.[7]

Note: The recommended MI:DCI (D-chiroinositol) ratio should be 40:1 in the composition given to the patient.

Melatonin

Melatonin promotes follicular maturation and ovulation through the protection of follicles against oxidative stress and their rescue from atresia. The melatonin level in the follicular fluid of PCOS women is notably lower than in healthy women, which could be related to ovulation problems. It is generally prescribed in doses of 1–2 mg/day.[22]

Other adjuvants include chromium, vitamin D, N-acetylcysteine, and minerals. The use of adjuvant therapies is usually empirical and finally based on physicians' personal views as there is no sufficient evidence to recommend their routine use **(Table 1)**.

Laparoscopic Ovarian Drilling

In PCOS women with CC resistance and high baseline LH levels, LOD can be recommended as a second-line management

TABLE 1: Adjuvants in PCOS.[23]

Adjuvant in PCOS	Application
Dexamethasone	• Beneficial in elevated DHEAS androgen levels • Highly effective adjunct to CC in PCOS women • Should be avoided in women with diabetes
Metformin	• Decreases the risk of OHSS when gonadotropins were used for ovulation induction • Increases the live birth rate (LBR) among women undergoing ovulation induction with gonadotropins
Myoinositol	• An insulin sensitizer that has beneficial effects on ovarian function and response to assisted reproductive technology (ART) in women with PCOS • No data on its effects on pregnancy rates (PR) and LBRs
Vitamin D	• Influences ovarian endocrine function and likelihood of pregnancy • Inverse associations with 25-hydroxy vitamin D levels and insulin resistance, features of hyperandrogenism, and circulating androgens in women with PCOS
N-Acetylcysteine	• Improves insulin sensitivity and decreases androgen level • Can improve the ovulation and pregnancy rates • May also have some beneficial impacts on endometrial thickness
Melatonin	• Regulates a variety of important central and peripheral actions related to circadian rhythms and reproduction • Powerful free radical scavenger and has a broad-spectrum antioxidant property • Melatonin deficiency seems to be involved in the pathophysiology of PCOS
Chromium polynicotinate	• Active component of glucose-tolerance factor, which is responsible for binding insulin to the cell membrane receptor sites • Improves insulin sensitivity • Stimulates the metabolism of sugar, fat, and cholesterol

(CC: clomiphene citrate; DHEAS: dehydroepiandrosterone sulfate; PCOS: polycystic ovarian syndrome; OHSS: ovarian hyperstimulation syndrome)

or as an alternative to gonadotropin therapy for couples who require laparoscopy to assess pelvic condition or those who cannot undergo an intensive USG during gonadotropin therapy. In LOD, electrocoagulation of the ovarian stroma reduces the ovarian androgen production, thus improving the function of the hypothalamus–pituitary–ovary axis. The advantages of LOD are unifollicular ovulation, low/no risk of OHSS or multiple pregnancies, and no need for regular intracycle USG monitoring. During the procedure, it is important to minimize the amount of diathermy to the lowest effective dose to minimize ovarian damage such as pelvic adhesions and decreased ovarian reserve. The recommended dosage for the procedure is four points per ovary for 4 seconds at 40 W. A large multicenter randomized controlled trial (RCT) included CC-resistant PCOS women undergoing OI with timed intercourse and randomized them into the LOD group and gonadotropin group (FSH). After 6 months, the cumulative pregnancy rate was 34% in the LOD group and 67% in the gonadotropin group. Reassessment after 12 months observed similar cumulative pregnancy rates of 67% in both groups. Thus, the study concluded that women undergoing LOD take a longer time to get pregnant and more than half (54%) required additional medications to induce ovulation.[18]

OVULATION INDUCTION PROTOCOLS

Letrozole

Standard Protocol

Letrozole is prescribed as a 5 mg/day dosage starting from day 1–5 of the menstrual cycle for 5 days. This is followed up with an USG after 7 days to check for a follicular response. If there is an adequate response, the woman is followed up with serial USG till the follicle size reaches 18 mm. Ovulation is then triggered with injectable human chorionic gonadotropin (hCG) (5,000 IU), and she is planned for IUI. In the absence of a dominant follicle (DF) on day 14 of the cycle and failure of signs of ovulation indicated by progesterone level (<3 ng/mL) and pelvic USG examination 7 days later (day 21), withdrawal bleeding is induced with progesterone **(Fig. 2)**.[24]

Stair-step Protocol

In stair-step protocol, letrozole is started at a dose of 2.5 mg/day for 5 days. If no response (all follicles <10 mm) is noted on USG after 1 week, the dose is increased to 5 mg/day for 5 days and follicular monitoring is repeated after 7 days. The same protocol is continued until a maximum dose of 7.5 mg letrozole is administered or until a dominant follicle is seen on USG **(Fig. 3)**.[25]

Extended Letrozole Protocol

In women who are resistant to the standard protocol, an extended letrozole protocol is recommended. In a recent study by Zhu et al., 69 PCOS women who were letrozole resistant were given a 7-day course of letrozole 5 mg/day. After 7 days, nonresponders were given an extended course of letrozole 5 mg/day for additional 10 days. The cumulative ovulation rate was 92.75% (64/69), cumulative clinical pregnancy rate was 31.88% (22/69), and cumulative live birth rate was 24.63% (17/69) with the two-step extended letrozole regimen.[26]

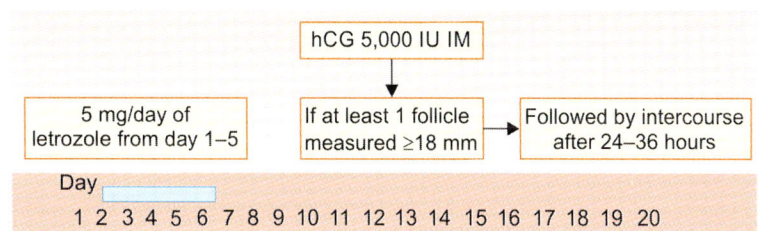

Fig. 2: Standard letrozole protocol. (hCG: human chorionic gonadotropin; IM: intramuscular)

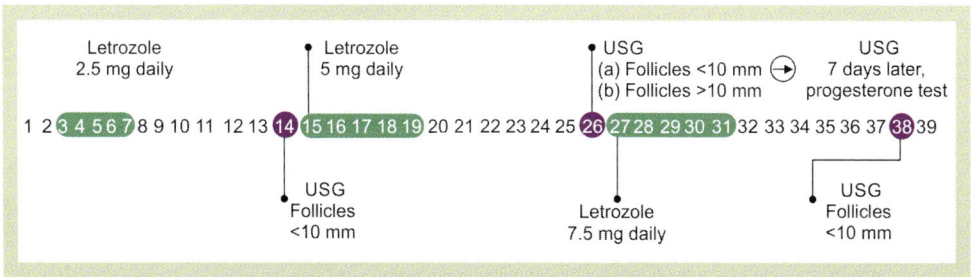

Fig. 3: Stair-step protocol of letrozole.[26] (USG: ultrasound)

Clomiphene Citrate

Standard Protocol

Clomiphene citrate is given orally in doses ranging between 50 and 150 mg starting from day 3 to 5 of the menstrual cycle for 5 days. CC dose required for induction is positively correlated with both bodyweight and obesity. A USG is performed 7 days after completion of treatment to check for follicular response. If there is an adequate response, the patient is followed up with serial USG till the follicle size reaches 18 mm and ovulation is triggered with injectable hCG (5,000 IU) and IUI is planned. In the absence of a dominant follicle on day 14 of the cycle or no signs of ovulation or serum progesterone level (<3 ng/mL), withdrawal bleeding is induced with progesterone.

Stair-step Protocol

In some women with CC resistance, this novel protocol can be used to achieve better ovulation rates. The protocol is described in **Figure 4**.[27]

The above protocol demonstrated significantly higher ovulation rates compared to the traditional regimen at the same dose with an additional advantage of reduced time to ovulation (32–53 days).[28]

Gonadotropin Hormone Regimen

Step-up Protocol

In this protocol, daily intramuscular (IM) injections of 75 IU of gonadotropin hormone (GtH) are given for 5 days from day 3 to 5 of the cycle along with USG monitoring of follicular growth. The dose of GtH is increased by 75 IU if no response is seen on USG. When the follicle size reaches 18 mm, the patient is triggered with 5,000 IU of Inj. hCG (IM) for ovulation.

Chronic Low-dose Step-up Protocol (Fig. 5)[29]

The most common protocol used in PCOS is the chronic low-dose step-up protocol

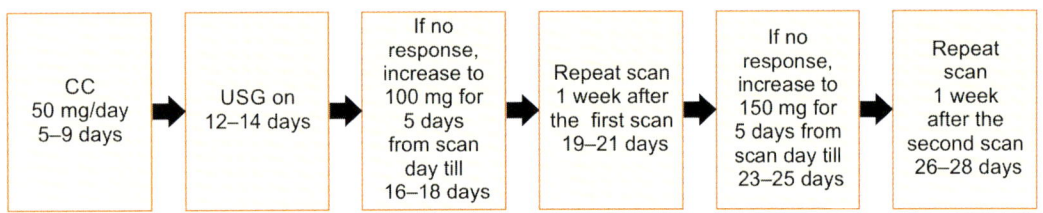

Fig. 4: Stair-step protocol of clomiphene citrate. (CC: clomiphene citrate; USG: ultrasound)

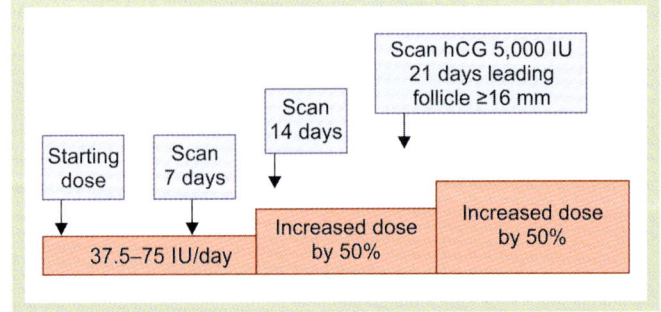

Fig. 5: Chronic low-dose step-up gonadotropin protocol for ovulation induction.[30] (hCG: human chorionic gonadotropin)

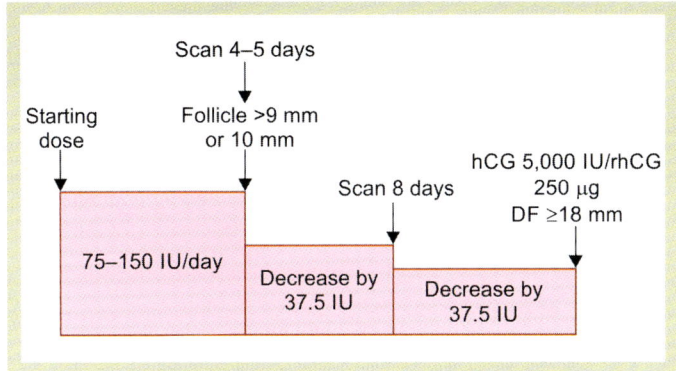

Fig. 6: Step-down protocol.[30] (DF: dominant follicle; hCG: human chorionic gonadotropin; rhCG: recombinant human chorionic gonadotropin)

starting on days 3–5 of menstrual cycle with a low dose of 37.5–75 IU units for 7–14 days. In case of absence of a response, a 50% dose increment of GtH dose is done every week and subsequently monitored with USG until the follicle size is 18 mm and then ovulation is triggered with injectable hCG 5,000 IU IM. The advantages with this protocol are the lower risk of OHSS and multiple pregnancy rates. The downside of this protocol is that it is impractical for clinical use considering the long days of stimulation and low rates of OI.

Step-down Protocol (Fig. 6)[29]

This protocol mimics the normal physiological pattern of FSH. It begins with 75–150 IU of GtH on day 2 or 3 of the menstrual cycle, which is continued for 4–5 days. The dose of GtH is reduced by 37.5 IU for 3 days on noting a follicular size >10 mm. Follicular growth is subsequently monitored with regular USG every 2–3 days and reducing GtH dose by 37.5 IU until the follicle size reaches 18 mm when ovulation is triggered with injectable hCG 5,000 IU IM. The long half-life of gonadotropins makes it difficult to judge the proper dosage for the maintenance of a lead follicle without the risk of OHSS. It is less commonly used in PCOS.

Sequential Protocol

The sequential protocol begins with an initial dose of gonadotropins at 37.5 IU for the first 14 days. Based on the USG findings, in case of absence of a follicular response (size <10 mm) the dose of GtH is increased by 50% for 7 days. Subsequent USG monitoring is carried out every 7 days and dose increment is continued till the follicle size reaches 14 mm. Following this, the GtH dose is sequentially decreased by 50% every 7 days till the follicle size reaches 18 mm when ovulation is triggered by injectable hCG 5,000 IU IM **(Fig. 7)**.[29]

When gonadotropins are used for OI, factors to be considered are the cost of treatment, necessary expertise for its use, and availability of regular USG monitoring facility to prevent multifollicular recruitment. Strict cancellation criteria when more than two follicles >14 mm in diameter are detected and advising avoidance of unprotected intercourse should be followed to reduce multiple pregnancies and OHSS rates.[7]

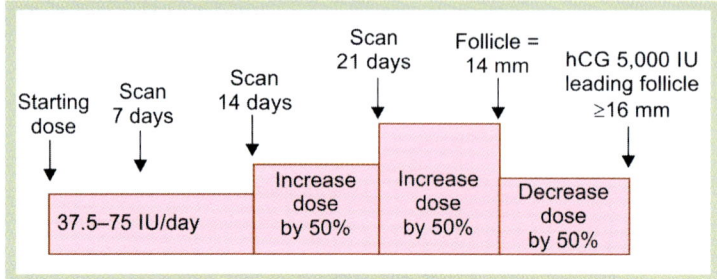

Fig. 7: Sequential protocol.[30] (hCG: human chorionic gonadotropin)

VAGARIES DURING OVULATION INDUCTION IN WOMEN WITH POLYCYSTIC OVARIAN SYNDROME

Hyper-response

The ovary in a PCOS woman is very sensitive to gonadotropin stimulation, thus mounting an exaggerated response to gonadotropins even with low doses and resulting in multifollicular development and higher ovarian steroid production. These women produce three times more follicles in comparison to non-PCOS women stimulated by a similar protocol putting them at a high risk of multiple gestation, OHSS, and cycle cancellation.[30]

The treatment options are as follows:
- *Coasting:* It is a commonly used strategy in fertility clinics where the gonadotropins are withdrawn for 2–3 days when there are more than two dominant follicles seen on USG. It lacks good-quality evidence for its routine use.
- *Conversion to in vitro fertilization (ad hoc in vitro fertilization):* Converting high-responder OI PCOS patients to IVF-embryo transfer (ET) avoids cycle cancellation. It also prevents the occurrence of associated complications such as OHSS and higher-order multiple pregnancies. The advantages of conversion to IVF include lesser gonadotropin dose, days of stimulation, and overall costs. Many studies found no statistical difference in the number of oocytes retrieved, number of mature oocytes, number of grade 1 embryos transferred, clinical pregnancy, and implantation rates between ad hoc IVF and conventional IVF cycles.[30]
- *Cycle cancellation:* It is a process of stopping further medications and withholding the ovulation trigger. A strict cancellation criterion is advised by the PCOS consensus guidelines when there are more than two follicles >14 mm.[7] Keeping in mind the financial impact and psychological distress it causes the couple, it is the last resort taken by clinicians.

No Response

About 15–40% of PCOS women experience resistance or failure to CC. This event is both unpredictable and unexplainable at times. Women with obesity, insulin resistance, and hyperandrogenism are at a higher risk of developing resistance to CC. A genetic predisposition was suggested as the cause in some women. Management in such situations includes changing the medication to letrozole, addition of adjuvants like metformin, myoinositol, glucocorticoids, CC with gonadotropins, stimulation with gonadotropins, or LOD.[31]

Thin Endometrium

Clomiphene citrate has an antiestrogenic effect on the cervical mucus and the endometrium. This negatively affects the endometrial receptivity resulting in low pregnancy rates as compared to letrozole. An RCT including 270 PCOS women studied the endometrial ultrasonic parameters such as the endometrial thickness, endometrial volume (EV), vascularization index (VI) along with integrin alpha V beta 3 ($\alpha_V\beta_3$), and vascular endothelial growth factor (VEGF) concentrations in uterine fluid in two groups receiving either CC or letrozole for OI. Results showed that all the above endometrial receptivity parameters were significantly better in the letrozole group compared with the CC group (p <0.05) resulting in a higher clinical pregnancy rate in the letrozole group.[32] Hence, changing the ovulation drug to letrozole is advisable in such cases.

INTRAUTERINE INSEMINATION: TIMING, SAMPLE COLLECTION FOR INSEMINATION AND PROCEDURE

In single insemination, IUI is performed only once after 36 hours of trigger, while in double insemination, the first IUI is performed 24 hours after trigger and the second IUI (postovulation) 36–40 hours after trigger. In a review by Cohlen et al., there is insufficient evidence that double IUI within the same cycle will lead to better pregnancy rates than a single IUI.[33] A recent Cochrane systematic review on the same concluded that there is low quality of evidence that double insemination improves live birth rates and reduces miscarriage rates. Hence, single insemination per cycle should be offered to women undergoing IUI.[34]

There is a lot of controversy in the literature regarding the time interval between semen sample collection, processing, and timing of insemination. If IUI is performed too soon after sperm preparation (<40 minutes), it might reduce the success rate due to reduced decondensation of sperm chromatin. If the preparation time is increased (>80 minutes), it may have a negative influence on pregnancy rates due to increased sperm deoxyribonucleic acid (DNA) fragmentation.[35,36] A study by Liang et al., including 191 IUI cycles, investigated the influence of the time interval from the end of semen processing to insemination on the clinical pregnancy rate. They divided the patients based on the incubation time as follows: 0–19, 20–39, 40–59, and 60–80 minutes, and again into another four groups according to the total progressively motile sperm count (TPMC): 0–9, 10–20, 21–30, and >30 million/mL. They found that the clinical pregnancy rate was significantly higher in the 20–39-minute group (18.3%) than the other groups.[37] The time interval from the end of sperm processing to insemination is a significant factor that influences the clinical pregnancy rate. Another study by Punjabi et al.[38] also found a significant difference in the odds of clinical pregnancies and live births when semen analysis was initiated in ≤21 minutes from the time of production, and the interval between the semen sample production and insemination was <107 minutes. Thus, the clinical pregnancy and live birth rates can be improved if the time interval between semen sample collection, analysis, and IUI is kept low.[38]

Regarding the type of IUI catheter to be used, a Cochrane review compared the use of soft versus stiff catheters for insemination and suggested that no specific conclusion can be made regarding the superiority of one catheter class over another.[39]

The role of cervical mucus in fertilization and the need for its removal during an IUI procedure is debatable. Cervical mucus is known to play an important role in natural fertilization, but in some cases, its undesirable properties could itself result in infertility. The hostile cervical mucus when introduced into the endometrial cavity by the insemination catheter negatively affects pregnancy rates by decreasing sperm motility and reducing/preventing sperm–oocyte interaction.[40] During the cervical mucus removal, touching the endocervix can stimulate uterine contractions and remove the lubricant effect of the mucus, thereby adversely affecting pregnancy rates. However, in a prospective randomized controlled study, which included 714 couples who were randomized into cervical mucus removal ($n = 361$) and no cervical mucus removal ($n = 353$) groups, the clinical pregnancy, ongoing pregnancy, and live birth rates in cervical mucus removal cycles were significantly higher than the no mucus removal group.[41] However, the removal of cervical mucus is still mired by controversy.

Literature on the role of bed rest after the IUI procedure as seen in an RCT and a few recent reviews observed that bed rest for at least 10–15 minutes after the IUI procedure improved the clinical pregnancy rates.[42,33] In a review comparing the effect of bed rest after IUI versus ET on assisted reproductive technology (ART) success, the authors found favorable effects after IUI ("moderate" quality evidence on clinical pregnancy) but no effect, and even possible unfavorable effects, after ET ("very low" quality evidence).[43]

FACTORS INFLUENCING INTRAUTERINE INSEMINATION OUTCOME

Factors that influence IUI success rates can be broadly divided into paternal factors, maternal factors, and cycle factors. The paternal factors adversely affecting IUI outcomes include advanced paternal age >40 years, a high body mass index (BMI), total motile sperm count <10 million/mL, post-wash sperm count <2 million, and a high DNA fragmentation index >30%.[44] Maternal factors adversely affecting IUI outcomes include advanced maternal age, high BMI, longer duration of infertility, and Hispanic and Asian origin.[44] Certain ovarian causes of infertility like endometriosis, poor ovarian reserve, etc., can also adversely affect IUI outcomes with the exception of ovulatory dysfunction which has the highest cumulative birth rate.[44]

A study by Guan et al. showed that overweight and obese women required more gonadotropin doses and longer days of stimulation when compared to normal BMI counterparts, but the clinical pregnancy rates remained the same irrespective of BMI.[45]

The cycle factors include the type of medications used and their associated side effects. The use of letrozole/CC/gonadotropins as a second-line agent can maximize pregnancy rates. Most pregnancies occur within the first four IUI cycles, after which IVF needs to be considered. Timing the insemination between 24 and 40 hours after hCG injection gives the best pregnancy rates. Single IUI is preferred to double IUI as both have comparable pregnancy rates.[44]

CONCLUSION

PCOS is the most common cause of ovulatory dysfunction. Management of infertility in PCOS should involve a stepwise approach starting with lifestyle modifications, followed by ovulation induction and finally proceeding to IVF if none of the simpler methods have succeeded. According to the recent PCOS consensus, ovulation induction is recommended as the first line management followed by IUI especially for anovulatory

PCOS. Letrozole is the drug of choice to produce a monofollicular growth.

Regarding the adjuvants, metformin and myoinositol have the largest body of evidence. Laparoscopic ovarian drilling is only reserved for women with CC resistance. Ovulation induction in PCOS can be tricky. Various protocols can be used for ovulation induction in PCOS, but one must be very careful about producing a hyper response which can lead to complications like OHSS and higher order multiple pregnancy. During ovulation induction, one must remember to make small and slow increments in gonadotropin doses with regular follicular monitoring. If there is multifollicular recruitment, early cancellation should be considered.

■ KEY LEARNING POINTS

- PCOS is the most common cause of anovulation, associated with endocrine and metabolic disturbances, all contributing to infertility.
- IUI is a simple, cost-effective, noninvasive treatment option for couples with PCOS and infertility prior to IVF/ICSI.
- Adequate tubal evaluation and semen analysis is a must prior to an IUI cycle.
- Ovulation induction with oral ovulogens is the recommended first-line therapy. If treatment with oral ovulogens fails, gonadotropins/LOD can be used as second-line therapy.
- Adequate monitoring using regular ultrasound, with strict cancellation criteria, is important to reduce multiple gestation and OHSS rates.
- Adjuvants, by acting on the various stages of altered metabolic pathways seen in patients with PCOS, can better the response to OI and produce better quality eggs.
- Vagaries of stimulation in a PCOS patient consist of a hyper-response (requiring coasting/ conversion to IVF/cycle cancellation), no follicular response, and thin endometrium.
- Regarding preparation prior to an IUI, the ideal duration between semen collection, processing, and insemination should range between 20 and 40 minutes. Longer semen processing time negatively affects pregnancy rates.
- Evidence on advantage of cervical mucus removal prior to insemination is debatable.
- Bed rest of 10–15 minutes after intrauterine insemination is recommended.
- There is no clear evidence showing the advantage of double insemination over a single insemination.
- Multiple factors such as maternal, paternal, and cyclical factors affect the success of IUI in PCOS women.

■ REFERENCES

1. Laven JSE, Imani B, Eijkemans MJC, Fauser BC. New approach to polycystic ovary syndrome and other forms of anovulatory infertility. Obstet Gynecol Surv. 2002;57(11):755-67.
2. Zhao H, Zhang J, Cheng X, Nie X, He B. Insulin resistance in polycystic ovary syndrome across various tissues: an updated review of pathogenesis, evaluation, and treatment. J Ovarian Res. 2023;16:9.
3. Toprak S, Yönem A, Cakir B, Güler S, Azal O, Ozata M, et al. Insulin resistance in nonobese patients with polycystic ovary syndrome. Horm Res. 2001;55(2):65-70.
4. Vyrides AA, El Mahdi E, Giannakou K. Ovulation induction techniques in women with polycystic ovary syndrome. Front Med (Lausanne). 2022;9:982230.
5. Sakumoto T, Tokunaga Y, Tanaka H, Nohara M, Motegi E, Shinkawa T, et al. Insulin resistance/hyperinsulinemia and reproductive disorders in infertile women. Reprod Med Biol. 2010;9(4):185-90.
6. Balen AH, Morley LC, Misso M, Franks S, Legro RS, et al. The management of

anovulatory infertility in women with polycystic ovary syndrome: An analysis of the evidence to support the development of global WHO guidance. Hum Reprod Update. 2016;22(6):687-708.
7. Teede HJ, Tay CT, Laven JJE, Dokras A, Moran LJ, Piltonen TT, et al.; International PCOS Network. Recommendations from the 2023 international evidence-based guideline for the assessment and management of polycystic ovary syndrome. Fertil Steril. 2023;120(4):767-93.
8. Gao Y, Jiang S, Chen L, Xi Q, Li W, Zhang S, et al. The pregnancy outcomes of infertile women with polycystic ovary syndrome undergoing intrauterine insemination with different attempts of previous ovulation induction. Front Endocrinol (Lausanne). 2022;13:922605.
9. Guideline Group on Unexplained Infertility; Romualdi D, Ata B, Bhattacharya S, Bosch E, Costello M, Gersak K, et al. Evidence-based guideline: unexplained infertility. Hum Reprod. 2023;38(10):1881-90.
10. National Collaborating Centre for Women's and Children's Health (UK). Fertility: Assessment and treatment for people with fertility problems. London: RCOG Press; 2004.
11. Yavas Y, Selub MR. Intrauterine insemination (IUI) pregnancy outcome is enhanced by shorter intervals from semen collection to sperm wash, from sperm wash to IUI time, and from semen collection to IUI time. Fertil Steril. 2004;82(6):1638-47.
12. Allahbadia GN. Intrauterine insemination: fundamentals revisited. J Obstet Gynaecol India. 2017;67(6):385-92.
13. Pandya MR, Patel K. A study of comparison of effectiveness of letrozole (5 mg) versus clomiphene citrate (100 mg) for ovulation induction among infertile women. J Obstet Gynecol Res India. 2021;8(4):553-8.
14. Legro RS, Brzyski RG, Diamond MP, Coutifaris C, Schlaff WD, Casson P, et al. Letrozole versus clomiphene for infertility in the polycystic ovary syndrome. N Engl J Med. 2014;371(2):119-29.
15. ACOG Committee Opinion No. 738: Aromatase inhibitors in gynecologic practice. Obstet Gynecol. 2018;131(6):1.
16. Lindheim SR, Glenn TL, Smith MC, Gagneux P. Ovulation induction for the general gynecologist. J Obstet Gynaecol India. 2018;68(4):242-52.
17. The Practice Committee of the American Society for Reproductive Medicine. Definitions of infertility and recurrent pregnancy loss: a committee opinion. Fertil Steril. 2013;99(1):63.
18. Li M, Ruan X, Mueck AO. Management strategy of infertility in polycystic ovary syndrome. Global Health J. 2022;6(2):70-4.
19. Weiss NS, Kostova E, Nahuis M, Mol BWJ, van der Veen F, van Wely M. Gonadotrophins for ovulation induction in women with polycystic ovary syndrome. Cochrane Database Syst Rev. 2019;1(1):CD010290.
20. Sharpe A, Morley LC, Tang T, Norman RJ, Balen AH. Metformin for ovulation induction (excluding gonadotrophins) in women with polycystic ovary syndrome. Cochrane Database Syst Rev. 2019;12(12):CD013505.
21. Darwish E, Elkassar YS, El-Agwany SA. Follicular phase dexamethazone administration in polycystic ovarian syndrome patients who are clomiphene citrate resistant. Reprod Clim. 2016;30(3):115-20.
22. Mojaverrostami S, Asghari N, Khamisabadi M, Heidari Khoei H. The role of melatonin in polycystic ovary syndrome: A review. Int J Reprod Bio Med. 2019;17(12):865-82.
23. The PCOS Society India. (2019). Module 4: Role of Adjuvants in Infertility Management: From Physiology to Therapeutics. [online] Available from: https://pcosindia.org/pdf/PCOS%20Module%204%20new%20logo.pdf [Last accessed January, 2024].
24. Badawy A, Mosbah A, Tharwat A, Eid M. Extended letrozole therapy for ovulation induction in clomiphene-resistant women with polycystic ovary syndrome: a novel protocol. Fertil Steril. 2009;92(1):236-9.
25. Chernukha GE, Kaprina EK, Golovanova AA. New perspectives on ovulation induction with letrozole in women with polycystic ovary syndrome. 2022;12:107-14.
26. Zhu X, Fu Y. Extending letrozole treatment duration is effective in inducing ovulation in women with polycystic ovary syndrome

and letrozole resistance. Fertil Steril. 2023; 119(1):107-13.
27. Abd Elsalam WY, Mohammed EM, Safwat HI. Clomiphene citrate "stair-step" protocol vs. traditional protocol in patients with polycystic ovary syndrome: a randomized controlled trial. New York Sci J. 2017;10(1): 113-9.
28. Hurst BS, Hickman JM, Matthews ML, Usadi RS, Marshburn PB. Novel clomiphene "stair-step" protocol reduces time to ovulation in women with polycystic ovarian syndrome. Am J Obstet Gynecol. 2009;200(5): 510.e1-e4.
29. In: Shah D, Ray S (Eds). Clinical Progress in Obstetrics and Gynecology. New Delhi: Jaypee Brothers Medical Publishers (P) Ltd; 2013.
30. Saleh SE, Ismail MT, Elshmaa N. The efficacy of converting high response–ovulation induction cycles to in vitro fertilization in patients with PCOS. Middle East Fertil Soc J. 2014;19(1):51-6.
31. EIkhateeb RR, Mahran AE, Kamel HH. Long-term use of clomiphene citrate in induction of ovulation in PCO patients with clomiphene citrate resistance. J Gynecol Obstet Hum Reprod. 2017;46(7):575-7.
32. Wang Li, Lv S, Li F, Bai E, Yang X. Letrozole versus clomiphene citrate and natural cycle: endometrial receptivity during implantation window in women with polycystic ovary syndrome. Front Endocrinol (Lausanne). 2021;11:532692.
33. Cohlen B, Bijkerk A, Van der Poel S, Ombelet W. IUI: review and systematic assessment of the evidence that supports global recommendations. Hum Reprod Update. 2018;24(3):300-19.
34. Rakic L, Kostova E, Cohlen BJ, Cantineau AE. Double versus single intrauterine insemination (IUI) in stimulated cycles for subfertile couples. Cochrane Database Syst Rev. 2021;7(7):CD003854.
35. Fauque P, Lehert P, Lamotte M, Bettahar-Lebugle K, Bailly A, Diligent C, et al. Clinical success of intrauterine insemination cycles is affected by the sperm preparation time. Fertil Steril. 2014;101(6):1618-23.e1-3.
36. Hammadeh ME, Strehler E, Zeginiadou T, Rosenbaum P, Schmidt W. Chromatin decondensation of human sperm in vitro and its relation to fertilization rate after ICSI. Arch Androl. 2001;47(2):83-7.
37. Liang JY, Li ZT, Yang XH, Huang ZC, Yang SF, Wang LH, et al. [Time interval from the end of sperm processing to artificial intrauterine insemination with husband's sperm correlates to the rate of clinical pregnancy]. Zhonghua Nan Ke Xue. 2015;21(6):532-5.
38. Punjabi U, Van Mulders H, Van de Velde L, Goovaerts I, Peeters K, Cassauwers W, et al. Time intervals between semen production, initiation of analysis, and IUI significantly influence clinical pregnancies and live births. J Assist Reprod Genet. 2021;38(2):421-8.
39. van der Poel N, Farquhar C, Abou-Setta AM, Benschop L, Heineman MJ. Soft versus firm catheters for intrauterine insemination. Cochrane Database Syst Rev. 2010;(11): CD006225.
40. Simsek E, Haydardedeoglu B, Hacivelioglu SO, Cok T, Parlakgumus A, Bagis T. Effect of cervical mucus aspiration before intrauterine insemination. Int J Gynecol Obstet 2008;103(2):136-9.
41. Maher MA, Sayyed TM, Elkhouly N. Cervical mucus removal prior to intrauterine insemination: a randomized trial. BJOG. 2018;125(7):841-7.
42. Yasser O, El-agwany AS, Darwish E, Salim N. The effect of bed rest after intrauterine insemination on pregnancy outcome. Middle East Fertil Soc J. 2015;20(1):11-5.
43. Blanchet C, Lavallée É, Babineau V, Ruchat SM. Do physical activity behaviours influence the success of assisted reproductive technology? A systematic review of the literature. J Obstet Gynaecol Can. 2018;40(3):342-50.
44. Starosta A, Gordon CE, Hornstein MD. Predictive factors for intrauterine insemination outcomes: A review. Fertil Res Pract. 2020;6(1):23.
45. Guan HJ, Pan LQ, Song H, Tang HY, Tang LS. Predictors of pregnancy after intrauterine insemination in women with polycystic ovary syndrome. J Int Med Res. 2021;49(5):3000605211018600.

CHAPTER 27

Intrauterine Insemination in Human Immunodeficiency Virus Serodiscordant Couples

Noushin Abdul Majid, Subhashini S

■ INTRODUCTION

Human immunodeficiency virus (HIV), a retrovirus, uses reverse transcriptase to transcribe ribonucleic acid (RNA) into deoxyribonucleic acid (DNA). The virus attaches itself to the surface of cells; usually helper clusters of differentiation 4 (CD4$^+$) T lymphocytes and gradually depletes these cells over time. If the CD4$^+$ count drops below 200 copies/mm^2, the development of acquired immunodeficiency syndrome (AIDS) can happen.[1] There were 39.0 million HIV-positive individuals in 2022.[2] Since the late 1990s, the progressive availability and success of highly active antiretroviral therapy (HAART) has reduced the risk of opportunistic infections and malignancies in people living with HIV, remarkably decreasing their morbidity and mortality.[3]

Furthermore, with the use of HAART, individuals living with HIV today have life expectancies comparable to those of HIV-negative individuals.[4] About >80% of HIV-positive individuals are between the ages of 15 and 44 years.[5] Globally, it has been reported that 20–50% of people with HIV desire children.[6] Human immunodeficiency virus-infected individuals started and maintained on HAART who achieve stable undetectable viral loads are no longer sexually infectious at viral load <50 copies/mL.[7]

■ EFFECT OF HUMAN IMMUNODEFICIENCY VIRUS ON FERTILITY

Infertility rates are higher in HIV-positive patients (both men and women) than in HIV-negative people. Human immunodeficiency virus infection causes decreased semen parameters and hypogonadism in males and higher incidence of tubal disease and pelvic infections in women, especially when the virus was acquired sexually.[8] Patients with HIV who are seeking assisted reproduction services should be highly motivated to become parents, have stable CD4 counts, undetectable plasma viral loads (<50 copies/mL), and adhere to HAART.[9]

■ HUMAN IMMUNODEFICIENCY VIRUS-POSITIVE MEN

Coincubation studies reveal the presence of HIV viral-like particles in spermatozoa and viral DNA and RNA can be found in the semen and spermatozoa of HIV-positive men; however, it has never been established that these particles are infectious HIV virions **(Table 1)**. Therefore, semen processing techniques are required to get rid of these contaminated cells.[3]

While most HIV-positive men have sperm counts that fall within the World Health Organization (WHO) normal range, the

TABLE 1: Presence of human immunodeficiency virus (HIV) in various cells.	
HIV	Presence
Sperm	No*
Oocytes	No
Placenta	Contradictory data
Breast milk	Yes
*Virions present.	

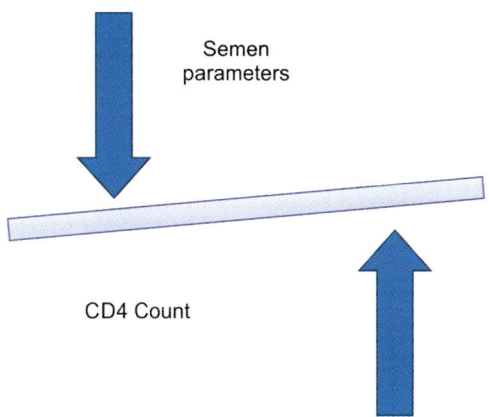

Fig. 1: Relationship between semen parameters and clusters of differentiation 4 (CD4) count.

motility and morphology of these counts are significantly reduced when compared to HIV-negative people and they have a negative correlation with CD4 cell count[6] (Fig. 1). This is likely due to the damaging effects of chronic disease on the male reproductive system.[10] Antiretroviral regimens that include the non-nucleoside reverse transcriptase inhibitor efavirenz was found to significantly reduce sperm motility, whereas regimens without efavirenz was not associated with significant semen changes.[11] Furthermore, sperm DNA integrity in HIV-positive men has been demonstrated to be impacted by antiretroviral therapy, which may be linked to high rates of miscarriage and low rates of natural and assisted reproduction.[8] Nonetheless, it is reassuring that in serodiscordant couples with a male partner testing positive for HIV, the efficacy of medically assisted conception is not affected.[3]

HUMAN IMMUNODEFICIENCY VIRUS-POSITIVE WOMEN

Viral DNA and RNA cannot be detected in oocytes when coincubation experiments with HIV are performed. Furthermore, no evidence of virus-like particles was discovered within the oocytes. HIV receptors could not be detected in the zona pellucida and granulosa cells of the oocytes. Therefore, the likelihood of the HIV virus binding to and infecting oocytes is unlikely[3] (Table 1).

However HIV-seropositive females may be vulnerable to two major categories of infertility. First, other sexually transmitted diseases are known to coexist with HIV, which may contribute to pelvic inflammatory disease (PID).[12] For this reason, tubal disease is a common cause of infertility in women who test positive for HIV.[13,14]

Secondly, research indicates that HIV could directly cause deleterious effects on the ovaries.[15] Numerous studies have revealed that HIV-affected females have a greater incidence of ovarian dysfunction,[16,17] diminished ovarian reserve, premature ovarian insufficiency, and amenorrhoea.[18] Human immunodeficiency virus-positive women are therefore more likely to experience tubal infertility and low ovarian reserve.[19] Oocytes from infertile HIV-infected HAART-treated women show decreased mitochondrial DNA content and this may account for their poor reproductive outcomes[20] (Fig. 2).

It should be noted that, in contrast to serodiscordant HIV-positive men, the efficacy

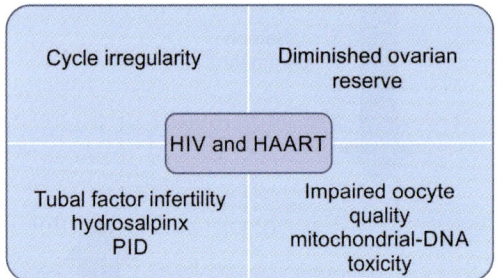

Fig. 2: Effect of HIV on female fertility. (DNA: deoxyribonucleic acid; HAART: highly active antiretroviral therapy; HIV: human immunodeficiency virus; PID: pelvic inflammatory disease)

of medically assisted conception may be impacted in serodiscordant couples with an HIV-positive female partner.[3]

RISK OF HUMAN IMMUNODEFICIENCY VIRUS SEXUAL TRANSMISSION

The risk of viral transmission during vaginal intercourse in serodiscordant couples who are trying to conceive depends on the following:
- Partner's plasma viral load
- Presence of sexually transmitted infections (STI)
- Frequency of sexual activity.

The risk of HIV transmission to an uninfected female partner in a stable relationship with an infected man who is not taking HAART is estimated to be between 0.1 and 0.3% for each act of sexual intercourse, assuming the couple is not engaged in any other high-risk activities. It is reported that the risk of transmission from female to male is lower at 0.03–0.09%.[21] When all of the following conditions are satisfied, the risk of HIV transmission from an HIV-positive man to his female partner during unprotected sexual activity is minimal.
- The man is compliant with HAART.
- The man has had a plasma viral load of <40 copies/mL or 50 copies/mL for >6 months.
- There are no other infections present.
- Unprotected intercourse is limited to the time of ovulation.

Risk Reduction Strategies

Male viral loads for the previous 6 months that are <200 copies/mL are usually accepted for assisted reproductive technology (ART).[22]

Preexposure Prophylaxis

Providing preexposure prophylaxis (PrEP) to HIV-uninfected adults in serodiscordant relationships has been shown to be associated with a 95% reduction in the risk of HIV transmission.[23] In serodiscordant couples, PrEP with daily doses of 200 mg of emtricitabine and 300 mg of tenofovir which are rapidly acting antiretroviral medications with long half-lives is recommended **(Table 2)**. Expert opinion with the Infectious Disease Control team will help to optimize patient outcomes.[24]

TABLE 2: Viral transmission during ART.

Virus	Transmission risk to partner	Vertical transmission	Breastfeeding risk	Risk reduction strategies
HIV	Little to none when on HAART	• <2% when on HAART • Cesarean section	• <2% when on HAART • Avoid breastfeeding	• Positive female—IUI/IVF • Positive male—sperm wash PrEP

(ART: assisted reproduction technique; HAART: highly active antiretroviral therapy; HIV: human immunodeficiency virus; IUI: intrauterine insemination; IVF: in vitro fertilization; PrEP: preexposure prophylaxis)

ROLE OF SPERM WASHING

Human immunodeficiency virus cannot attach itself to or infect sperm, but it is mostly found in seminal fluid. Sperm wash techniques that separate motile sperm from the round cells and seminal fluid fractions can reduce HIV levels before insemination markedly.[24] Sperm wash techniques that involve a double density gradient (DDG) centrifugation step followed by a sperm swim-up step have been used to separate HIV-positive somatic cells from motile sperm.[25,26]

According to the National Institute for Health and Care Excellence Clinical Guideline (NICE CG156), if a man has had a plasma viral load of <50 copies/mL for >6 months, sperm washing may not further reduce the risk of transmission and may further decrease the likelihood of a successful pregnancy. But still, sperm washing may be offered to those couples who despite counseling, perceive the risk of HIV transmission through sexual intercourse to be unacceptable or if the man is not compliant with HAART or his plasma viral load is 50 copies/mL or more; however, it has to be noted that sperm washing reduces but does not completely eliminate the risk of HIV transmission.[7]

Sperm Wash Procedure

History

Sperm washing was first proposed in 1992 by Dr Augusto Enrico Semprini, several years before the introduction and development of ART.

Steps

- In accordance with the European Society of Human Reproduction and Embryology (ESHRE) 2021 guidelines for medically assisted reproduction in patients with viral infection, for semen preparation, dilute the sperm sample 1:1 in HEPES [4-(2-hydroxyethyl)-1-piperazineethanesulfonic acid] buffered medium prior to performing the density gradient and pellet the sperm by centrifugation. (This optional first step removes the most amounts of virus particles by removing the excess seminal plasma right before sperm is processed). Following suspension, the pellet is subjected to density gradient centrifugation.[3]
- Sperm is prepared at a minimum through a density gradient (80–40% or 90–(50)45%) centrifugation [400 g (10–20 minutes)] after which the pellet is washed two times by adding 5 mL of HEPES buffered medium the first time, 2.5 mL the second time.[3]
- Following these two washes, the pellet can be resuspended 1:1 in HEPES buffered medium and swim-up can be performed (1 hour, angle of 45° at 37°C)[3]
- Postpreparation semen samples are tested for HIV RNA and/or DNA.[3] Quantitative assessment of HIV in semen before and after the double-tube gradient method indicates that >99.99% of HIV-1 RNA is removed[25] **(Fig. 3)**.

The latest guidance of the American Society for Reproductive Medicine (ASRM) 2023 mentions a modified method for limiting contamination of the sperm during the gradient separation. It is the double-tube method using ProInsert (Nidacon) as a product. This product has an additional tube that acts as a channel to remove the sperm pellet away from the gradient material that runs along the tube's sidewalls, which could be contaminated with free virus or white blood cells[24] **(Fig. 4)**.

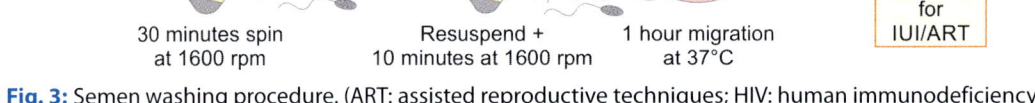

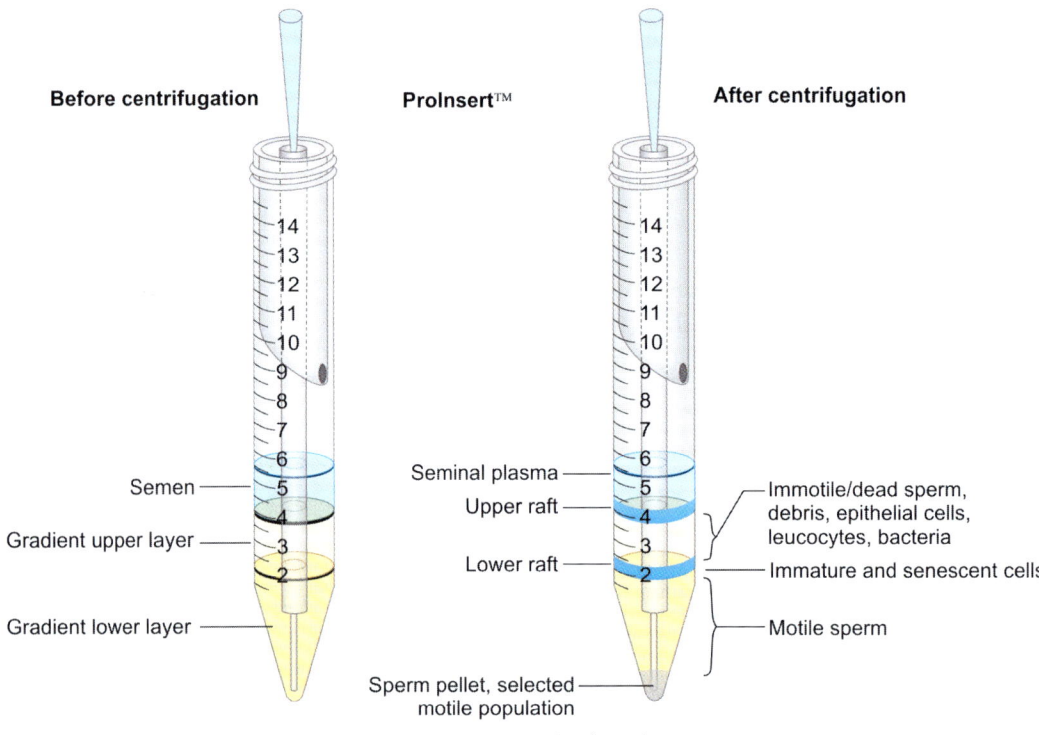

Fig. 3: Semen washing procedure. (ART: assisted reproductive techniques; HIV: human immunodeficiency virus; IUI: intrauterine insemination; PCR: polymerase chain reaction; RNA: ribonucleic acid)

Fig. 4: Proinsert (Nidacon).

A meta-analysis of 11,585 cycles of assisted reproduction using washed semen among 3,994 women revealed no cases of infection of the female partner when sperm washing is performed. There were no cases of vertical transmission reported in studies measuring

TABLE 3: Effectiveness of semen washing to prevent HIV transmission.

Parameters	Number of cycles
ART cycles with semen washing initiated	12,079
ART cycles with semen washing completed	11,915
ART cycles where female HIV status known posttreatment (%)	3994/4257 (93.8%)
Number of HIV seroconversions per (95%):	
• Completed ART cycle with semen washing	0/11,585 (0–0.0001)
• Women's-HIV status posttreatment known	0/3994 (0–0.0004)
• Completed cycle in couples where the man is not virally through HAART	0/2863 (0–0.0006)
(ART: assisted reproduction technique; HAART: highly active antiretroviral therapy; HIV: human immunodeficiency virus)	

HIV transmission to infants. Overall, the use of washed semen resulted in a clinical pregnancy in 56.3% of couples (2,357/4,184)[27] **(Table 3)**.

ADDITIONAL STRATEGIES

- It is strongly advised to perform sexual health screening on both partners. HIV-1 transmission can be accelerated by bacterial vaginosis, herpes simplex virus type 2, *Trichomonas vaginalis*, *Chlamydia trachomatis*, *Neisseria gonorrhoeae*, and *Treponema pallidum* infections, all of which need to be treated. If the viral load of an HIV-positive partner is high or if there is concurrent genital infection, inflammation, or abrasions in an HIV-negative partner, there is a significant increase in the risk of viral transmission.[24]
- Given that multiple pregnancies raise the risk of obstetric complications and vertical transmission in HIV-affected females, aggressive ovarian stimulation is best avoided.[28]
- Trauma to the cervix or uterus during the intrauterine insemination (IUI) procedure must be minimized.[24]
- As an extra precaution, virologic testing of the sperm fraction for detectable HIV virus residue before using it for insemination can be performed, since 5–10% of samples may still have virus after this preparation. As a result, some centers test-washed sperm using a polymerase chain reaction (PCR) assay to see if the virus is present. However, the utility and effectiveness of this added step have been questioned by other centers that have eliminated PCR from their protocols. (ESHRE recommends testing the postpreparation sample for HIV PCR, irrespective of the semen processing method).[28]
- Throughout fertility treatments and pregnancy, the uninfected partner in a serodiscordant couple should get tested for HIV every 3 months.[24]

HUMAN IMMUNODEFICIENCY VIRUS SEROCONCORDANT COUPLES

It is crucial to at least talk to the couple about the possibility of HIV superinfection, even though HIV-seroconcordant couples do not have to worry as much about transmission to their partner as serodiscordant couples do. There are growing reports that an

HIV-positive partner can pass on their specific strain of the virus to another partner who is also infected, despite the incompleteness of the data. In a situation where both partners have completely suppressed viral loads due to effective antiretroviral therapy, the risk of such an event is expected to be very low. This would be the best way to minimize this risk while maximizing outcomes for the couple and their offspring.[8]

HUMAN IMMUNODEFICIENCY VIRUS AND HEALTH PROFESSIONAL

Human immunodeficiency virus-positive individuals and couples should not be denied access to reproductive services because there is very little chance of viral transmission to medical staff if standard precautions are followed.[8]

MANAGEMENT OF CRYOPRESERVED TISSUE

It is strongly advised that the processing and culturing of gametes from viral carriers be carried out in a specific area within the laboratory to enable the separation of these samples and minimize the risk of cross-contamination, even though there is no record of cross-contamination of cryopreserved stored human tissue. Although there is very little chance of cross-contamination, samples in liquid nitrogen storage tanks may become contaminated by HIV, hepatitis C virus (HCV), hepatitis B virus HBV, and possibly other viruses. For this reason, keep the samples in different canisters within the same tank.

Use cryopreservation devices guaranteed by the manufacturer to withstand freezing temperatures and thawing cycles. Utilize sealing methods or a closed-system vitrification apparatus to keep cryopreservation equipment away from liquid nitrogen. Storage sample in liquid nitrogen vapor as opposed to nitrogen's liquid phase.[3]

Alternative Strategy

A study involving male-positive serodiscordant couples who were on HAART and PrEP in conjunction with condom-free intercourse timed to ovulation found that no seroconversions occurred and that 75% of the couples became pregnant. This finding highlights the potential benefits of this combination in reducing the risk of HIV infection.[29]

The risk of HIV infection spreading from an HIV-positive man to an HIV-negative woman is minimal if the right risk-reduction measures are taken, such as using HAART, PrEP, and sperm washing, according to Centers for Disease Control and Prevention (CDC) data from 2017. As per recent research, discordant couples may think about condom-free sex timed to coincide with ovulation, IUI, or in vitro fertilization (IVF) combined with sperm washing after discussing the advantages and disadvantages of each procedure with the doctor. Although this method may not be as safe as homologous insemination, it is still an option that clinicians should emphasize. There are no head-to-head comparison studies between timed intercourse and homologous insemination.[30]

This CDC recommendation endorsing condomless intercourse in serodiscordant HIV couples is a larger shift from prior recommendations. This furthered the Prevention Access Campaign's undetectable equals untransmissable (U = U) initiative, encouraging the use of antiretroviral therapy and supporting condomless intercourse around the time of ovulation window for HIV serodiscordant couples as a method to conceive if the viral load is undetectable

CHAPTER 27: Intrauterine Insemination in Human Immunodeficiency Virus Serodiscordant Couples

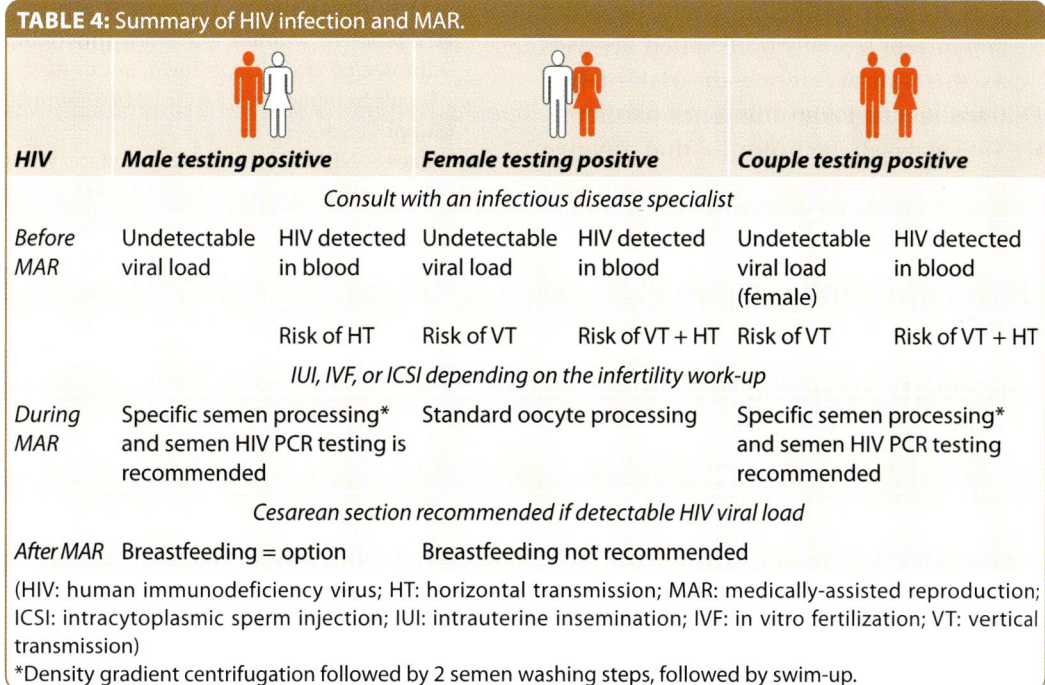

TABLE 4: Summary of HIV infection and MAR.

	Male testing positive		Female testing positive		Couple testing positive	
HIV						
	Consult with an infectious disease specialist					
Before MAR	Undetectable viral load	HIV detected in blood	Undetectable viral load	HIV detected in blood	Undetectable viral load (female)	HIV detected in blood
	Risk of HT	Risk of VT	Risk of VT + HT	Risk of VT	Risk of VT + HT	
	IUI, IVF, or ICSI depending on the infertility work-up					
During MAR	Specific semen processing* and semen HIV PCR testing is recommended		Standard oocyte processing		Specific semen processing* and semen HIV PCR testing recommended	
	Cesarean section recommended if detectable HIV viral load					
After MAR	Breastfeeding = option		Breastfeeding not recommended			

(HIV: human immunodeficiency virus; HT: horizontal transmission; MAR: medically-assisted reproduction; ICSI: intracytoplasmic sperm injection; IUI: intrauterine insemination; IVF: in vitro fertilization; VT: vertical transmission)
*Density gradient centrifugation followed by 2 semen washing steps, followed by swim-up.

on treatment to minimize infection of the partner and pregnancy **(Table 4)**.[31]

CONCLUSION

When it comes to HIV-discordant couples who want to have children, semen washing seems to dramatically lower the risk of transmission. Sperm wash procedures have been used to separate HIV-positive somatic cells from motile sperm. These procedures consist of a density-gradient centrifugation step and a sperm swim-up step.[3] It is highly recommended that the processing and culture of gametes from virus carriers be done in a designated area of the laboratory in order to facilitate sample separation and reduce the possibility of cross-contamination. Semen samples obtained after preparation are examined for HIV DNA and/or RNA.[3]

KEY LEARNING POINTS

- Fertility services should not be withheld from individuals with chronic viral infections, including HIV infection.
- Infertility rates are higher in HIV-positive patients, mainly due to HIV associated decreased semen parameters and hypogonadism in males as well as a higher incidence of tubal disease and pelvic infections in women, particularly when the virus was acquired sexually.
- As per CDC 2017, in HIV serodiscordant couples, who take antiretroviral therapy as prescribed and achieve and maintain an undetectable viral load (<50 copies/mL) have effectively no risk of transmitting HIV through sex.
- Providing preexposure prophylaxis to HIV-uninfected partners further decreases the risk of transmission.

- It is strongly advised to check for other concurrent sexually transmitted diseases as this can accelerate the risk of HIV transmission to the uninfected partner.
- Sperm wash techniques that involve a density-gradient centrifugation step followed by a sperm swim-up step have been used to separate HIV-positive somatic cells from motile sperm.
- It is strongly advised that the processing and culturing of gametes from viral carriers be carried out in a specific area within the laboratory to enable the separation of these samples and minimize the risk of cross-contamination.
- Postpreparation semen samples are tested for HIV RNA and/or DNA.

REFERENCES

1. In: Gardner DK, Weissman A, Howles CM, Shoham Z (Eds). Textbook of assisted reproductive techniques, 4th edition. Clinical perspectives. Florida: CRC press; 2012.
2. UNAIDS. (2023). Fact sheet. [online] Available from: https://www.unaids.org/sites/default/files/media_asset/UNAIDS_FactSheet_en.pdf [Last accessed January, 2023].
3. Mocanu E, Drakeley A, Kupka MS, Lara-Molina EE, Le Clef N, Ombelet W, et al. ESHRE guideline: medically assisted reproduction in patients with a viral infection/disease. Hum Reprod Open. 2021;2021(4):hoab037.
4. INSIGHT START Study Group; Lundgren JD, Babiker AG, Gordin F, Emery S, Grund B, et al. Initiation of antiretroviral therapy in early asymptomatic HIV infection. N Engl J Med. 2015;373(9):795-807.
5. Beyeza-Kashesya J, Ekstrom AM, Kaharuza F, Mirembe F, Neema S, Kulane A. My partner wants a child: a cross-sectional study of the determinants of the desire for children among mutually disclosed sero-discordant couples receiving care in Uganda. BMC Public Health. 2010;10(1):247.
6. Mantell JE, Exner TM, Cooper D, Bai D, Leu CS, Hoffman S, et al. Pregnancy intent among a sample of recently diagnosed HIV-positive women and men practicing unprotected sex in Cape Town, South Africa. J Acquir Immune Defic Syndr. 2014;67 Suppl 4 (Suppl 4):S202-9.
7. Wilkes S. NICE CG156: fertility update. What it means for general practitioners. J Fam Plann Reprod Health Care. 2013;39(4):241-3.
8. Ethics Committee of the American Society for Reproductive Medicine. Human immunodeficiency virus and infertility treatment: an Ethics Committee opinion. Fertil Steril. 2021;115(4):860-9.
9. Estes SJ, Ginsburg ES. (2019). Use of assisted reproduction in HIV- and hepatitis-infected couples. [online] Available from: https://pro.uptodatefree.ir/show/7394 [Last accessed January, 2024].
10. Nicopoullos JD, Almeida PA, Ramsay JW, Gilling-Smith C. The effect of human immunodeficiency virus on sperm parameters and the outcome of intrauterine insemination following sperm washing. Hum Reprod. 2004;19(10):2289-97.
11. Frapsauce C, Grabar S, Leruez-Ville M, Launay O, Sogni P, Gayet V, et al. Impaired sperm motility in HIV-infected men: an unexpected adverse effect of efavirenz? Hum Reprod. 2015;30(8):1797-806.
12. Sobel JD. Gynecologic infections in human immunodeficiency virus-infected women. Clin Infect Dis. 2000;31(5):1225-33.
13. Santulli P, Gayet V, Fauque P, Chopin N, Dulioust E, Wolf JP, et al. HIV-positive patients undertaking ART have longer infertility histories than age-matched control subjects. Fertil Steril. 2011;95(2):507-12.
14. Nurudeen SK, Grossman LC, Bourne L, Guarnaccia MM, Sauer MV, Douglas NC. Reproductive outcomes of HIV seropositive women treated by assisted reproduction. J Womens Health (Larchmt). 2013;22(3):243-9.
15. Savasi V, Mandia L, Laoreti A, Cetin I. Reproductive assistance in HIV serodiscordant couples. Hum Reprod Update. 2013;19(2):136-50.
16. Clark RA, Mulligan K, Stamenovic E, Chang B, Watts H, Andersen J, et al. Frequency of

anovulation and early menopause among women enrolled in selected adult AIDS clinical trials group studies. The Journal of infectious diseases. 2001;184(10):1325-7.
17. Englert Y, Lesage B, Van Vooren JP, Liesnard C, Place I, Vannin AS, et al. Medically assisted reproduction in the presence of chronic viral diseases. Hum Reprod Update. 2004;10(2):149-62.
18. Seifer DB, Golub ET, Lambert-Messerlian G, Springer G, Holman S, Moxley M, et al. Biologic markers of ovarian reserve and reproductive aging: application in a cohort study of HIV infection in women. Fertil Steril. 2007;88(6):1645-52.
19. Adegoke AA, Anthony E, Olumide AB, Folake O, Idowu AA. Hysterosalpingographic tubal abnormalities in retroviral (HIV) positive and negative infertile females. Journal of clinical and diagnostic research. J Clin Diagn Res. 2013;7(1):35-8.
20. López S, Coll O, Durban M, Hernàndez S, Vidal R, Suy A, et al. Mitochondrial DNA depletion in oocytes of HIV-infected antiretroviral-treated infertile women. Antivir Ther. 2008;13(6):833-8.
21. Fakoya A, Lamba H, Mackie N, Nandwani R, Brown A, Bernard EJ, et al. British HIV Association, BASHH and FSRH guidelines for the management of the sexual and reproductive health of people living with HIV infection 2008. HIV Med. 2008; 9(9):681-720.
22. Jindal SK, Rawlins RG, Muller CH, Drobnis EZ. Guidelines for risk reduction when handling gametes from infectious patients seeking assisted reproductive technologies. Reprod Biomed Online. 2016;33(2):121-30.
23. Baeten JM, Heffron R, Kidoguchi L, Mugo NR, Katabira E, Bukusi EA, et al. Integrated delivery of antiretroviral treatment and pre-exposure prophylaxis to HIV-1–serodiscordant couples: a prospective implementation study in Kenya and Uganda. PLoS Med. 2016;13(8):e1002099.
24. Practice Committee of the American Society for Reproductive Medicine. Recommendations for reducing the risk of viral transmission during fertility treatment with the use of autologous gametes: a committee opinion. Fertil Steril. 2023;99(2):340-6.
25. Politch JA, Xu C, Tucker L, Anderson DJ. Separation of human immunodeficiency virus type 1 from motile sperm by the double tube gradient method versus other methods. Fertil Steril. 2004;81(2):440-7.
26. Semprini AE, Levi-Setti P, Bozzo M, Ravizza M, Taglioretti A, Sulpizio P, et al. Insemination of HIV-negative women with processed semen of HIV-positive partners. Lancet. 1992;340(8831):1317-9.
27. Zafer M, Horvath H, Mmeje O, van der Poel S, Semprini AE, Rutherford G, et al. Effectiveness of semen washing to prevent human immunodeficiency virus (HIV) transmission and assist pregnancy in HIV-discordant couples: a systematic review and meta-analysis. Fertil Steril. 2016;105(3):645-55.e2.
28. Marina S, Marina F, Alcolea R, Expósito R, Huguet J, Nadal J, et al. Human immunodeficiency virus type 1—serodiscordant couples can bear healthy children after undergoing intrauterine insemination. Fertil Steril. 1998;70(1):35-9.
29. Vernazza PL, Graf I, Sonnenberg-Schwan U, Geit M, Meurer A. Preexposure prophylaxis and timed intercourse for HIV-discordant couples willing to conceive a child. AIDS. 2011;25(16):2005-8.
30. McCray E, Mermin J. National Gay Men's HIV/AIDS Awareness Day. [online] Available from: https:// www.cdc.gov/hiv/library/dcl/dcl/092717.html [Last accessed January, 2023].
31. Bhatt SJ, Douglas N. Undetectable equals untransmittable (U = U): implications for preconception counseling for human immunodeficiency virus serodiscordant couples. Am J Obstet Gynecol. 2020;222(1):53.e1-4.

CHAPTER 28

Intrauterine Insemination in Unexplained Infertility

Sandeep Talwar, Rohit Gutgutia, Sonia Malik

■ UNEXPLAINED INFERTILITY

Infertility is a disease historically defined by the failure to achieve a successful pregnancy after 12 months or more of regular, unprotected sexual intercourse or due to an impairment of a person's capacity to reproduce either as an individual or with her/his partner. In absence of any relevant history or clinical findings, evaluation of infertility should be initiated at 12 months in women <35 years of age, at 6 months in >35 years, and immediately in >40 years ASRM March 2020—American Society for Reproductive Medicine (ASRM); evidence-based treatments for couples with unexplained infertility: A guideline (2020).

Approximately, 30% of infertile couples are considered to experience "unexplained infertility" (UI) ASRM February 2020—American Society for Reproductive Medicine (ASRM); evidence-based treatments for couples with unexplained infertility: A guideline (2020).

The diagnosis of UI is made when no abnormalities of the female and male reproductive systems are identified. UI is inevitably a diagnosis by exclusion, following otherwise "standard" investigations. However, a consensual standardization of the diagnostic workup is still lacking.[1]

■ DEFINITION OF UNEXPLAINED INFERTILITY

The International Committee for Monitoring Assisted Reproductive Technologies (ICMART) defined UI as "infertility in couples with apparently normal ovarian function, fallopian tubes, uterus, cervix, and pelvis and with adequate coital frequency; and apparently normal testicular function, genitourinary anatomy, and a normal ejaculate. The potential for this diagnosis is dependent upon the methodologies used and/or those methodologies available."[2]

■ WORKUP OF COUPLE WITH UNEXPLAINED INFERTILITY

A medical, reproductive, and sexual history should be routinely taken from both the male and female partner.

Ovarian Reserve

In women with regular menstrual cycles, ovarian reserve testing is not required to identify the etiology of infertility or to predict the probability of spontaneous conception over 6–12 months.[3]

A regular menstrual cycle is considered to be of 24–38 days, up to 8 days in duration, and shortest to longest cycle variation of <7–9 days.[4]

Ovarian function can be measured by serum anti-Müllerian hormone (AMH) and antral follicle count on ultrasound.

Confirmation of Ovulation

In women with regular menstrual cycles, tests for confirmation of ovulation are not routinely recommended.

In women with regular menstrual cycles, if confirmation of ovulation is warranted, tests such as urinary luteinizing hormone (LH) measurements, ultrasound monitoring, or midluteal progesterone measurement can be used.

Oocyte/Corpus Luteum Quality

In women with regular menstrual cycles, it is suggested not to routinely measure midluteal serum progesterone levels.

In women investigated for infertility, endometrial biopsy for histological examination is not recommended in the absence of other indications.

Tubal Patency

All tests are focused on patency of tubes. Tubal patency does not reflect on tubular function. Ciliary dysfunction and tubal flexibility cannot be assessed.

Hysterosalpingo contrast sonography (HyCoSy) and hysterosalpingography (HSG) are valid tests for tubal patency compared to laparoscopy and chromopertubation.

Hysterosalpingography and HyCoSy are comparable in diagnostic capacity; thus, selection of the technique depends on the preference of the clinician and the patient.

Chlamydia antibody testing (CAT) for tubal patency could be considered a noninvasive test to differentiate between patients at low and at high risk for tubal occlusion.

In patients at high-risk for tubal abnormality, such as previous history of pelvic inflammatory disease (PID), positive CAT test, history of tubal surgery, peritonitis, and endometriosis, a visual demonstration of tubal patency is necessary.[3,4]

Uterine Factor

A simple transvaginal sonography (TVS) in a regularly menstruating woman is sufficient for uterine evaluation.

Ultrasound, preferably three dimensional (3D), is recommended to exclude uterine anomalies in women with UI.

Magnetic resonance imaging (MRI) is not recommended as a first-line test to confirm a normal uterine structure and anatomy in women with UI.

If ultrasound assessment of the uterine cavity is normal, no further evaluation is needed.

Cochrane review has not shown any benefit for routine hysteroscopy over HyCoSy procedures in women with normal ultrasonography findings. Considering availability and cost profile of HyCoSy compared to hysteroscopy, these less invasive methods should be prioritized in cases where further assessment for uterine cavity is needed.

Laparoscopy

Routine diagnostic laparoscopy is not recommended for the diagnosis of UI.

Cervical/Vaginal Factor

The postcoital test is not recommended in couples with UI.

Vaginal microbiota testing could be considered in couples with UI only in research settings.

Semen Analysis

Routine semen analysis by the World Health Organization (WHO) 2021 criteria (6th edition) is advocated.

Measuring deoxyribonucleic acid (DNA) fragmentation index (DFI), sperm oxidative stress or sperm aneuploidy is not advocated in patients of UI.

At least one basic semen examination should be done according to the WHO criteria (6th edition), performed by a laboratory which subscribes to an external quality control program. If the result from first basic semen analysis is below the lower 5th percentile reference limit, a second analysis should be performed after a 3-month interval.

Testicular imaging, testing for antisperm antibodies, and sperm DNA fragmentation are not recommended when semen analysis according to the WHO criteria is normal.

Adequate Coital Frequency

In couples seeking to conceive, it could be reasonable to advise to increase sexual intercourse to at least every 2–3 days within the fertility window to the extent that such suits their own preference. The guideline development group (GDG) of the European Society of Human Reproduction and Embryology (ESHRE) 2023 suggests that such timing and frequency of intercourse can sometimes be stressful for individuals.[5]

Additional Tests for Systemic Conditions

- Testing for antisperm antibodies in serum of either males or females with UI is not recommended.
- Testing for celiac disease in women with UI can be considered.
- Testing for thyroid antibody and other autoimmune conditions (apart from celiac disease) in women with UI is not recommended.
- Thyroid-stimulating hormone (TSH) measurement is considered good practice in preconception care.
- No additional thyroid evaluation in women is recommended if TSH is within the normal range.
- Testing for thrombophilia in women with UI is not recommended.

■ MANAGEMENT

Couples can be classified into three groups:
1. Mechanical issues such as sex/coital act dysfunction or tubal dysfunction (often due to subtle endometriosis)
2. Quality issues such as sperm or egg not being of optimum quality
3. Rarest of rare uterine receptivity issues.

When to Start Treatment

It is known that couples presenting with UI can achieve spontaneous pregnancy. Models have been developed to predict the chance of spontaneous pregnancy, such as the Hunault model.[6] These models use a validated set of prognostic factors shown to impact the chance of spontaneous pregnancy.

The most important prognostic factors are:
- Age
- Duration of infertility
- Previous treatment
- Previous pregnancy.

Young women with a short duration of infertility have a high prognostic index and the added benefit of active treatment is small. However, with longer duration of infertility and older age, the prognostic index decreases and the benefit of active treatment increases.

One randomized controlled trial (RCT) comparing ovarian stimulation (OS) and intrauterine insemination (IUI) to expectant management in good-prognosis patients found no difference in live birth rate (LBR),[7] while another RCT investigating the same treatment comparison in poor-prognosis patients reported a striking benefit of treatment (OS and IUI) over expectant management.[8]

Treatment of Unexplained Infertility

- Expectant management
- Active management—OS and IUI
- In vitro fertilization (IVF)/intracytoplasmic sperm injection (ICSI)
- Mechanical–surgical procedures
- Hysteroscopy.

While deciding if expectant management can be tried or to directly go for active treatment, female age and the duration of infertility should be considered as important factors in making the decision of treatment modality to be followed.

Expectant Management

Expectant management has a role in good-prognosis patients. However in poor-prognosis patients, expectant management is inferior to active treatment.

Pregnancy rates were significantly higher after timed intercourse with Clomiphene citrate (CC) and human chorionic gonadotropin (hCG) compared to placebo without hCG [7/37 (19%) vs. 0/36 (0%)].[9]

Letrozole with timed intercourse (± ovulation trigger) versus expectant management: Evidence—no relevant studies were identified comparing letrozole with timed intercourse (± ovulation trigger) with expectant management in couples with UI.

Gonadotropins with timed intercourse (± ovulation trigger) versus expectant management: Evidence—no relevant studies were identified comparing OS with gonadotropins and timed intercourse (± ovulation trigger) with expectant management in couples with UI.

Intrauterine insemination in a natural cycle versus expectant management: Live birth rate was not significantly different between IUI and expectant management in a natural cycle [38/165 (23%) vs. 26/167 (16%)].[10]

Evidence—one RCT compared IUI in a natural cycle with expectant management in couples with UI. RCT shows no significant evidence that CC is either more efficient or cheaper than expectant treatment. Similar findings were reported for IUI in a natural cycle versus expectant management.[8]

Active Treatment

Ovarian stimulation with intrauterine insemination versus expectant management: Evidence strongly suggests that IUI with OS is recommended in preference to expectant management, particularly for couples with poor prognosis. Although IUI involves obviously more invasive treatment, the difference in LBRs between these two alternatives provides justification for its use. The latest (mainly European) studies suggest that only a low-dose regimen should be employed when using gonadotropins for OS, since it can greatly reduce the multiple pregnancy rate without significantly reducing the LBR.

Evidence—a systematic review and meta-analysis compared OS combined with IUI and expectant management in couples with UI. The odds ratio (OR) for cumulative LBR in couples with poor prognosis was 4.48 [95% confidence interval (CI) 2.00–10.01; one RCT,

201 women). The OR for LBR in couples with moderate prognosis was 0.82 (95% CI 0.45–1.49; one RCT, 253 women). The OR for multiple pregnancy rate was 3.01 (95% CI 0.47–19.28; two RCTs, 454 women).[11]

In a retrospective cohort study which analyzed data of couples with UI who underwent two to three IUI cycles, the inclusion criteria were age 20–40 years, failure to conceive for at least 2 years of unprotected intercourse, ovulation, normal semen analysis, and tubal patency. Total of 578 IUI cycles of 286 couples with UI were included in the final analyses.

Results: Approximately, 30% of couples achieved pregnancy and 25% gave live birth following two cycles of OS and IUI. The LBR per IUI cycle was calculated as 13.1% for couples with at least 2 years of UI.[12]

A Cochrane systematic review that examined the outcome of IUI in couples with UI showed that IUI without controlled OS (COS) does not improve pregnancy outcomes, while adding COS to IUI significantly increases LBRs (OR = 2.07; 95% CI 1.22–3.50; n = 396).[13]

Justification of ovarian stimulation with intrauterine insemination: The efficacy of COS-IUI in improving fertility is suggested to stem from the combined impact of OS resulting in more than one follicle and the placement of prepared sperm into the uterus around the time of ovulation. Furthermore, the aim of IUI is to increase the sperm density by sperm preparation.

Intrauterine insemination with OS with CC, letrozole, and gonadotropins: Huang et al. (2018) concluded that similar LBRs were achieved with letrozole, CC, or gonadotropins. Moreover, they observed that multifollicular growth did not improve pregnancy outcome, but it increased the multiple pregnancy rates (OR = 22.4).[14] Hence, routine use of gonadotropins for stimulation is not indicated for IUI cycles.

Measuring Midluteal Serum Progesterone in Intrauterine Insemination Cycles

No studies conclusively document a minimum midluteal serum progesterone level required for the occurrence of pregnancy. Even if the presence of a threshold of midluteal serum progesterone level below which pregnancy and LBRs are decreased is assumed, there is no evidence showing an increase in LBRs with exogenous progesterone administration in any form.

In Vitro Fertilization versus Intrauterine Insemination

Evidence: A systematic review and meta-analysis compared IVF with IUI in a natural cycle.

Live birth rate was higher with IVF compared to unstimulated IUI (OR 2.47; 95% CI 1.19–5.12, two RCTs, 156 women). There was no evidence of a difference in multiple pregnancy rate (OR 1.03, 95% CI 0.04–27.29, one RCT, 44 women).[15]

Another systematic review and meta-analysis, including eight RCTs with 1,497 couples with UI, compared efficacy and safety of IVF and IUI with OS[15]—LBR was significantly higher after IVF compared to IUI with OS [relative risk (RR) 1.54, 95% CI 1.04–2.28, seven RCTs, 1,391 women]. No significant difference between groups was found for multiple pregnancy rate (RR 0.83, 95% CI 0.50–1.38, six RCTs, 507 women) or ovarian hyperstimulation syndrome (OHSS) (RR 1.77, 95% CI 0.49–6.37, three RCTs, 981 women).

In a sensitivity analysis including only studies with women without previous treatment, no significant difference in LBR was found in women.

According to the Belgian Register of Assisted Reproduction from 2017, the delivery rate per cycle for patients over 40 years was 1.7% for IUI and 9.5% for IVF–ICSI.[16]

Course of Management in Unexplained Infertility

- American Society for Reproductive Medicine (ASRM) guidelines
- ESHRE guidelines.

American Society for Reproductive Medicine Guidelines

According to the latest guidelines of the ASRM for UI, the best initial therapy for most couples is recommended a course (typically three or four cycles) of OS with oral medications and IUI (OS–IUI) followed by IVF for those unsuccessful with OS–IUI treatments.[17]

The decision to go for IVF is decided by patient's characteristics such as age, duration of infertility, previous treatment, and previous pregnancy.

European Society of Human Reproduction and Embryology 2023 Guidelines

- IUI with OS is recommended as a first-line treatment for couples with UI.
- The GDG advices to base the decision to start active treatment on prognosis in couples with UI.

Active treatment—European Society of Human Reproduction and Embryology 2023 guidelines

- IUI with OS is recommended as a first-line treatment for couples with UI.
- To avoid multiple pregnancies and OHSS, care is needed by using gonadotropin treatment only in a low-dose regimen with adequate monitoring.
- IVF is probably not recommended over IUI with OS in couples with UI.
- It is expected that the decision to use IVF is individualized by patient characteristics such as age, duration of infertility, previous treatment, and previous pregnancy.
- ICSI is not recommended over conventional IVF in couples with UI.

Mechanical–Surgical Procedures

- *Hysteroscopy* for the detection and possible correction of intrauterine abnormalities not seen at routine imaging is not recommended.
- *HSG* (i.e., tubal flushing) with an oil-soluble contrast medium is preferable over a water-soluble contrast medium. Risks and benefits of tubal flushing with oil-soluble contrast medium should be discussed with all couples with UI.
- If incidentally minimal-to-mild endometriosis is found at laparoscopy, then this is not further considered UI.
- Endometrial scratching should not be offered for UI.

Alternative Therapeutic Approaches

- Adjunct oral antioxidant therapy to women undergoing fertility treatment is probably not recommended.
- Adjunct oral antioxidant therapy to males undergoing fertility treatment is probably not recommended.
- Acupuncture in women is probably not recommended.
- Inositol supplementation in women is probably not recommended.

- Psychological support, including psychotherapy, is recommended for patients when needed.
- A healthy diet and regular exercise, supported by behavioral therapy, when necessary, are recommended.

CONCLUSION

- UI is inevitably a diagnosis by exclusion, following otherwise "standard" investigations.
- A consensual standardization of the diagnostic work-up is still lacking.
- History of prior treatment taken is very important to decide their further course of management.
- Patients have to be categorized according to their prognosis based on predictor models (Hunault Model).
- Expectant management has a role only in good-prognosis patients.
- In patients with intermediate or poor prognosis, active management should be started which comprises IUI with OS.
- The decision to go for IVF depends on their age, previous treatment taken, and history of previous pregnancy.
- Additional procedures such as hysteroscopy are not routinely recommended.
- Alternate therapeutic treatment modalities have a limited role in management.

KEY LEARNING POINTS

- Prevalence of UI
- Definition of UI
- When to label a couple with UI?
- Diagnosis of UI
- Possible causes of UI
- IUI or IVF or ICSI—What to offer to which patient of UI?
- Prognosticating success of treatment in patients of UI
- Role of endoscopy in UI.

REFERENCES

1. Zegers-Hochschild F, Adamson GD, Dyer S, Racowsky C, de Mouzon J, Sokol R, et al. The international glossary on infertility and fertility care, 2017. Fertil Steril. 2017; 108(3):393-406.
2. Zegers-Hochschild F, Adamson GD, Dyer S, Racowsky C, de Mouzon J, Sokol R, et al. The international glossary on infertility and fertility care, 2017. Hum Reprod. 2017;32:1786-801.
3. Gaskins AJ, Sundaram R, Buck Louis GM, Chavarro JE. Predictors of sexual intercourse frequency among couples trying to conceive. J Sex Med. 2018;15:519-28.
4. Munro MG, Critchley HOD, Fraser IS; FIGO Menstrual Disorders Committee. The two FIGO systems for normal and abnormal uterine bleeding symptoms and classification of causes of abnormal uterine bleeding in the reproductive years: 2018 revisions. Int J Gynaecol Obstet. 2018;143:393-408.
5. WHO. WHO laboratory manual for the examination and processing of human semen, 6th edition. Geneva: WHO; 2021.
6. Hunault CC, Habbema JD, Eijkemans MJ, Collins JA, Evers JL, te Velde ER. Two new prediction rules for spontaneous pregnancy leading to live birth among subfertile couples, based on the synthesis of three previous models. Hum Reprod. 2004;19(9):2019-26.
7. Steures P, van der Steeg JW, Hompes PG, Habbema JD, Eijkemans MJ, Broekmans FJ, et al.; Collaborative Effort on the Clinical Evaluation in Reproductive Medicine. Intrauterine insemination with controlled ovarian hyperstimulation versus expectant management for couples with unexplained subfertility and an intermediate prognosis: a randomised clinical trial. Lancet. 2006; 368(9531):216-21.
8. Farquhar CM, Liu E, Armstrong S, Arroll N, Lensen S, Brown J. Intrauterine insemination with ovarian stimulation versus expectant management for unexplained infertility (TUI): a pragmatic, open-label, randomised, controlled, two-centre trial. Lancet. 2018; 391(10119):441-50.

9. Fisch P, Casper R, Brown S, Wrixon W, Collins J, Reid R, et al. Unexplained infertility: evaluation of treatment with clomiphene citrate and human chorionic gonadotropin. Fertil Steril. 1989;51(5):828-32.
10. Battacharya S, Harrild K, Mollison J, Wordsworth S, Tay C, Harrold A, et al. Clomiphene citrate or unstimulated intrauterine insemination compared with expectant management for unexplained fertility: pragmatic randomised controlled trial. BMJ. 2008;337:a716.
11. Ayeleke RO, Asseler JD, Cohlen BJ, Veltman-Verhulst SM. Intra-uterine insemination for unexplained subfertility. Cochrane Database Syst Rev. 2020;3(3):CD001838.
12. Osmanlıoğlu Ş, Şükür YE, Tokgöz VY, Özmen B, Sönmezer M, Berker B, et al. Intrauterine insemination with ovarian stimulation is a successful step prior to assisted reproductive technology for couples with unexplained infertility. J Obstet Gynaecol. 2022;42(3):472-7.
13. Veltman-Verhulst SM, Hughes E, Ayeleke RO, Cohlen BJ. Intra-uterine insemination for unexplained subfertility. Cochrane Database Syst Rev. 2016;2:CD001838.
14. Huang S, Du X, Wang R, Li R, Wang H, Luo L, et al. Ovulation induction and intrauterine insemination in infertile women with polycystic ovary syndrome: a comparison of drugs. Eur J Obstet Gynecol Reprod Biol. 2018;231:117-21.
15. Nandi A, Raja G, White D, Tarek ET. Intrauterine insemination + controlled ovarian hyperstimulation versus in vitro fertilisation in unexplained infertility: a systematic review and meta-analysis. Arch Gynecol Obstet. 2022;305(4):805-24.
16. Ombelet W, Van der Auwera I, Bijnens H, Onofre J, Kremer C, Bruckers L, et al. Improving IUI success by performing modified slow-release insemination and a patient-centred approach in an insemination programme with partner semen: a prospective cohort study. Facts Views Vis Obgyn. 2021;13(4):359-67.
17. Practice Committee of the American Society for Reproductive Medicine. Evidence-based treatments for couples with unexplained infertility: a guideline. Fertil Steril. 2020; 113(2):305-22.

CHAPTER 29

Cost-effective Intrauterine Insemination

Rita Bakshi, Riva Kiran KC

INTRODUCTION

Intrauterine insemination (IUI) is an assisted conception technique that involves the deposition of a processed semen sample in the upper uterine cavity, overcoming natural barrier to sperm ascent in the female reproductive tract. The IUI treatment may include the following:

- *Natural cycle IUI:* It involves monitoring a woman's menstrual cycle without any additional fertility medications or hormones. The goal is to time the IUI procedure with the woman's natural ovulation, making it a less invasive and lower-cost option.
- *Modified natural cycle IUI:* In this, minimal fertility medication may be used to stimulate the development of a single dominant follicle. This approach can help improve the timing of the IUI and increase the chances of success while still being relatively low intervention.
- *Ovulation induction:* It involves the use of fertility medications to stimulate the development of multiple follicles (structures containing eggs) in the ovaries. This is typically done when natural ovulation is irregular or unpredictable. There are two main types of ovulation induction drugs:
  1. *Oral ovulation induction drugs:* These are oral medications, such as clomiphene citrate (CC) or letrozole, that are often used to induce ovulation by regulating hormone levels.
  2. *Injectable gonadotropins:* These are hormones [follicle-stimulating hormone (FSH) and luteinizing hormone (LH)] that are administered through injections. They are used to stimulate the ovaries and induce the development of multiple follicles. This method is more potent and typically requires close monitoring.

Combined ovulation induction: In some cases, a combination of oral and injectable medications may be used to optimize follicular development and improve the chances of success.

The choice of which IUI treatment option to use depends on various factors, including the patient's medical history, the cause of infertility, and the patient's response to previous treatments. Typically, treatment is tailored to meet the specific needs of each patient, aiming to maximize the chances of a successful pregnancy while minimizing risks and costs.

PREREQUISITES FOR INTRAUTERINE INSEMINATION

- Age of the couple
- Shorter duration of infertility
- At least one patent fallopian tube with good tubo-ovarian relationship

- Sperm count of >10 million/mL prewash or a postwash count of >5 million motile sperms.

INDICATIONS OF INTRAUTERINE INSEMINATION

- Unexplained infertility including mild endometriosis
- Mild-to-moderate male factor infertility
- A hostile cervical condition including cervical mucus problem
- Immunological
- Ejaculatory dysfunction

In addition, donor insemination is considered effective in following conditions:
- Severe deficits in semen quality in couples who do not wish to undergo intracytoplasmic sperm injection (ICSI)
- Risk of transmission of genetic disorder to the offspring
- Single women starting family or lesbian couples.

NATURAL CYCLE INTRAUTERINE INSEMINATION/UNMEDICATED INTRAUTERINE INSEMINATION CYCLE

Natural cycle IUI is a simple and cost-effective choice, provided that the candidates are properly selected.
- *Regular cycles:* Natural cycle IUI is best suited for women with regular menstrual cycles in which ovulation can be predicted reliably. In such cases, monitoring the natural cycle without additional medications is a straightforward and effective approach.
- *Irregular cycles:* For women with irregular cycles, predicting ovulation can be more challenging. It may take a longer time to detect ovulation, making the timing of IUI more uncertain. In these cases, other IUI treatment options, such as modified natural cycle IUI or ovulation induction, may be considered.
- *Monitoring and timing:* Women undergoing natural cycle IUI typically come in for a scan between day 8 and day 10 of their menstrual cycle to check for follicular growth. Once the LH surge is detected, which indicates that ovulation is imminent, the IUI procedure is scheduled for the following day. Timing is critical to maximize the chances of success.

Natural cycle IUI is simple, requiring fewer interventions and investigations. It also involves fewer clinic visits which can help decrease the overall financial burden on the patient. This makes it an attractive option for those with regular cycles.

MODIFIED NATURAL INTRAUTERINE INSEMINATION

In modified natural cycle, we administer human chorionic gonadotropin (hCG) for triggering ovulation. A study conducted by Ji-Peng Wan, which included 5,610 natural IUI cycles with donor sperm in normoovulatory women without tubal infertility, provides valuable insights into the use of hCG for triggering ovulation in modified natural cycle IUI. The key findings of the study were as follows:
- *Improved clinical pregnancy rates:* The study found that in the group of women who received hCG to trigger ovulation, there was a significantly higher clinical pregnancy rate (27.40%) compared to the group where ovulation occurred spontaneously (22.73%).
- *Higher live birth rates (LBR):* The LBR was also significantly higher in the hCG-triggered ovulation group (24.52%) when compared to the spontaneous LH group (20.13%).

These findings suggest that among women undergoing natural cycle IUI with donor sperm, using hCG to trigger ovulation offers benefits in terms of both clinical pregnancy rates and LBR. The use of hCG can help improve the timing of insemination, which may increase the chances of successful conception.

It is important to note that while this study provides promising results for this specific population, the applicability of hCG-triggered ovulation in IUI may vary based on individual patient characteristics and the underlying causes of infertility.

Ovulation Induction

Which medication is most effective for inducing ovulation during IUI? The term "best agent" can be defined in three ways in this context:
1. The agent with the highest cumulative LBR
2. The agent with the lowest likelihood of multiple pregnancy and ovarian hyperstimulation syndrome (OHSS)
3. The least expensive agent.

The best agent should be selected based on the patient's exact diagnosis, medical history, and response to previous therapies, as well as the patient's specific goals. Proper patient selection and the selection of the optimal ovulation induction method are critical to a cost-effective IUI cycle.

■ ORAL OVULOGENS

Clomiphene Citrate

Clomiphene citrate is a selective estrogen receptor modulator (SERM). CC interferes with the feedback mechanism of endogenous estrogen on the pituitary and hypothalamus by competitively inhibiting estrogen receptors in the hypothalamus and pituitary. As a result, the pituitary gland secretes more FSH and LH, stimulating the formation of ovarian follicles and ovulation. Pregnancy rates with CC are poor due to its antiestrogenic effect on tubal motility, cervical mucus, and endometrium.

Tamoxifen

Tamoxifen is a nonsteroidal SERM with a similar structure as CC. Because it acts as an agonist on estrogen receptors (ERs) in the vaginal mucosa and endometrium, it improves endometrium and cervical mucus, resulting in higher conception rates.

Letrozole

Letrozole operates peripherally by blocking the activity of the enzyme aromatase, which is responsible for the process of aromatization—the conversion of androgens into estrogens—in contrast to the central activities of CC and tamoxifen. Pituitary gonadotropin secretion increases in response to a decrease in central estrogen feedback action caused by inhibition of ovarian follicular estradiol synthesis.

Clomiphene with Intrauterine Insemination versus Letrozole with Intrauterine Insemination

In general, it is observed that ovulation induction by letrozole is superior to CC in terms of improved ovulation, pregnancy, and LBR.[1-3] Letrozole has no adverse antiestrogenic effect on the endometrium or cervical mucus and is safer due to shorter half-life. Monofollicular ovulation with letrozole leads to reduced rate of multiple pregnancy and OHSS.

Fei Qin[4] in a systematic review and meta-analysis concluded that compared to clomiphene, letrozole is an effective treatment in the IUI cycle, has a likelihood to improve dominant follicles ($p = 0.0003$), and reduces the miscarriage rate ($p = 0.03$) with no significant differences between the two groups in terms of total pregnancy rate, pregnancy rate per cycle, multiple pregnancy, and endometrial thickness.

In a study of 214 patients with unexplained infertility by Fouda et al.,[5] the pregnancy rate per cycle and cumulative pregnancy rate were significantly greater in extended letrozole group (18.96% vs. 11.43% and 37.73% vs. 22.86%, respectively).

Injectable Gonadotropins

The use of gonadotropins supports the growth of entire cohort of developing preantral follicles, thereby increasing the pregnancy rates but are costlier compared to oral ovulogens. Available gonadotropins are:
- Urinary menotropins or human menopausal gonadotropin (hMG)
- Purified or highly purified urinary FSH
- Recombinant

Human menopausal gonadotropin products contain an equal mixture of FSH and LH and are extracted from the urine of postmenopausal women. It has the advantage of being cheaper but also has high levels of urinary impurities and LH which may be detrimental especially in patients with high LH levels such as polycystic ovary syndrome (PCOS). No significant difference has been found regarding pregnancy rate and reproductive outcomes with urinary hMG and highly purified hMG. Hence, the cheaper hMG can be used in IUI cycles to make it cost-effective **(Table 1)**.

Recombinant gonadotropins have some advantages over the urinary products in terms of purity, batch-to-batch consistency, limitless source and supply, predictable bioactivity, and safety, but the major drawback is its cost.

Gonadotropins with Intrauterine Insemination versus Clomiphene Citrate with Intrauterine Insemination

In Chitra et al. trial,[6] a total of 224 patients were randomized to CC/IUI (100 mg) or hMG/IUI (75 IU) group. This study concluded that low-dose hMG have a better pregnancy rate (31.2%) in comparison to CC (16.9%) when used for ovulation induction with IUI in patients with unexplained infertility and mild male factor infertility.

The diamond et al. trial[7] also showed a statistically significant difference in LBR, with 32.2% in the gonadotropin group compared with 23.3% in the clomiphene group.

Bordewijk et al.[8] in their randomized controlled trial (RCT) found gonadotropins to be more effective (LBR 52% vs. 41%) and more expensive {€4,495 vs. €3,006, cost difference of €1,475 [95% confidence interval (CI) €1,457–1,493]} than CC.

Gonadotropins with Intrauterine Insemination versus Letrozole with Intrauterine Insemination

The diamond trial[7] showed a significantly higher LBR in the gonadotropin group (32.2%) compared with the letrozole group (18.7%). The letrozole group had 9 twin pregnancies and no higher-order multiples, compared with 24 and 10, respectively, in the gonadotropin group. In contrast to this, other studies[9,10] reported that the efficacy of IUI using letrozole was comparable with that using gonadotropins.

Combined Treatment

Better number of follicles and improved endometrial thickness resulted in higher pregnancy rate in letrozole-hMG protocol when compared to letrozole alone protocol

TABLE 1: Injectable gonadotropins in IUI.

	hMG	*hMG HP*	*uFSH*	*uFSH HP*	*rFSH*
Full name	Human menopausal gonadotropins	Human menopausal gonadotropins highly purified	Urinary FSH	Highly purified urinary FSH	Recombinant FSH
Source	Urine from postmenopausal women	Urine from postmenopausal women	Urine from postmenopausal women	Urine from postmenopausal women	Genetically modified cells from Chinese hamster ovary
Ingredients	FSH + LH	FSH + LH	FSH	FSH	FSH
Purity	<5%	>70%	<5%	>95%	>99%
Administration	IM	IM or SC	IM	IM or SC	IM or SC
Brands	Humog Menogon	Menopur Puregraf	Metrodin	Metrodin HP	Gonal-F

(FSH: follicle-stimulating hormone; IM: intramuscular; LH: luteinizing hormone; SC: subcutaneous)

(35.48% vs. 10.81%; *p* = 0.013).[11] The addition of letrozole to gonadotropins decreases gonadotropin requirements, increases the number of preovulatory follicles, and decreases endometrial thickness, without a negative effect on pregnancy rates.[12]

Yu et al.[13] in their study of 1,005 IUI cycles concluded that the letrozole + hMG protocol of ovulation stimulation in IUI can improve follicular development, increase the thickness of endometrium, and significantly increase the LBR but not significantly increase the multiple pregnancy rate. Letrozole + hMG group was found to have better chemical (31.3% vs. 18.4%) and clinical (26.51% vs. 12.64%) pregnancy rates compared to CC + hMG group with fewer side effects.[14]

Relevance of Use of Cetrorelix in Intrauterine Insemination

Addition of gonadotropin-releasing hormone (GnRH) antagonists to controlled ovarian stimulation IUI significantly decreases the incidence of premature luteinization and increases the clinical pregnancy rates and LBR.[15] Routine use of cetrorelix in IUI is not recommended, but in patients with premature follicular rupture, its addition can be cost-effective.

■ DETERMINATION OF COSTS

The entire cost of any infertility therapy consists of the following:
- Total number of clinic appointments
- Laboratory and radiographic investigations
- Drug prices
- If necessary, hospitalization.

Every failing cycle and subsequent consequences (several pregnancies, OHSS, and early delivery) increase the cost strain.

■ HOW TO MAKE THE INTRAUTERINE INSEMINATION CYCLE COST-EFFECTIVE?

Efficient commissioning of healthcare to optimize population health outcomes while minimizing resource utilization is a crucial factor in any health care system. Optimizing

IUI outcomes and lowering patient costs can be achieved by carefully evaluating each of the ensuing stages.

Proper Patient Selection

Important prognostic indicators of success with IUI include:
- Age of patient (<35 years in women and <40 years in men)
- Duration of infertility (<5 years)
- Infertility etiology
- Number of cycles
- Timing of insemination
- Semen parameters (total motile sperm count >10 million/mL)

Intrauterine insemination is cost-effective for selected patients with:
- Functionally normal tubes
- Infertility due to a cervical factor
- Anovulation
- Mild-to-moderate male factor
- Unexplained infertility
- Immunological factor
- Ejaculatory disorders

Couples presenting at younger age with lesser duration of infertility and unexplained infertility are good candidates for IUI. It, however, has limited use in patients with severe endometriosis, severe male factor infertility, and tubal factor infertility where direct offer to in vitro fertilization (IVF) proves to be more cost-effective.

Performing Only Necessary Investigations

A complete couple workup that includes patient history, physical examination, and clinical and laboratory investigations is mandatory to justify the choice in favor of IUI. It is important to individualize the investigations depending on the particular case. Performing a battery of infertility investigation profile prior to embarking upon any form of treatment causes unnecessary financial burden to the couple.

- Semen analysis is a simple test and should be performed in all cases.
- A baseline transvaginal ultrasonography is just an extension of the internal examination of the female partner.
- It is not mandatory to perform tubal patency test in all females before IUI. Patients with no prior history of tuberculosis or any tubal pathology or tubal surgeries, with regular cycles can be directly offered IUI without hysterosalphingography (HSG). Only in cases of IUI failure or prior history related to tubal pathology, HSG can be considered.
- Young females with regular cycles and sonography showing good ovarian reserve do not require hormonal analysis. Assessment of serum FSH is advocated in case of advanced age, irregular scanty menses, poor response in previous cycles, or in those patients who are being taken up for assisted reproductive technology (ART).

Choosing the Right Intrauterine Insemination Protocol

- Couples with mild male factor infertility, cervical mucus hostility, and donor cycles should be offered natural cycle IUI if women have regular cycles and are ovulating.
- Adding hCG trigger to the same yields better result in terms of pregnancy rate and LBR.[16]
- Advanced aged couple with longer duration of infertility, previous failed natural cycles, and irregular cycles should be offered stimulated IUI.
- In stimulated cycle, it is observed that ovulation induction by letrozole is

superior to CC in terms of improved ovulation, pregnancy, and LBR.[1-3]
- The more costly low-dose hMG was found to have a better pregnancy rate compared to oral ovulogens when used for ovulation induction with IUI in patients with unexplained infertility and mild male factor infertility.[6-10]
- The addition of letrozole to gonadotropins is found to be a cost-effective alternative as it decreases gonadotropin requirements, increases the number of preovulatory follicles, and decreases endometrial thickness, without a negative effect on pregnancy rates.[12]

In nutshell, strict patient selection criteria and individualized stimulation protocols tailored according to the age and etiology of the patient with a strict cycle cancelation policy will help to decrease the financial burden of the patient with promising success rates with IUI.

Monitoring

Usually for IUI, only transvaginal ultrasound close monitoring of follicular growth and endometrial development is needed. It is a simple, noninvasive, repeatable, and reliable method of follicular monitoring during IUI cycles. Transvaginal sonography (TVS)-guided follicular study helps in the following:
- Evaluation of infertility
- To count the number of follicles
- To monitor the growth of follicles
- To evaluate the right time for injecting ovulation trigger drugs
- To analyze the best time for IUI procedure
- To monitor changes in the endometrium (uterine lining) for successful implantation
- To monitor the effectiveness of drugs used for the treatment
- To monitor drug side effects such as OHSS.

For those at risk of hyperstimulation, serum estradiol can be beneficial.

In natural cycle IUI, *single TVS at 8th or 10th day of cycle* is enough. In stimulated cycles, a baseline scan on day 2/3 followed by scan on day 10/12 can be done. This decreases the number of visits to the clinic, making it more cost-effective to the couple.

Right Timing of Ovulation Trigger and Insemination

- The right time of ovulation trigger is when at least one follicle reaches 18 mm size and IUI is performed anytime between 24–40 hours after hCG injection.
- IUI in a natural cycle should be performed 1 day after LH surge or positive ovulation test.

Semen Washing: Laboratory Aspects

Proper collection and processing of the semen sample is must. Abstinence <3 days or >10 days does not yield a good sample. If the semen is viscous, it is ideal to collect it in a bottle with media. The choice of the type of semen preparation technique whether swim up (cheaper) or density gradient is dictated by the nature of semen sample.

Semen parameters that must be considered in an IUI program include:
- Semen processing time
- Processed total motile sperm count
- Rapid progressive motility after processing
- Sperm morphology before and after processing
- Inseminating motile sperm count (IMSC)
- IUI insemination time
- 24-hour sperm survival.

Delaying semen processing from 30 minutes up to 1 hour and/or delaying IUI from 90 minutes up to 2 hours after collection compromises the pregnancy outcome in IUI cycles.[16]

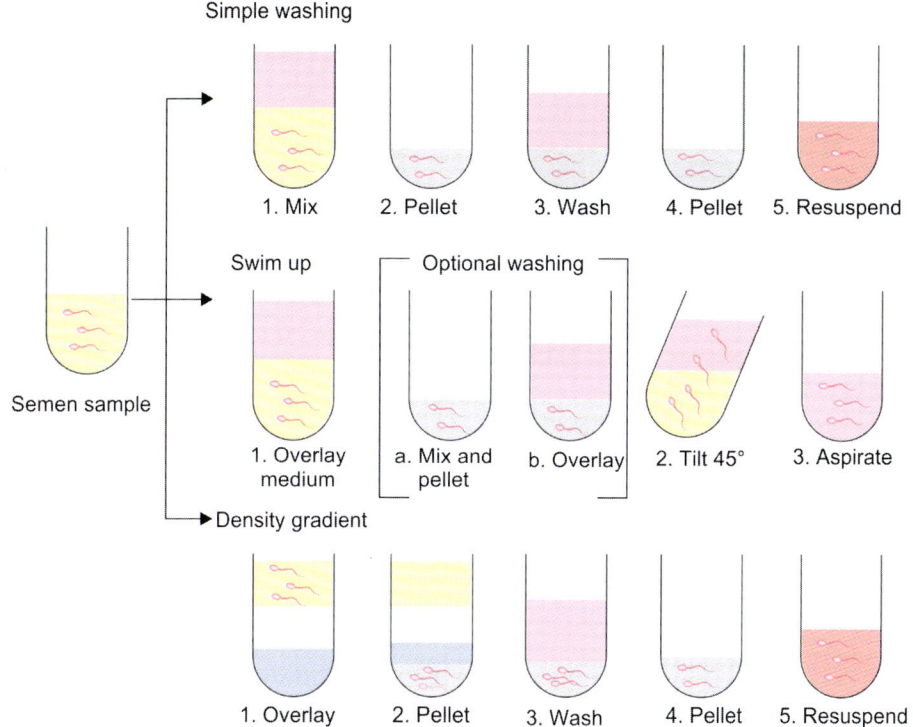

Fig. 1: Semen preparation techniques.

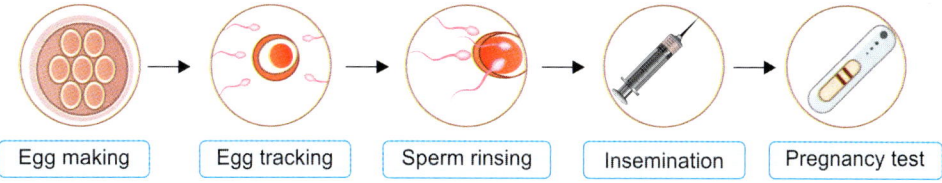

Fig. 2: Intrauterine insemination (IUI) process.

It has been found that fresh samples are better than frozen samples in IUI **(Fig. 1)**.

Procedure Itself

The possibilities of infection are eliminated by strict quality control, standardized equipment, clean air, and laboratory sterility maintenance.

In IUI, it is crucial to deposit the appropriate amount of processed semen sample at the appropriate time and location.

Throughout the process, trauma and bleeding must be prevented.

It is advised to stay in bed for 10–20 minutes following the operation **(Fig. 2)**.

Number of Intrauterine Insemination Cycles

The number of IUIs needed to achieve a successful pregnancy has long been a contentious topic. On the other hand, the European Society of Human Reproduction

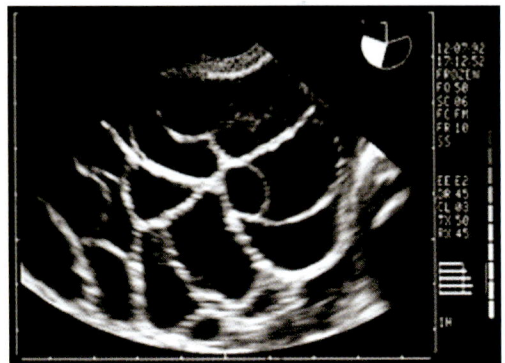

Fig. 3: Ovarian hyperstimulation syndrome (OHSS) in transvaginal sonography (TVS) scan.

and Embryology (ESHRE) advises providing at least three IUI cycles. Certain centers provide a more advantageous package to the couple that covers all visits, TVS monitoring, medications, and procedures for up to three cycles.

Avoiding Complications

Ovarian hyperstimulation syndrome and multiple pregnancy are known complications of gonadotropins. Careful TVS monitoring to rule out possibility of OHSS and cancellation of the cycle showing ominous signs remain keystone in IUI treatment **(Fig. 3)**.

■ CONCLUSION

Cost-effective IUI is a viable and accessible option for individuals and couples dealing with infertility. Proper patient selection, thoughtful treatment protocols, and medication choices can help make IUI both affordable and successful. Additionally, emotional support, realistic expectations, and financial assistance programs can contribute to a positive and hopeful experience throughout the fertility treatment journey. Cost-effective IUI offers a path to parenthood that is within reach for many, providing an opportunity to realize the dream of starting or expanding a family.

■ KEY LEARNING POINTS

- *Proper patient selection:* Selecting the right patients for IUI is crucial. This typically involves assessing factors such as age, fertility issues, and the underlying cause of infertility. Patient selection ensures that IUI is an appropriate treatment option for them.
- *Timely results:* Providing results as quickly as possible is important because it can help reduce the overall cost of achieving pregnancy. Prompt results enable healthcare providers to make necessary adjustments to the treatment plan or explore other options if IUI is unsuccessful.
- *Gonadotropins:* They are hormones that stimulate the ovaries to produce multiple eggs. It is noted that pregnancy rates tend to be higher in women who receive gonadotropin stimulation during the IUI process.
- *Letrozole addition:* Letrozole is sometimes added to IUI cycles to reduce the requirement for gonadotropins. This can lead to the development of more preovulatory follicles, which may improve the chances of success while potentially reducing costs.
- *Choice of gonadotropins:* The choice between recombinant or urinary-derived gonadotropin products can impact the cost of IUI. It is mentioned that there is no significant difference in ongoing pregnancy rates between these options, but urinary products are typically more cost-effective.
- *Patient-centric approach:* Implementing strict patient selection criteria and individualized stimulation protocols

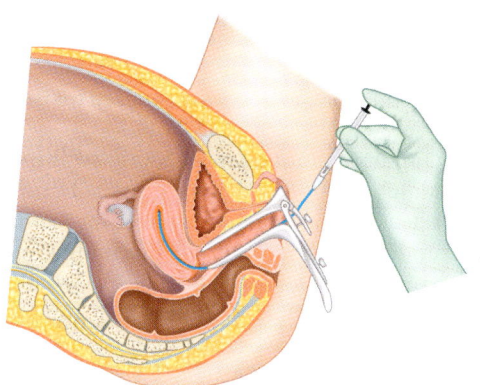

Fig. 4: Intrauterine insemination (IUI).

are important for optimizing success rates with IUI. Additionally, having a clear policy for cycle cancellation, when necessary, can help manage the financial burden on patients.

In summary, the success of IUI in achieving pregnancy while minimizing costs depends on several factors, including patient selection, timely monitoring, the use of gonadotropins, the addition of letrozole, and cost-effective choices for medications. Customizing the approach to each patient's specific needs and circumstances is essential in maximizing the chances of success with IUI **(Fig. 4)**.

■ REFERENCES

1. Liu Z, Geng Y, Huang Y, Hu R, Li F, Song Y, et al. Letrozole Compared With Clomiphene Citrate for Polycystic Ovarian Syndrome: a systematic review and meta-analysis. Obstet Gynecol. 2023;141(3):523-34.
2. Maji A, Ramani MV, Kiran K. Clomiphene versus letrozole: a better agent for ovulation induction. Int J Reprod Contracept Obstet Gynecol. 2020;9(10):4145-9.
3. Legro RS, Brzyski RG, Diamond MP, Coutifaris C, Schlaff WD, Casson P, et al. Letrozole versus clomiphene for infertility in the polycystic ovary syndrome. N Engl J Med. 2014;371(2):119-29.
4. Qin F, Zhou Y, Huan L, Gui W. Comparison of clomiphene and letrozole for superovulation in patients with unexplained infertility undergoing intrauterine insemination: a systematic review and meta-analysis. Medicine (Baltimore). 2020;99(31):e21006.
5. Fouda UM, Sayed AM. Extended letrozole regimen versus clomiphene citrate for superovulation in patients with unexplained infertility undergoing intrauterine insemination: a randomized controlled trial. Reprod Biol Endocrinol. 2011;9:84.
6. Thyagaraju C, Naidu A, Chaturvedula L. Comparison of low-dose human menopausal gonadotropins with clomiphene citrate for ovarian stimulation in intrauterine insemination: a randomized clinical trial. Int J Infertil Fetal Med. 2022;13(2):47-51.
7. Diamond MP, Legro RS, Coutifaris C, Alvero R, Robinson RD, Casson P, et al. Letrozole, gonadotropin or clomiphene for unexplained infertility. N Engl J Med. 2015;373:1230-40.
8. Bordewijk EM, Weiss NS, Nahuis MJ, Bayram N, van Hooff MHA, Boks DES, et al. Gonadotrophins versus clomiphene citrate with or without IUI in women with normogonadotropic anovulation and clomiphene failure: a cost-effectiveness analysis. Hum Reprod. 2019;34(2):276-84.
9. Berker B, Kahraman K, Taskin S, Sukur YE, Sonmezer M, Atabekoglu CS. Recombinant FSH versus clomiphene citrate for ovulation stimulation in couples with unexplained infertility and male subfertility undergoing intrauterine insemination: a randomized trial. Arch Gynecol Obstet. 2011;284(6):1561-6.
10. Dankert T, Kremer JA, Cohlen BJ, Hamilton CJ, Pasker-dejong PC, Straatman H, et al. A randomized clinical trial of clomiphene citrate versus low dose recombinant FSH for ovarian hyperstimulation in intrauterine insemination cycles for unexplained infertility and male subfertility. Hum Reprod. 2007;22(3):792-7.

11. Malhotra N, Karmakar D, Kumar S. Letrozole alone or letrozole gonadotropin combination as first line for superovulation in women with unexplained infertility undergoing intrauterine insemination: a prospective randomized trial. Fertil Steril. 2012;98(3):494.
12. Oglak SC, Sakar MN, Ege S, Otcu SMO, Obut M, Kahveci B, et al. Comparison of the efficacy of letrozole and gonadotropin combination versus gonadotropin alone in intrauterine insemination cycles in patients with unexplained infertility. East J Med. 2020;25(3):427-33.
13. Yu X, Cao Z, Hou W, Hu W, Yan G. Effects of letrozole combined with human menopausal gonadotrophin in ovarian stimulation for intrauterine insemination cycles. Ann Transl Med. 2019;7(23):771.
14. Pourali L, Ayati S, Tavakolizadeh S, Soleimani H, Teimouri Sani F. Clomiphene citrate versus letrozole with gonadotropins in intrauterine insemination cycles: a randomized trial. Int J Reprod Biomed. 2017;15(1):49-54.
15. Gopal L, Sudhakar P, Kandaswami D, Manivannan S. Addition of gonadotropin releasing hormone antagonist for women undergoing intrauterine insemination: a randomized controlled trial. Int J Reprod Contracept Obstet Gynecol. 2023;12(4):1101-5.
16. Wan J-P, Wang Z-J, Sheng Y, Chen W, Guo Q-Q, Xu J, et al. Effect of HCG-Triggered Ovulation on Pregnancy Outcomes in Intrauterine Insemination: An Analysis of 5,610 First IUI Natural Cycles with Donor Sperm in China. Front Endocrinol. 2020;11:423.

SECTION 12: Recent Updates

30. **Artificial Intelligence and Intrauterine Insemination**
    Rashmika Gandhi, Sunita Tandulwadkar

31. **Intrauterine Insemination Guidelines**
    Mily Pandey

CHAPTER 30

Artificial Intelligence and Intrauterine Insemination

Rashmika Gandhi, Sunita Tandulwadkar

INTRODUCTION

Infertility represents a significant life crisis that can result in psychological distress and intense stress for couples struggling with this condition. Advances in infertility treatment have introduced various methods to address the needs of infertile couples. One such method is intrauterine insemination (IUI), which proves effective in treating infertility attributed to male, cervical, ovarian, immunological factors, and unexplained causes, accounting for approximately 40% of infertility cases.[1] Unlike some other fertility treatments, IUI is cost-effective, straightforward to administer, and minimally invasive, with numerous studies reporting a considerable success rate.[2] Infertility treatments are not only time-consuming but also place substantial financial and psychological burdens on affected couples. The ability to select the most appropriate treatment protocol and predict the outcomes of assisted reproduction can significantly alleviate these challenges, reducing both costs and time required to achieve pregnancy. As the success of IUI is influenced by a multitude of factors, accurately predicting its outcomes remains a complex task. Various studies have explored the impact of different factors on IUI success, often utilizing conventional statistical methods and considering either sperm parameters or female-related factors in isolation. However, these studies have demonstrated that relying solely on individual sperm parameters or female factors does not suffice for accurately predicting IUI success.[3,4] Given the intricate interplay of several influential factors, leveraging machine-learning algorithms can represent a more effective approach. Machine-learning techniques, such as artificial neural networks (ANNs), exhibit notable promise for predicting the success of IUI due to their efficiency and rapid computational capabilities.[5,6] Recent years have witnessed an increasing number of studies employing machine-learning algorithms to predict in vitro fertilization (IVF) outcomes, indicating the potential applicability of these approaches to the field of IUI.

TYPES OF ARTIFICIAL INTELLIGENCE RELEVANT TO HEALTHCARE

Artificial intelligence (AI) encompasses a diverse array of technologies, each with its own unique relevance to the healthcare field. While these technologies hold immense potential, their specific applications and functions can vary widely. Some of the key AI technologies that are highly significant in the healthcare domain are as follows:[7]

- *Machine learning: Neural networks and deep learning:*
  - Machine learning is a statistical technique used to develop models based

on data, allowing systems to "learn" from the data they are trained on.
- In healthcare, traditional machine learning is often applied to precision medicine, which involves predicting effective treatment protocols for individual patients based on various attributes and the context of their treatment.
- Neural networks, a more complex form of machine learning, have been employed in healthcare research for several decades and are used for tasks like disease prediction and patient classification.
- Deep learning, a subset of neural networks, is increasingly applied in healthcare for tasks such as recognition of potentially cancerous lesions in radiology images.

■ *Natural language processing (NLP):*
- NLP focuses on making sense of human language and includes applications like speech recognition, text analysis, and language translation.
- It helps in processing unstructured clinical notes, generating reports, transcribing patient interactions, and facilitating conversational AI.

■ *Rule-based expert systems*:
- Expert systems based on "if-then'" rules are widely used in healthcare for clinical decision support.
- These systems require human experts to construct a set of rules within a specific knowledge domain. They work well for simpler tasks but can become unwieldy and less effective when dealing with a large number of conflicting rules.

■ *Physical robots:* These are used for various tasks, from industrial applications to healthcare, such as assisting in surgeries, including gynecologic, prostate, and head and neck surgeries.

■ *Robotic process automation (RPA):* It involves using computer programs to automate structured digital tasks for administrative purposes, like claims processing, clinical documentation, revenue cycle management, and medical records management.

■ *Diagnosis and treatment applications:* AI is employed for diagnosis and treatment purposes, using machine-learning models for tasks such as radiological image analysis, retinal scanning, and genomic-based precision medicine.

■ *Patient engagement and adherence applications:*
- AI can personalize and contextualize care, engaging patients to take a more active role in their health management.
- Machine learning and business rule engines are used to trigger nuanced interventions and provide messaging alerts and targeted content to drive desired patient actions.

Incorporating AI into the healthcare workforce has the potential to enhance patient care and administrative processes. Integration challenges, regulatory issues, and the unique nature of healthcare tasks slow the adoption of AI.

USE OF ARTIFICIAL INTELLIGENCE IN REPRODUCTIVE MEDICINE

In the realm of assisted reproductive techniques (ARTs), the integration of AI methods commenced as early as 1997 when ANNs were first employed to predict IVF outcomes based on clinical data.[8] Subsequent research efforts incorporated support vector machines (SVM), ANNs, and random forest models, combining patient-specific clinical characteristics with embryo morphological data. These efforts demonstrated superior predictive capabilities compared to traditional statistical methods. Nonetheless, their clinical utility often remained limited due to a lack of external validation.[9,10] Recent years have witnessed a surge of interest in the application of AI in medically assisted reproduction.

Annual congresses of prominent reproductive medicine societies, such as the American Society for Reproductive Medicine (ASRM) and the European Society for Human Reproduction and Embryology (ESHRE), have featured an increasing number of abstracts dedicated to AI in this field, predominantly focusing on the assessment and selection of embryos.[11] Khosravi et al. conducted significant work in this field by utilizing Google's Inception Model for embryo image analysis in conjunction with decision trees that incorporated visual and clinical data. Their study demonstrated that AI algorithms surpassed embryologists in predicting blastocyst quality and IVF outcomes.[12]

While research specifically focusing on the application of AI in IUI procedures is lacking, some studies have explored the predictive value of various clinical parameters to enhance the success of the procedure. Lemmens et al. established that in the first finished IUI episode, a positive relationship was found for ≤4% of morphologically normal spermatozoa and a moderate number of inseminated progressively motile sperms (NIPMS) (5–10 million). Low NIPMS showed a negative relation (≤1 million). The total progressively motile sperm count (TPMSC) had no predictive value. The multivariable model (i.e., sperm morphology, NIPMS, female age, male age, and the number of cycles in the episode) had a moderate discriminatory accuracy. However, in contrast, a meta-analysis by Kohn et al. concluded that sperm morphology had no significant effect on IUI success rates.[13] Michau et al. conducted an evaluation encompassing the clinical characteristics of both male and female partners. They found that the highest live birth rates were observed in patients with anovulatory infertility compared to other indications, including endometriosis, unexplained infertility, and unilateral tubal factor.[14] Furthermore, factors such as the female partner's age and the number of preovulatory follicles exhibited noteworthy predictive value, alongside sperm parameters, reinforcing the validity of predictive models. Additionally, Lee et al. explored the timing of IUI procedures, revealing that performing IUI >36 hours after ovulation triggering led to superior results.[15]

Nejc Kozar et al. conducted a retrospective observational study including 1,029 cycles of IUI performed in 413 couples between 2017 and 2020 at a single tertiary infertility center. The standard course of treatment for couples with either unexplained infertility, anovulatory infertility, mild endometriosis, or mild male factor consisted of one to four cycles of IUI with either gonadotropin stimulation, clomiphene citrate, or, in some cases, even letrozole or natural cycles. A database was created based on the demographics of both partners, previous treatment, and infertility workup, including the cause of infertility, body mass index (BMI), and hormonal analysis. Respective IUI cycles were also recorded with respect to the stimulation type and dosage, type of trigger, follicle measurements, and detailed sperm analysis. The exclusion criteria were women >42 years old and follicle-stimulating hormone (FSH) >15 IU/L, severe endometriosis, severe male factor infertility, and cycles with no or over-response to ovarian stimulation. Therefore, the population consisted mainly of younger women with expected good ovarian reserve, which is consistent with indications for the IUI procedure. Out of the 1,029 IUI cycles, 528 were performed in couples with unexplained infertility, 331 in isolated female factor infertility, and 89 in isolated male factor infertility. In the women's group, 617 IUI cycles were performed for unexplained infertility, 147 for anovulatory infertility, 53 for unilateral tubal damage, 53 for endometriosis, 63 for a combination of different causes, and 69 for other reasons. In the male partners, 864 IUI cases tested as normozoospermia. All 32 variables were statistically analyzed to determine the individual correlation values. Prior to model building, the data were split into training and testing sets by randomly allocating 70% of cases to the training set. The statistical analysis demonstrated that the age of the females, BMI, day of the trigger, number of follicles (>17 mm), sperm concentration, motile spermatozoa concentration, total sperm count, number of successive IUI procedures, and stimulation type were statistically significant (p <0.05).[16]

Assisted reproductive technique encounters significant barriers in the form of cost, convenience, and access. IUI is marked by a lack of standardization. The approach to IUI cycle timing is characterized by a mix of costly ultrasounds, multiple qualitative urinary luteinizing hormone (LH) testing, and diverse serum laboratories, leading to varied expenses. On average, a natural IUI cycle can cost between USD 500 and 4,000, with a considerable portion allocated to ultrasounds and bloodwork.[17]

Notably, Youngster et al. have adopted a unique approach, targeting IUI cycle timing as their problem of interest and proposing a method that not only enhances efficiency but also directly reduces expenses. In their research, Youngster et al. introduced a machine-learning algorithm that relies solely on a limited set of laboratory values to determine the optimal timing for ovulation and insemination, thereby eliminating the need for imaging techniques. This innovative algorithm was trained on a dataset of natural IUI cycles, encompassing all cycle data, including ultrasounds. It underwent rigorous testing against two distinct benchmarks, one involving expert physician determinations of ovulation timing and another based on the disappearance of the leading follicle on consecutive ultrasounds. Impressively, the algorithm exhibited a remarkable accuracy rate, suggesting insemination 1 or 2 days before the predicted ovulation time in 93% of cases and requiring, on average, fewer than three laboratory draws.[18] It is important to note that, like any newly developed AI solution, this algorithm operates within specific parameters. Its training data originated from natural cycle IUI, and its applicability is primarily limited to patients with regular menstrual cycles. Nevertheless, despite some instances of missed ovulation or incorrect insemination timing (7% of cases), the algorithm is a pivotal step forward. Its capacity to reduce or eliminate the need for ultrasounds in IUI cycles has the potential to significantly cut costs and alleviate the burden on patients, especially those residing far from their healthcare facilities.[17]

Furthermore, there is excitement regarding the future potential of this AI tool to integrate with at-home fertility hormone testing. The algorithm relies solely on LH, estradiol, and progesterone levels to predict ovulation and insemination timing. Preliminary studies already indicate that at-home spot urinary measurements of these hormones can offer comparable accuracy to serum measurements, accurately predicting cycle timing. The integration of these at-home tests with the algorithm could enable patients to undergo IUI without the necessity of clinic visits prior to insemination.

As we contemplate the various scenarios in which this algorithm could be implemented, it becomes clear that its implications reach far beyond individual patients. It has the potential to address a bottleneck that the ART industry grapples with—limited access to clinicians. Simultaneously, it enhances accessibility while lowering costs. Although the transition from a conceptual algorithm to a rigorously tested and prospectively validated product requires further steps, it is imperative to embrace and encourage advancements of this nature. These innovations have the capacity to transform the field, making ART more accessible and affordable, ultimately benefiting both patients and the healthcare industry as a whole.

■ CONCLUSION

Due to the intricate decisions that clinicians and embryologists encounter regularly in the field of reproductive medicine, it comes as no surprise that there is a growing enthusiasm for applying machine-learning techniques to ART. Although we are still in the early stages of exploring this potential, several studies have already generated encouraging outcomes. In the realm of embryology, image-based algorithms have proven capable of effectively emulating the tasks traditionally performed by embryologists. While the integration of machine-learning algorithms into IVF decision-making processes may hold the potential for enhanced patient outcomes, we maintain the view that if these algorithms can guide decisions resulting in pregnancy outcomes that are at least as good as those achieved without their aid, this would represent a noteworthy and commendable achievement. It is important to note that cost remains one of the most significant obstacles to accessing fertility care. Doctors invest a substantial amount of time in making crucial decisions related to stimulation protocols, day of trigger, and success of pregnancy. If machine-learning algorithms can assist and streamline these decisions, while still producing comparable outcomes, it holds promise as a cost-effective and efficient innovation.

■ KEY LEARNING POINTS

Intrauterine insemination is a cost-effective and minimally invasive infertility treatment applicable to various causative factors. The prediction of IUI success is intricate due to multiple influencing factors, often defying accurate estimation using conventional methods. AI and machine learning offer a promising avenue for enhancing the predictability of IUI outcomes. The chapter explores how AI can transform the IUI decision-making process, reduce costs, and streamline treatment for infertility patients.

■ REFERENCES

1. Sperof L, Fritz, M. The Clinical Gynecologic Endocrinology and Infertility, 7th Edition. Philadelphia: Lippincott Williams & Wilkins. 2005.
2. Ruiter-Ligeti J, Agbo C, Dahan M. The impact of semen processing on sperm parameters and pregnancy rates with intrauterine inseminations. Minerva Ginecol. 2017; 69(3):218-24.
3. Lemmens L, Kos S, Beijer C, Brinkman JW, van der Horst FA, van den Hoven L, et al. Predictive value of sperm morphology and progressively motile sperm count

for pregnancy outcomes in intrauterine insemination. Fertil Steril. 2016;105(6):1462-8.
4. Mohammadi F, Mehdinia Z, Ghasemi S, Zolfaghari Z, Amjadi FS, Ashrafi M. Relationship between sperm parameters and clinical outcomes of intra uterine insemination (IUI). Caspian J Intern Med. 2021;12(1):70-6
5. Blank C, Wildeboer RR, DeCroo I, Tilleman K, Weyers B, De Sutter P, et al. Prediction of implantation after blastocyst transfer in vitro fertilization: a machine-learning perspective. Fertil Steril. 2019;111(2):318-26.
6. Güvenir HA, Misirli G, Dilbaz S, Ozdegirmenci O, Demir B, Dilbaz B. Estimating the chance of success in IVF treatment using a ranking algorithm. Med Biol Eng Comput. 2015;53:911-20.
7. Davenport T, Kalakota R. The potential for artificial intelligence in healthcare. Future Healthc J. 2019;6(2):94-8.
8. Kaufmann SJ, Eastaugh JL, Snowden S, Smye SW, Sharma V. The application of neural networks in predicting the outcome of in-vitro fertilization. Hum Reprod. 1997; 12(7):1454-7.
9. Uyar A, Bener A, Ciray H, Bahceci M. A frequency based encoding technique for transformation of categorical variables in mixed IVF dataset. Annual Int Conf IEEE Eng Med Biol Soc. 2009;2009:6214-7.
10. Siristatidis C, Pouliakis A, Chrelias C, Kassanos D. Artificial intelligence in IVF: a need. Syst Biol Reprod Med. 2011;57(4): 179-85.
11. Curchoe CL, Bormann CL. Artificial intelligence and machine learning for human reproduction and embryology presented at ASRM and ESHRE 2018. J Assist Reprod Genet. 2019;36(4):591-600.
12. Khosravi P, Kazemi E, Zhan Q, Malmsten JE, Toschi M, Zisimopoulos P, et al. Deep learning enables robust assessment and selection of human blastocysts after in vitro fertilization. NPJ Digit Med 2019;2(21).
13. Kohn TP, Kohn JR, Ramasamy R. Effect of sperm morphology on pregnancy success via intrauterine insemination: a systematic review and meta-analysis. J Urol. 2018;199(3):812-22.
14. Michau A, El Hachem H, Galey J, Le Parco S, Perdigao S, Guthauser B, et al. Predictive factors for pregnancy after controlled ovarian stimulation and intrauterine insemination: a retrospective analysis of 4146 cycles. J Gynecol Obstet Hum Reprod. 2019;48(10):811-5.
15. Lee J, Hwang S, Lee J, Yoo J, Jang D, Hwang K, et al. Effect of insemination timing on pregnancy outcome in association with female age, sperm motility, sperm morphology and sperm concentration in intrauterine insemination. J Obstet Gynaecol Res. 2018;44(6):1100-6.
16. Kozar N, Kovač V, Reljič M. Can methods of artificial intelligence aid in optimizing patient selection in patients undergoing intrauterine inseminations? J Assist Reprod Genet. 2021;38(7):1665-73.
17. Hariton E, Andrusier MA, Khorshid A, Timing intrauterine inseminations: do we need an ultrasound, or can artificial intelligence do the trick? Fertil Steril. 2023; 120(5):985-6.
18. Youngster M, Luz A, Baum M, Hourvitz R, Reuvenny S, Maman E, et al. Artificial intelligence in the service of intrauterine insemination and timed intercourse in spontaneous cycles. Fertil Steril. 2023; 120(5):1004-12.

CHAPTER 31

Intrauterine Insemination Guidelines

Mily Pandey

■ INTRODUCTION

Intrauterine insemination (IUI) is the direct placement of processed, highly motile, concentrated sperm, washed free of seminal plasma and other cells into the uterus, near the medial ends of the fallopian tubes. This procedure greatly reduces the distance that the sperm must travel and increases the number of spermatozoa available to the oocyte. The number of sperms that reach the fallopian tubes is increased as much as 25% with IUI.

Intrauterine insemination, both in spontaneous and in ovulation induction cycles, is recommended as the first-choice option of assisted conception techniques since the procedure is noninvasive and also much more cost-effective.

INDICATIONS OF INTRAUTERINE INSEMINATION

Male Partner

- Anatomic defects of penis (hypospadias)
- Sexual or ejaculatory dysfunctions where semen is collected using vibrator or electroejaculation
- Retrograde ejaculation
- Erectile dysfunction
- Immunological factor—sperm agglutination or autoantibodies
- Serodiscordant couples
- Donor sperm insemination.

Female Partner

- Psychological and psychogenic sexual dysfunction, e.g., vaginismus
- Cervical factors
- Ovulatory dysfunction
- Unexplained infertility where pregnancy is not achieved with other medical intervention
- Minimal-to-mild endometriosis
- Antisperm antibodies in the cervix.

■ INITIAL WORKUP

Before beginning IUI, couples should be informed of the expected course, the technique aspects of the procedures, the risks of complications, and expected outcomes. They should be offered to speak with a psychotherapist/social worker who specializes in infertility. Counseling must be adequate and realistic expectations for pregnancy rate should be explained.

■ INVESTIGATIONS

Male Partner

- Physical examination—systemic and local
- Semen analysis
  - Morphological and functional test
  - Culture
  - Antisperm antibody
- Screening for infection including syphilis, hepatitis B, human immunodeficiency virus (HIV), and anti-hepatitis C (anti-HCV)

- If needed, appropriate endocrinological investigations and therapy.

The investigations should be carried out within span of 2 months before collection of semen for IUI.

Female Partner

- Physical examination—systemic and local
- Detection and timing of ovulation by basal body temperature (BBT), cervical mucus study. Ultrasonography (USG) monitoring of follicular growth
- Assessment of tubal patency—hysterosalpingography (HSG), laparoscopy, and hysteroscopy
- Screening for local factors including cervical mucus
- Screening for reproductive tract infections including syphilis, chlamydia, tuberculosis, hepatitis B, and HIV
- Appropriate endocrinological investigation
  - Follicle-stimulating hormone (FSH)/day 3 of cycle
  - Luteinizing hormone (LH)/day 3 of cycle
  - Progesterone/day 21
  - Thyroid-stimulating hormone (TSH)
  - Prolactin
  - Glycated hemoglobin (HbA1c).

Women with evidence of vaginitis or pelvic inflammatory diseases should not be taken for IUI. In case it is present, procedure should be postponed and condition should be treated by appropriate local and systemic chemotherapeutic agents.

TIMING OF INTRAUTERINE INSEMINATION

A well-timed IUI is "must" and is a "critical key" to success because spermatozoa survive for a limited period in the female reproductive tract and oocytes are fertilizable for only 12–16 hours; hence, the timing of IUI becomes more important. Good pregnancy rate depends on the correct identification of LH surge or on an ovulatory human chorionic gonadotropin (hCG) injection given when follicles reach 18–22 mm with a single-planned insemination 36–38 hours later.

STIMULATION PROTOCOLS AND MONITORING OF THE CYCLE

In natural cycle, ovulation is monitored carefully by either serial ultrasound examination of dominant ovarian follicle or by urinary, plasma, or dipstick methods of LH assay. IUI is usually performed 24 hours after LH surge. When in a woman who has ovulatory cycles but fails to become pregnant after 4–6 cycles of IUI, ovulation induction may provide an effective adjunct to therapy. In stimulated cycle, different protocols are used to activate ovary to produce more than one mature oocyte, thus increasing the changes of fertilization and therapy pregnancy. The regimens may vary depending upon patient's response to the drugs.

Different ovarian stimulation drugs used are:
- Clomiphene citrate (CC)
- CC + hCG
- CC + FSH/human menopausal gonadotropin (HMG) + hCG
- FSH/HMG + hCG
- Gonadotropin hormone-releasing hormone agonist (GnRHa) + FSH/HMG + hCG.

LABORATORY SETUP—ASSISTED REPRODUCTIVE TECHNOLOGY LEVEL 1 CLINIC

- A room should be provided for the production and collection of semen. The room should be comfortable and furnished with any material that is

thought necessary to aid production of semen such as magazines and video films.
- Trained laboratory personnel and basic equipment requirements should be fulfilled.
- Outpatient clinic facilities and insemination room.

EQUIPMENT FOR THE INTRAUTERINE INSEMINATION UNIT

- Centrifuge machine
- Carbon dioxide incubator
- Carbon dioxide cylinders (medical grade)
- Light microscope
- Laminar air flow hood
- Class 2 cabinet
- Makler sperm counting chamber/Neubauer chamber
- Pasteur pipettes
- Pipette controller
- Refrigerator
- Test tube rack
- Culture medium/sperm washing kit/Percoll, PureSperm, or ISolate gradient
- Sterile sperm–semen specimen container
- 1 mL insulin syringe (disposable)
- Insemination catheter.

STEPS OF INTRAUTERINE INSEMINATION

1. Well-lit room with gynecological examination table.
2. Women to lie in dorsal lithotomy position after emptying the bladder (table may have slight degree of Trendelenburg).
3. Under strict aseptic conditions and precautions, the semen sample washed and prepared for insemination, to be loaded in IUI catheter.
4. Perform bimanual examination to assess uterine size and position.
5. Speculum is inserted to visualize the cervix.
6. Clean the cervical os if any discharge is present with dry sterile swab or swab dipped in normal saline.
7. Thread the preloaded catheter through the cervix. Do not use force.
8. A tenaculum does not usually need to be used, except with a marked degree of ante- or retroflexion.
9. A stiffer catheter may be necessary in the presence of cervical stenosis.
10. Bring prepared specimen into the room in sterile wrapper. The name should be written on the wrapper.
11. Slowly inject the specimen for over 30–60 seconds to avoid flushing the uterus too fast and causing retrograde flow. Be careful that the catheter does not act as an outflow wick. Injecting the solution too rapidly can force semen through the tubes into the peritoneum and cause considerable pain.
12. Remove the catheter with slight twist to avoid any spillage.
13. Inject 0.5 cc of air to clear the catheter of any remaining specimen; be careful not to inject air into the uterus.
14. Leave the woman in a comfortable reclining position for 15–20 minutes.
15. Instruct the woman to call if any abdominal pain, cramps, or fever develops; with the onset of menses or if menses is 2 or 3 days late, she should call to arrange for a pregnancy test and for further instructions.
16. If the catheter traumatizes the lining of the uterus and bleeding occurs, the chance of fertilization is reduced because immunoglobulins may be secreted from the endometrium.

RISKS OF INTRAUTERINE INSEMINATION

Risks of intrauterine insemination are very few and rarely severe.
- Uterine cramping (pain)—5%
- Spotting (1%)
- Gastrointestinal upset (0.5%)
- Infection (0.2%)
- Risks of controlled ovarian stimulation—severe ovarian hyperstimulation syndrome (1%), multiple gestation, and ectopic gestation.

HUMAN REPRODUCTION UPDATE (2018)[1]

Summary recommendations for the development of global, evidence-based guidelines of IUI based upon methodology established by the World Health Organization (WHO) are as follows:

- **What are the indications of expectant management versus IUI versus intercourse for management of infertile couples?**
  In couples with unexplained infertility with a prognosis of becoming pregnant without assistance within the next 12 months (estimate >30%), IUI could be postponed for at least 6 months. In couples with unexplained infertility and men with a total motile sperm count (TMSC) >10 million and a prognosis of spontaneous pregnancy <30% in a year, it is recommended to do IUI + ovarian stimulation (OS) is the treatment of choice.[1] In couples with solely a poor sperm quality in the male partner, it is not recommended either for or against use of IUI.

- **When is OS required in an IUI cycle?**
  In couples with unexplained infertility and men with a TMSC above 10 million, IUI should be combined with OS to improve live birth rates.

- **How is IUI outcome affected by semen quality? What is the threshold level for successful IUI?**
  Clear lower cutoff levels of pre- or post-wash sperm parameters below which IUI should be withheld cannot be defined.

- **When is the best timing of insemination in an IUI cycle? What is the optimal method of timing in natural or stimulated IUI cycles?**
  Providers can determine the method of triggering in IUI-stimulated cycles with gonadotropins as there is no evidence to recommend for or against a method. Providers can determine the method of timing IUI in natural cycles as there is no evidence to recommend for or against a method. If hCG injection is used, single IUI can be performed any time between 24 and 40 hours after hCG injection without compromising pregnancy rates. IUI in a natural cycle should be performed 1 day after LH rise.

- **What is the role of "fallopian sperm perfusion" (FSP)?**
  The intervention of FSP should not be the treatment of choice.

- **What is optimal number of inseminations per cycle?**
  There is insufficient evidence that the intervention, a double IUI, within the same cycle will lead to better pregnancy rates than a single IUI, in both unexplained and male factor infertility. Women undergoing IUI should be offered a single insemination per cycle.

- **What is the role of bed rest after IUI?**
  Women should have 10–15 minutes of bed rest following insemination.

- **What is the number of consecutive IUI cycles in which pregnancy rates still increase significantly?**
  There is insufficient evidence to recommend a maximum number of IUI

treatment cycles. At least three consecutive IUI cycles should be performed.
- **Which semen preparation technique used yields the best results (in terms of pregnancy rates) for IUI?**
  It is not possible to recommend any semen preparation technique over another (swim-up, gradient, wash, and centrifugation), as per recent recommendation.
- **What is the cost-effectiveness of IUI versus in-vitro fertilization (IVF)/intracytoplasmic sperm injection (ICSI)?**
  In couples with unexplained infertility and men with a TMSC of >10 million and a prognosis of a pregnancy without assistance <30% within a year, at least three cycles of IUI–OS are the most effective option.
- **How can you prevent infections in a IUI laboratory?**
  Good practice point—couples and individuals undergoing IUI and their partner should be screened for infectious agents based on local, regional, and national standards and regulations.
- **What is the perinatal outcome for IUI pregnancies?**
  These individuals are at increased risk for preterm birth and low birthweight in singletons and twin pregnancies.

NATIONAL INSTITUTE FOR HEALTH AND CARE EXCELLENCE GUIDELINE (2017)[2]

Consider unstimulated intrauterine insemination as a treatment option in the following groups as an alternative to vaginal sexual intercourse:
- Couples who are finding it difficult to, or are unable to, have vaginal intercourse because of a physical disability or psychosexual problem.
- People with conditions requiring specific consideration in relation to methods of conception (for example, after sperm washing where the man is HIV positive).
- People in same-sex relationships.
- For people who have not conceived after six cycles of donor or partner insemination, despite evidence of normal ovulation, tubal patency and semen analysis, offer further six cycles of unstimulated intrauterine insemination before IVF is considered.
- In couples with unexplained infertility, mild male factor infertility, or mild endometriosis who are having regular unprotected sexual intercourse.
- Intrauterine insemination, either with or without ovarian stimulation, should not be routinely offered (in exceptional circumstances, for example, when people have social, cultural, or religious objections to IVF).
- Advise them to try to conceive for a total of 2 years before considering IVF (2016).

EUROPEAN SOCIETY OF HUMAN REPRODUCTION AND EMBRYOLOGY 2023

- IUI with ovarian stimulation is recommended as a first-line treatment for couples with unexplained infertility—strong evidence.
- To avoid multiple pregnancies and ovarian hyperstimulation syndrome (OHSS), care is needed by using gonadotropin treatment only in a low-dose regimen with adequate monitoring.[3-6]

CONCLUSION

Intrauterine insemination (IUI) with or without ovarian stimulation is a common treatment for infertility. Keeping in mind the low success rate of IUI (10–20%), proper patient selection is crucial for positive result.

■ KEY LEARNING POINTS

- IUI is simple, easy to perform and relatively inexpensive treatment modality for couples with unexplained or mild male factor infertility.
- When coupled with ovarian stimulation to achieve modest results, there are high multiple pregnancy rates, which makes it no more than a poor substitute for IVF treatment.

■ REFERENCES

1. Cohlen B, Bijkerk A, Van der Poel S, Ombelet W. IUI: review and systematic assessment of the evidence that supports global recommendations. Hum Reprod Update. 2018;24(3):300-19.
2. National Institute for Health and Care Excellence (NICE). (2017). Fertility problems: assessment and treatment. [online] Available from: https://www.nice.org.uk/guidance/cg156 [Last accessed January, 2024].
3. Fisch P, Casper RF, Brown SE, Wrixon W, Collins JA, Reid RL, et al. Unexplained infertility: evaluation of treatment with clomiphene citrate and human chorionic gonadotropin. Fertil Steril. 1989;51:828-33.
4. Bhattacharya S, Hamilton MP, Shaaban M, Khalaf Y, Seddler M, Ghobara T, et al. Conventional in-vitro fertilisation versus intracytoplasmic sperm injection for the treatment of non-male-factor infertility: a randomised controlled trial. Lancet. 2001; 357:2075-9.
5. Ayeleke RO, Asseler JD, Cohlen BJ, Veltman-Verhulst SM. Intra-uterine insemination for unexplained subfertility. Cochrane Database Syst Rev. 2020;3:Cd001838.
6. Pandian Z, Gibreel A, Bhattacharya S. In vitro fertilisation for unexplained subfertility. Cochrane Database Syst Rev. 2015;2015:Cd003357.

SECTION 13

Frequently Asked Questions

32. **Frequently Asked Questions**
    Sunita Tandulwadkar, Mily Pandey

CHAPTER 32

Frequently Asked Questions

Sunita Tandulwadkar, Mily Pandey

Intrauterine insemination (IUI) is a fertility treatment procedure that involves placing sperm directly in the uterus to facilitate fertilization.

Here are some frequently asked questions (FAQ) about IUI:

Q1. What is IUI?
Intrauterine insemination is a fertility treatment in which prepared sperm is introduced into a woman's uterus to increase the chances of fertilization. It is often used for couples with mild male factor infertility, unexplained infertility, or with cervical factor.

Q2. How does IUI work?
During IUI, a fertility specialist will place sperm into the uterus near the time of ovulation. This process helps sperm bypass the cervix and enter the fallopian tubes more easily, increasing the chances of fertilization.

Q3. Who is a good candidate for IUI?
Intrauterine insemination may be suitable for couples with unexplained infertility, mild male fertility issues, or difficulties related to cervical mucus. It is typically not recommended for severe male factor infertility or tubal blockages.

Q4. How is the sperm prepared for IUI?
Before the procedure, sperm is washed and concentrated in the laboratory to remove impurities and increase the number of motile sperm. This helps improve the chances of successful fertilization.

Q5. When is the best time for IUI?
Intrauterine insemination is performed around the time of ovulation. Ovulation can be predicted using various methods, including ovulation predictor kits or ultrasound monitoring.

Q6. Are fertility medications used with IUI?
In some cases, fertility medications such as clomiphene citrate or gonadotropins are prescribed to stimulate the ovaries and increase the eggs produced, improving the chances of successful fertilization.

Q7. Is IUI painful?
Intrauterine insemination is generally not a painful procedure and is often compared to a Pap smear. Some women may experience mild discomfort, but it is usually well tolerated without the need for anesthesia.

Q8. What is the success rate of IUI?
Intrauterine insemination success can vary depending on factors such as the woman's age, the cause of infertility, the quality of sperm, and the number of IUI cycles attempted. On average, the success rate per cycle is around 10–20%.

Q9. How many IUI cycles are typically recommended?
The number of IUI cycles recommended can vary, but it is common for couples to try

3–6 cycles before considering other fertility treatments such as in vitro fertilization (IVF).

Q10. What are the risks and side effects of IUI?
The risks and side effects of IUI are generally minimal. Common side effects include mild cramping, spotting, or discomfort. There is increased risk of multiple pregnancies due to the stimulation of the ovaries, so this is carefully monitored.

Q11. Can same-sex couples or single individuals use IUI?
Yes, IUI is a fertility treatment option for same-sex couples and single individuals who want to have children, using donor sperms.

Q12. How much does IUI cost?
The cost of IUI can vary depending on factors such as location, clinic, and whether fertility medications are used. It is essential to inquire about the costs and potential insurance coverage.

Q13. Are there any lifestyle changes to improve IUI success?
Healthy lifestyle such as eating well, exercising regularly, and managing stress can help improve your overall fertility and chances of success with IUI.

Q14. What postprocedure guidelines should patients follow?
Patients can usually resume normal activities after IUI, but they should be advised to avoid strenuous exercise or sexual intercourse for a specific period. A pregnancy test is typically performed about 2 weeks Before giving a sperm sample, male partner must abstain from ejaculation for 2–3 days to maximize his sperm count and motility.

Q15. Are there any specific positions patients should lie in after IUI?
There are no specific position patients need to maintain after IUI. Lying down or sitting up is generally a matter of personal comfort.

Q16. Should patients abstain from sexual intercourse after IUI?
It is typically recommended to abstain from sexual intercourse for a brief period after IUI, usually for about 24–48 hours. This helps minimize any potential discomfort and the risk of infection.

Q17. Are there any restrictions on exercise or physical activity after IUI?
While strenuous exercise is best avoided immediately after IUI, patients can engage in light-to-moderate physical activity, such as walking or gentle yoga, if they are comfortable.

Q18. How soon can patients return to work after IUI?
Patients can generally return to work the same day as the IUI procedure as it does not require an extended recovery period.

INDEX

Page numbers followed by *b* refer to box, *f* refer to figure, *fc* refer to flowchart, and *t* refer to table

A

Abortions, multiple
    spontaneous 52
Acanthosis nigricans 52
Acarbose 122
Accessory sex gland function,
        biochemical assays
        for 169
Acne 52
Acquired immunodeficiency
        syndrome 258
    development of 258
Acrosome reaction 166, 167
    steps of 168*f*
Activin 7
Adenosine monophosphate 44
Advanced sperm function
        testing 57
Agonists 141*f*
    disadvantages of 138
Air-handling unit 187
Alcohol consumption 64
Alpha-glucosidase
        inhibitors 117, 122
Alpha-lipoic acids 124
Amenorrhea 51
    exercise-induced 227
    hypothalamic 95
American College of Obstetricians
        and Gynecologists 245
American Society for
        Reproductive Medicine
        100, 238, 261, 268, 291
    guidelines 273
    practice committee of 57
    revised 233
Aminoglutethimide 110, 230
Anastrozole 110, 115, 230
Androgen, role of 5
Anemia 121
Aneuploid oocytes 219
Angina 121
Anorexia 119
Anovulation 70, 281
    chronic 228*f*
    normoestrogenic 53
    normogonadotropic 53

Antagonists 139*f*, 141*f*
    advantages of 140
    indications of 140
Anti-hepatitis C 295
Anti-Müllerian hormone 55, 56,
        58, 59, 123*f*, 216, 229,
        243, 269
Antioxidant 182
    action 181
    properties 181
    support 181
Antisperm antibody 58, 295
    test 172
Antitubercular treatment 58
Antral follicle count 55, 55*f*, 56,
        58, 80, 81, 216
    low 55*f*
Arimidex 230
Aromasin 230
Aromatase enzyme,
        function of 109*f*
Aromatase inhibitors 100, 108,
        109, 110*f*, 114, 115, 245
    advantages of 110
    classification of 109, 110*t*,
        230, 230*t*
Artificial intelligence 289
    types of 259
    use of 290
Artificial neural networks 289
Assisted reproductive techniques
        12, 31, 51, 56*b*, 61, 139,
        147, 165, 181, 184, 248,
        254, 260, 260*t*, 262*f*, 263,
        281, 290, 292, 296
    Act 184, 194
    clinic 195
    cycles 33, 34, 81
Astral follicles 55*f*
Autoantibodies 295
Autoimmune disorders 52
Azoospermia 68

B

Balanced diet 181
Basal body temperature 45, 54,
        99, 296

Basalis membrane 123*f*
Baseline score calculation 81*t*
Basic semen examination,
        temporal outline of 157
Beta-human chorionic
        gonadotropin 86
Biguanides 117
Bilateral tubal block 68
Bimanual pelvic vaginal
        examination 53
Biomedical waste
    categories of 186*f*
    management of 186
Biopsy, endometrial 54, 57
Biosafety cabinet 188*f*
Bloating, abdominal 99
Blood
    flow, endometrial 27
    pressure assessment 52
B-mode ultrasound image 78*f*,
        82*f*, 84*f*, 85*f*, 87*f*
Body mass index 52, 64, 69, 80,
        81, 95, 120, 216, 230,
        254, 291
Bone fractures 121
Breast
    cancer therapy 93
    discomfort 99
    examination 52
    milk 259
Breastfeeding 121
    risk 260
Bulbourethral glands 157

C

Cancer
    disorders, hereditary 52
    ovarian 99
Carbon dioxide
    cylinders 297
    incubator 297
Cardiac disease 121
Cardiac failure 118
    congestive 118
Cell membrane structure 182
Centers for Disease Control and
        Prevention 264

Index

Centrifugation 176, 177
  methods 177
Centrifuge 178
  machine 297
Cervical factors 68, 69, 226, 269, 295
  infertility 226
Cervical mucus 45, 226
Cervicitis 68
Cervix 295
Cetrorelix, relevance of use of 280
Chemical composition 93
Chlamydia
  antibody 58
    testing 269
  trachomatis 58, 263
Cholesterol transport 23
Chromium 247
  picolinate 117, 122
  polynicotinate 248
Chymotrypsin 71
Clinical Establishment Act 186
Clinical pregnancy rate 140, 180, 208, 277
Clomiphene 95, 97, 98, 102, 103, 119-121, 231, 232, 278
  action of 94f
  citrate 32, 33, 82, 93, 96, 96f, 102, 108, 120, 129, 142, 203, 208, 227, 245, 248, 250, 250f, 253, 271, 276, 278, 279, 296
  cycles 33, 208
  stair-step protocol of 250f
  treatment monitoring 98
  failure 97
  role of 101
  structure of 93f
  use of 97
Coital frequency, adequate 270
Collagen synthesis 182
Combined ovulation induction 276
Computer-assisted semen analysis 62
Conception, nature of 52
Condoms, nonspermicidal 189
Conical test tubes 178
Contraception requirements 121
Controlled ovarian hyperstimulation 46, 209, 233
Controlled ovarian stimulation 136, 207, 233, 234
  risks of 298

Conventional semen analysis 165
Corpus luteum 21, 25, 207, 209
  Doppler evaluation of 26
  endocrine
    autocrine regulation of 22
    paracrine regulation of 22
  quality 269
Cowper's glands 157, 158
Cryopreservation 156
Cyclic adenosine monophosphate 22
Cyst
  fimbrial 217f
  ovarian 95

D

D-chiro-inositol 122, 123f, 245
Dehydration 118
Dehydroepiandrosterone 247
  sulfate 98, 248
Density gradient centrifugation 177
Deoxyribonucleic acid 61, 253, 258, 260f, 270
  fragmentation
    index 71, 171, 218
    test 57, 172
Dexamethasone 248
Diabetes mellitus 243
  gestational 52
  noninsulin-dependent 121
Diarrhea 119
Direct swim-up technique 179
Discomfort, abdominal 99
Discontinuous density gradient technique 178
Distention, abdominal 99
Distilled water 189
Donor intrauterine insemination 68, 72
Donor sperm insemination 295
Doppler 82
Double density gradient 261
Double stimulation protocol 114f
Douglas pouch 217, 217f
Dydrogesterone 209, 210

E

Ectopic pregnancy, previous 244
Edema 121
Ejaculate
  collection 157

  macroscopic appearance of 158
  odor 159
  pH 159
Ejaculation, retrograde 68, 295
Ejaculatory
  abstinence 201
  disorders 281
  dysfunction 68, 70, 226, 277, 295
Electroejaculation 295
Embryo transfer 136
Enclomiphene 231
Endocrine
  disorders 52
  gland 22
Endogenous luteinizing hormone, prevention of 12, 13
Endometrial
  microbiome metagenomic analysis 59
  pattern 26
  preparation 101
  scratching 218
  thickness 26, 253
  vascularity 86t
  volume 85, 253
Endometrioma 239
Endometriosis 69, 70, 137f, 238-241, 244
  fertility index 239
  mild 68, 233
  minimal 233
  minimal to mild 226, 295
  peritoneal 59
Endometritis 68
  infectious chronic 59
Endometrium 84f, 85f, 86, 86f, 86t, 87, 87f, 149
  B-mode features of 83
  Doppler features of 84
  triple layer 149f
End-organ failure 227
Enhanced follicle-stimulating hormone
  action 5
  receptor expression 6
Enzymes 182
  proteolytic 9
Epidermal growth factor 7, 31
Epididymis 157
  secretory markers of 169
Erectile dysfunction 295

Estradiol 33, 42, 43*f*, 57, 123*f*
   concentration of 7
   elevation, duration of 7
   levels 45
Estrogen 210
   antagonist effects 96
   biphasic regulation of 7
   levels 43
   negative feedback effect of 5
   receptors 31, 93, 278
   role of 5
   synergistic effect of 6
Estrone-3-glucoronide 45
Eugonadotropic hypogonadism 227
European Medicines Agency 121
European Society of Human
      Reproduction and
      Embryology 70, 133,
      215, 233, 238, 261, 270,
      291, 299
   guidelines 273
Exemestane 110, 230

F

Fadrozole 110, 230
Fallopian sperm perfusion, role
      of 298
Fatal growth restriction 52
Female fertility 68, 260*f*
Female infertility
   causes of 59
   evaluation of 58
Fertility 51, 258
Fertilization, steps of 165*f*
Fibroblast growth factor 31
Final oocyte maturation,
      triggering of 17
Flatulence 119
Flexible continuous dose
      protocol 139*f*
Flow index 84*f*
Fluorescence in situ
      hybridization 219
Follicle 81, 86, 86
   color Doppler image of 79*f*
   luteinization 21
   phase 3, 207
   rupture 13
   stimulating hormone 3, 5, 9,
      6, 10*f*, 12, 16*f*, 31, 42, 55,
      57, 62, 79, 94, 94*f*, 108,
      118, 138, 147, 155, 208,
      243, 245, 246*f*, 276, 280,
      291, 296
      recombinant 81, 280

Follicular phase, endocrinology
      of 3, 12
Folliculogenesis
   dynamic 11
   gonadotropin
      dependent 4, 11
      independent 3, 11
Food sources 181, 182
Formestane 110, 230
Fragile X premutation carriers 227
Fragmentation index 270
Freezing media 189
Frozen embryo transfer 101

G

Gelatinous bodies 159
Genetic
   abnormalities 62, 219
   disorders 52
Genital tract 156
   bleeding 68
   infection 68
Geriatric 122
Gestation
   ectopic 298
   multiple 298
Glucagon-like peptide-1 122
   analogs 122
Glucocorticoids 97, 245, 247
Glucose production 118
Glycerophosphocholine 169
Gonadal dysgenesis 227
Gonadotropin 98, 120, 121, 129,
      139*f*, 142, 179, 227, 232,
      246, 271, 272, 279, 284
   choice of 284
   cycles 208
   dose modification chart 82*fc*
   exogenous 12
   injectable 276, 279, 280*t*
   regimen 113*f*
   stimulation 130
      drawbacks of 131
      effect of 208
   therapy 129
Gonadotropin hormone-releasing
      hormone 32, 42, 94*f*, 95,
      109, 109*f*, 110*f*, 117, 132,
      137, 149, 204, 227, 228,
      240, 246*f*, 280
   agonist 114*f*, 138, 150, 296
      effect of 34
      trigger, types of 150
   analogs 12, 137

   antagonist 138
      administration 14
      protocol 139
      deficiency, idiopathic 227
      use of 136
Granulosa cell 16*f*, 22, 30, 44
   stimulation 6
Growth hormone 228
Gynecology 119

H

Headache 99
Heart failure 121
Hemizona assay 167, 173
Hemoglobin, glycated 296
Hepatic disease 122
Hepatic impairment 118
Hepatitis
   B 295
      surface antigen 68, 191
   C virus 191, 264, 296
Highly active antiretroviral therapy
      258, 260, 260*f*, 263
High-resistance uterine artery
      flow waveform 87*f*
Hirsutism 52
Hormonal test 57
Hormone 132
   adrenocorticotropic 228
   regulation of 182
   replacement therapy 228
Hot flushes 99
Human chorionic gonadotropin
      6, 12, 22, 31, 35, 46, 98,
      99, 102*f*, 113*f*, 149, 203,
      207, 249, 249*f*-251*f*, 252,
      271, 277, 296
   agonist, effect of 35
   effect of 35
   recombinant 251
   supplementation 36
Human corpus
      luteum 27, 30
Human follicle-stimulating
      hormone 132
Human immunodeficiency virus
      68, 72, 191, 258-260,
      260*f*, 261, 263, 264, 264*f*,
      265, 295
   effect of 258, 260*f*
   infection 265
   risk of 260
   transmission 263*t*

Index

Human menopausal
    gonadotropin 15, 98,
    108, 114f, 130, 202, 229,
    245, 246, 279, 296
Human reproduction update 298
Human serum albumen 190
Hyaluronan-binding assay 167, 168
Hyaluronic acid 168
    binding 167
Hydroxyeicosatetraenoic acids 44
Hydroxylation 16f
Hydroxyprogesterone 32
Hydroxysteroid dehydrogenase
    16f, 30
Hyperandrogenemia 118, 246
Hyperinsulinemia 118,
    123, 244fc
Hypersensitivity 95, 118
Hypertension 52
Hypoglycemia 119, 122
Hypogonadism
    hypergonadotropic 227
    hypogonadotropic 95, 227
Hypogonadotropic hypogonadal
    anovulation 53
Hypo-osmotic swelling test 172
Hypospadias 68, 70, 295
Hypospermia 68, 70
Hypothalamic dysfunction 227
Hypothalamic failure 227
Hypothalamic ovulatory
    disorder 228
Hypothalamic pituitary-ovarian
    axis 94f, 138, 226
Hysterolaparoscopy 217
Hysterosalpingo-contrast-
    sonography 244, 269
Hysterosalpingography 56, 217,
    233, 244, 269, 281, 296
Hysteroscopy 57, 273, 296

I

Immature germ cells 162
Immune
    dysregulation 64
    factors 64, 66
Immunoglobulin G 58
Implantation, window of 31, 58
Impotence 68
In vitro fertilization 63, 81, 95,
    102f, 112, 124, 136, 147,
    170f, 177, 208, 215, 219,
    225, 243, 252, 260, 264,
    265, 272, 281, 289, 299
    cycles 102
    mild stimulation 101
    treatment 207
    witness system 178
Infection 298
    severe 118
Infertility 51, 52, 61, 66, 101, 117,
    165, 207, 215, 225,
    268, 289
    anovulatory 95
    causes of 69, 69t, 225
    duration of 69, 215, 225, 270
    etiology 69
    evaluation of 282
    idiopathic 95
    immunological 57, 68
    male 68, 101
    management of 243, 254
    rates 258
    tests 57b
    treatment 119
    unexplained 57, 68, 69, 95,
        100, 110, 226, 233, 268,
        273, 281, 295
Inflammation 64
Inflammatory markers 64, 66
Inositide triphosphate 123f
Inositols 122
    types of 122
Insemination 282
    best timing of 203, 298
    catheter 297
    number of 203
    per cycle, optimal number
        of 298
Insulin 123f
    receptor 123f
    sensitizers 117
        novel molecules for 122
International Committee for
    Monitoring Assisted
    Reproductive
    Technologies 268
International Federation of
    Gynecology and
    Obstetrics 54, 227f
Intracytoplasmic sperm injection
    172, 215, 219, 244, 265,
    277, 299
    physiological 168
Intrauterine adhesions 68
Intrauterine insemination 51, 61,
    68, 75, 77, 81, 98, 111,
    129-131, 136, 137, 137f,
    139f, 142, 147, 170f, 172,
    176, 179, 183, 184, 194,
    196, 197, 201-203, 207,
    208, 215, 223, 225, 227,
    238, 243, 245, 253, 258,
    260, 262f, 263, 265, 268,
    271, 272, 276, 278-280,
    280t, 285f, 289, 293,
    295, 299
    artificial 68
    cannula 202
    catheters 189
    contraindications of 68, 68b
    cost-effective 276
    cycles 102, 136, 137f, 139, 140,
        148, 217, 272, 277, 298
        causes of 137f
        cost-effective 280
        fail 69, 136
        monitoring of 77
        number of 283
    devices 203
    double 234
    guidelines 295
    indications of 68, 68b, 277, 295
    laboratory, setting up 184
    outcome 202, 215, 254
    preparation for 180
    prerequisites for 244, 276
    procedure 180, 201
        timing of 179
    process 283
    program 203
    protocol 65, 67, 281
    results 215
    risks of 298
    role of 233, 243
    selection for 68
    steps of 297
    therapy 151
    timing of 216, 219, 226,
        282, 296
    unit, equipment for 297
Isopropyl alcohol 189

J

Joint consultations 65

K

Kallmann syndrome 227
Karyotype 57, 63
Ketoacidosis, diabetic 121
Kisspeptins 150

L

Lactic acidosis 118
Laminar air flow hood 178, 297
Laparoscopic ovarian drilling 110, 120, 247
Laparoscopy 57, 269, 296
Late follicular phase 6
    serum progesterone levels 15
Letrozole 100, 101, 110-113, 113*f*, 114, 115, 129, 131, 142, 227, 230, 232, 245, 249, 252, 271, 272, 276, 278, 279, 284
    induced cycles 208
    mechanism of action of 246*f*
    protocol 112*f*, 249, 249*f*
Leukemia inhibitory factor 32
Leukocytes 168
Leuprolide acetate 150
Light microscope 297
Lipoprotein
    low-density 23
    high-density 23
Liquefaction 158
Live birth 52
    rate 218, 248, 271, 272
        higher 277
Liver disease 95
Low-resistance perifollicular flow, pulse Doppler image of 83*f*
Luteal estradiol biosynthesis 24
Luteal phase 3, 23, 30*f*, 32-34, 35, 207, 209
    defect 32, 33*fc*, 34, 36
    deficiency 207, 210
    endocrinology of 21, 30
    endometrium, Doppler evaluation of 26
    laboratory assessment of 26
    physiology of 207
    support 205, 207, 208
Luteal progesterone synthesis 23
Luteal steroidogenic cells 23
Luteinized unruptured follicle syndrome 23, 53, 149
Luteinizing hormone 3, 7, 16*f*, 21, 31, 42, 43*f*, 45, 53, 57, 62, 94, 94*f*, 113, 117, 132, 136, 137*f*, 147, 203, 207, 216, 226, 243, 244, 269, 276, 280, 292, 296
    ceiling 9
    induced progesterone, physiological significance of 8
    onset of 148*f*
    pulses 23
    receptors, completion of 9
    recombinant 150
    role of 6, 14
    surge 8, 23, 132, 147
        critical determinants of 7
        initiation of 8
        midcycle 9
Luteolysis 24

M

Machine learning 289
Magnetic resonance imaging 269
Makler's chamber 188*f*, 297
Malignancy 95
Malignant disorders 52
Matrix metalloproteinase 32, 44
Maturation 148
Mature follicle 86*t*
    B-mode ultrasound image of 82*f*
Medroxyprogesterone acetate 114*f*
Mekler's chamber 160
Melatonin 247, 248
Menarche 51
Menopause, early 52
Menstrual bleeding 15
Menstrual cycle 207
    irregular 207
    normal 30*f*, 147
Metabolic acidosis
    acute 118
    chronic 118
Metalloproteinases, tissue inhibitors of 44
Metformin 117-120, 124, 245, 247, 248
    treatment, rationale for 119
    use of 97, 119
Microfluidic devices 181
Microfluidic technology, overview of 181
Micronized vaginal progesterone, dose of 209
Midluteal serum progesterone 272
Mild stimulation
    protocol 102*f*
    regimen 95
Miscarriage
    clinical 52
    rates 180
Mitochondrial dysfunction tests 172
Monitoring ovarian stimulation 79
Morphologically ideal spermatozoa 161
Morphology 156, 161
Motility 159, 176
Mucus, enzymatic digestion of 71
Müllerin anomalies 56
Multifollicular growth, induction of 12
Multiple infertility etiologies 68
Multiple pregnancy 99, 110
    prevention of 203
    rate 180, 203, 245
Myocardial infarction, recent 118
Myoinositol 117, 122, 123*f*, 245, 247, 248
    role of 123*f*

N

N-acetylcysteine 247, 248
National Institute for Health and Care Excellence 69, 244
    clinical guideline 261, 299
Natural intrauterine insemination 276, 277
    modified 276, 277
Natural killer cells 36, 59
Natural progesterone, oral formulations of 209
Nausea 99, 119
Neck swelling, midline 52
Neisseria gonorrhoeae 263
Neubauer chamber 297
Neutralizing free radicals 182
Neutrophils 168
New York Heart Association 121
Nitric oxide synthase, inducible 25
Nonsperm cells 162
Nonsteroidal inhibitor 230
Nonsteroidogenic luteal cells 22
Normozoospermia 202
Nuclear chromatin decondensation test 172

O

Obesity 53, 246
Obstructive sleep apnea 243
Occasional metallic taste 119
Odor 158

Index

Oligoasthenospermia,
  very severe 68
Oligomenorrhea 51
Omega-3 fatty acids 182
Oocyte 259, 269
  cumulus complex 7
    expulsion of 9
  granulosa cells regulatory
    loop 6, 7, 10, 11
  maturation 12, 151
    inhibitor 7, 44
  pickup 113f
  quality 56b
  quantity 56b
Optimizing sperm
  preparation 176
Oral ovulation induction
  drugs 276
Oral ovulogens 91, 245b, 278
Orozole 230
Ovarian dysfunction 69
Ovarian failure 68
Ovarian function 21
Ovarian hyperstimulation
  syndrome 72, 77, 100,
  110, 119, 141f, 203, 231,
  245, 248, 278, 284,
  284f, 299
  severe 298
Ovarian insufficiency,
  primary 227
Ovarian physiology 118
Ovarian reserve 59, 215, 268
  testing 54
Ovarian stimulation 12, 15, 17,
  56, 100, 115, 129, 130,
  166, 208, 215, 220, 271,
  298, 299
  drugs for 216
  justification of 272
  protocol 111fc, 226
    used for 111
  several 129
Ovarian stromal flow,
  measurement of 80
Ovary 55f, 118, 123f
  B-mode ultrasound
    image of 80f
  color Doppler image of 78f
  three orthogonal diameters
    of 78f
Ovulation 3, 42, 43, 43f, 45, 45t
  confirmation of 269
  detection of 45
  disorders of 53, 54, 228f
  endocrinology of 42
  induction 108, 207, 229, 243,
    245, 245f, 247, 250f, 252,
    276, 278
    injectable drugs for 245b
    protocols 91, 127, 249
    prediction tests 54
    promotion of 8
    therapeutic triggering of 46
    trigger 46, 145, 147, 149, 151
      right timing of 282
Ovulatory disorders 226, 227t
  classification 54, 227f
Ovulatory dysfunction 53, 68,
  226, 295
  assessment of 53t
  causes of 53t
  presentation of 53t
Ovulatory factor 53
Ovulatory phase 7
Ovulatory status, assessment
  of 59
Oxidative stress 169
Oxygen levels 176

P

Pain 298
Papanicolaou stain 162
Pasteur pipette 178, 297
Peak systolic velocity 79, 81,
  86, 148
Pelvic inflammatory disease 244,
  259, 260f, 269
Penis, anatomic defects of 295
Perifollicular
  flow 83f
  vascularization index 83
  vessels 79f
pH 158
  levels 176
Phospho-inositide
  phosphate 123f
Pinhead spermatozoa 161
Pioglitazone 117, 121
Pituitary ovulatory disorder 228
Placenta 259
Placental disease 52
Plasmin 71
Plasminogen activator
  production 9
Polycystic ovarian syndrome
  52-54, 58, 99, 100, 108,
  117, 120, 130, 140, 150,
  208, 226, 227, 227f,
  229-232, 243, 244, 244fc,
  248, 252, 279
  adjuvants in 248t
  pathogenesis of 117b
  pathophysiology of 117
Polymerase chain reaction 262f, 263
Polymorphonuclear
  leukocytes 168
Polyp 68
  endometrial 218f
POSEIDON'S stratification 56b
Post-coital test 57, 226
Post-intrauterine insemination
  monitoring 180
Postsperm preparation steps 179
Power Doppler 86
Preconception and Prenatal
  Diagnostic Techniques
  185, 186
Preexposure prophylaxis 260
Pregnancy 52, 95
  biochemical 52
  cycles 69
  ectopic 52
  loss
    recurrent 207
    subclinical 96
  medical termination of 186
  rates 69, 142t, 201, 271
Pregnanediol 3-glucuronide 45
Preimplantation genetic
  testing 63, 72
Preintracytoplasmic sperm
  injection 166
Premature luteinizing hormone
  surge 136
  prevention of 102
Premature ovarian failure 227
Preovulatory follicle, development
  of 42
Progesterone 15, 16f, 30f, 33, 42,
  57, 123f, 209, 210, 296
  choice of 209
  hydroxylated 16f
  production 8
  receptors 21
    classic 21
  serum 45
  synthesis 16f
Prolactin 296
  disorder 53
Prostaglandins 9
Prostate, secretory markers of 169

Protein kinase A 123*f*
Psychiatric disorders 52
Pulsatility index 86
Pulse Doppler image 83*f*, 87*f*

Q

Quality-controlled reagents 183

R

Raloxifene 231
Randomized controlled trial 69, 96, 132, 140, 248, 271
Rash 119
Reactive oxygen species 168, 178, 201
    levels 169
Registration certificate 184, 194, 195
Reproductive
    function, male 156
    gamete, male 155
    medicine 290
Retrovirus 258
Ribonucleic acid 258, 262*f*
Rivizor 230
Robotic process automation 290
Rogletimide 110, 230
Rosiglitazone 117, 121, 122
    combination therapy of 121
Round bottom test tubes 178
Routine semen analysis 165
Rule based expert systems 290

S

Second follicle-stimulating hormone peak 8
Selective estrogen receptor modulators 63, 93, 99, 100, 102, 103, 111, 230, 245, 278
    development of 93
    use of 101
Selenium 181, 182
Semen 196
    analysis 59, 62, 66, 155, 155*f*, 156*t*, 162, 165, 218, 270
    collection 189
        jar 189
    culture 168
    examination 156
    parameters 71, 156, 259*f*
    poor quality of 169

preparation
    methods 202
    techniques 283*f*
processing 215
    time 282
volume 156, 158
washing 282
    effectiveness of 263*t*
    procedure 262*f*
Seminal fluid 59
Seminal reactive oxygen species test 172
Seminal vesicles, secretory markers of 169
Serum luteal progesterone 54
Sex hormone binding globulin concentration 119
Sexual dysfunction 51, 295
    psychogenic 295
    psychological 295
Sexually transmitted infections 260
Sheehan's syndrome 227
Simple wash technique 179
Single-cell gel electrophoresis assay 171
Sonosalpingography 56
Specific sperm defects 162
Sperm 155, 196, 259
    acrosome reaction 219
    agglutination 295
    analysis 179
    binding 167
    chromatin
        dispersion test 166, 171
        structure assay 166, 171
    clumping, assessment of 162
    concentration 156
    count 277
    deoxyribonucleic acid
        fragmentation 170, 218
        indications of 170*f*
        tests 170, 171
    examination 157
    function tests 166, 166*fc*, 171, 172*fc*, 173
        importance of 165
    functional assay 165
    health 181
        essential nutrients for 181
    motility 176, 181, 182
    parameters, subnormal 68
    penetration assay 166
    preparation 156, 176, 183

    process, overview of 176
    techniques 177, 226
processing 189
production 181
protection 182
quality 181
    significance of 176
selection device 168
survival test 192
viability 176, 178
vitality 160
wash 261
    procedure 261
    role of 261
    wash kit 297
zona pellucida binding assays 166
Spermatozoa 157, 159, 160
Spermifuge 178
Sterile tissues 189
Steroid biosynthesis 22
Steroidal inhibitor 230
Steroidogenic acute regulatory protein 23, 31
Stillbirth 52
Stress 227
Stromal vessels 78*f*
Subfertility 225
    female 225, 234
Supraphysiologic progesterone levels 34
Swim-up technique 177
Syphilis 295

T

Tamoxifen 100, 101, 203, 231, 278
Test tube 189
    rack 297
Testosterone 62, 123*f*
Theca cells 16*f*, 30, 31, 44
Thiazolidinediones 117, 121
Thin endometrium 253
Thrombophilia testing 57
Thyroid
    disorder 53
    dysfunction 59
        severe 118
    stimulating hormone 53, 58, 59, 228, 270, 296
Total motile sperm count 71, 203, 245, 253, 291, 298
Toxin exposure 64

Toxoplasmosis, rubella, cytomeg-
	alovirus, and herpes
	simplex virus test 57
Transforming growth factor 7
Transvaginal route 77
Transvaginal sonography 202,
	269, 282
	scan 284*f*
Treponema pallidum 263
Trichomonas vaginalis 263
Triptorelin acetate 150
Troglitazone 121
Tubal factor 69, 71
	infertility 55
Tubal patency 269
	assessment of 296
Tuberculosis 218*f*
Tumor
	necrosis factor-alpha 23, 64
	pituitary 227
Turner syndrome 227
Two-cell two-gonadotropin
	theory 4, 5, 11, 14

U

Ultrasound 45, 85, 243, 249*f*, 250*f*
	monitoring 54
Unexplained infertility 57, 68, 69,
	95, 100, 110, 226, 233,
	268, 273, 281, 295
	treatment of 271

United States Food and Drug
	Administration 231
Urinary gonadotropins 133, 245
Urinary luteinizing hormone 54
Uterine
	abnormalities 56
	cramping 298
	factor 269
	microbiome 59
	pathology 68

V

Vaginal factor 269
Vaginal microbiota testing 269
Vaginal preparations 209
Vaginal progesterone 209, 210
Vaginismus 68, 295
Varicocele 63
	assessment 66
	management 66
Vascular endothelial growth factor
	22, 30, 253
Vascularization index 84*f*, 253
Viability 156, 176
Viral transmission 260*t*
Virtual organ computer-aided
	analysis 84*f*, 85
Virus 260
Viscosity 159
Visual disturbances 95
Visual symptoms 99

Vitamin
	B_{12}, malabsorption of 119
	C 181, 182
	D 182, 247, 248
	E 182
Vomiting 99, 119
Vorozole 110

W

Weakness 119
Weight
	loss 119
	management 64
World Health Organization 111,
	155, 156, 165, 201, 225,
	227*t*, 243, 270, 298

Y

Y-chromosome microdeletion
	analysis 63

Z

Zinc 169, 181
Zona
	pellucida 58, 166
	sperm binding 167
Zuclomiphene 231
Zygote 155